Respiratory Disease Series: Diagnostic Tools and Disease Managements

Series Editors
Hiroyuki Nakamura, Professor Emeritus, Tokyo Medical University, Tokyo, Japan
Kazutetsu Aoshiba, Visiting Professor, Tokyo Medical University Ibaraki Medical Center, Ibaraki, Japan

This book series cover a variety of topics in respiratory diseases, with each volume providing an overview of the current state of knowledge, recent discoveries and future prospects for each disease. In each chapter the editors pose critical questions, which are often unresolved clinical issues. These are then discussed by the authors, providing insights and suggestions as to which developments need to be addressed. The series offers new information, which will inspire innovative ideas to further develop respiratory medicine. This collection of monographs is aimed at benefiting patients across the globe suffering from respiratory disease.

Edited by established authorities in the field and written by pioneering experts, this book series will be valuable to those researchers and physicians working in respiratory medicine. The series is aimed at a broad readership, and the books will also be a valuable resource for radiologists, emergency medicine physicians, pathologists, pharmacologists and basic research scientists.

Kazuo Chin
Editor

The Current State of Sleep Disordered Breathing in Japan and Around the World

Springer

Editor
Kazuo Chin
Department of Sleep Medicine
and Respiratory Care
Division of Sleep Medicine
Nihon University of Medicine
Itabashi-ku, Tokyo, Japan

ISSN 2509-5552 ISSN 2509-5560 (electronic)
Respiratory Disease Series: Diagnostic Tools and Disease Managements
ISBN 978-981-96-6032-2 ISBN 978-981-96-6030-8 (eBook)
https://doi.org/10.1007/978-981-96-6030-8

This Springer imprint is published by the registered company Springer Nature Singapore Pte Ltd.
The registered company address is: 152 Beach Road, #21-01/04 Gateway East, Singapore 189721, Singapore

Preface

Sleep disordered breathing (SDB) includes adult and pediatric obstructive sleep apnea (OSA), central sleep apnea, sleep-related hypoventilation disorders, etc [1]. Through managing SDB, we can not only induce a healthy life but improve quality of life and mortality. While treating SDB, we provide guidance regarding lifestyle issues such as reducing body weight among those who are overweight or obese. In addition, sometimes medical devices are used such as for continuous positive airway pressure (CPAP), noninvasive positive pressure ventilation, adaptive servo ventilation, oral appliances, and provision of oxygen as well as any applicable new instruments according to patients' pathophysiology. To use this equipment properly, medical staff must have knowledge of the pathophysiology of various forms of SDB. It is also important to recognize changes related to the occurrence of cardiovascular diseases and changes in energy and metabolism following CPAP treatment because the number of patients receiving CPAP treatment is now over 20 million.

Among SDBs, the prevalence of adult OSA is as high as ever reported with significance [2–4], and pediatric OSA is increasing because of the gains in body weight of children that have been reported worldwide. Three main factors related to the occurrence of OSA are obesity, aging, and male sex. Also, among east Asians, facial morphology is an important factor to be aware of regarding both adult and pediatric OSA [5]. Therefore, to gain information on the prevalence and characteristics of OSA in Japan, data on Japanese patients should be analyzed. In the recent past we were given much information on the prevalence and characteristics of OSA from cohort data of Western countries such as in the Sleep Heart Health Study and Wisconsin Sleep Cohort Study. Now we are going to acquire big cohort data on Japanese with SDB [3, 4].

By achieving control of SDB especially that of OSA, we could reduce not only incidences of cardiovascular diseases but social problems such as traffic and occupational accidents due to hypersomnolence and cognitive impairment caused by OSA.

Recently, telemedicine has become an important area for improvement of medical management overall. CPAP remote monitoring systems are well developed. This enables great opportunities to advance healthcare in this field such as not only improving CPAP adherence but teaching strategies for body weight loss and controlling blood pressure [6]. Since sleep medicine, including managing SDB, is an interdisciplinary branch of medicine, advances in sleep medicine by telemonitoring systems would be a key factor in improving health worldwide in the future.

In Japan, it is an important issue on how to manage transitional care for patients with intractable diseases from childhood to adolescence to adulthood. In respiratory care, congenital central alveolar hypoventilation syndrome (CCHS) is one such disease. In patients with CCHS, central nervous system autonomic dysfunction is present, most often due to a mutation of the *PHOX2B* gene. In this book, although we mainly focused on several issues about sleep apnea, we have included CCHS as a topic.

Sleep Apnea Syndrome (SAS) Clinical Practice Guidelines 2020 was published in Japanese in 2020 and in English in 2022 [7, 8]. In addition to summarizing these guidelines, we introduce development, progress, and perspective of sleep medicine focusing SDBs in this book.

Funding This book is partly based on funds from a project, JPNP23019, subsidized by the New Energy and Industrial Technology Development Organization (NEDO), and grants from the Intractable Respiratory Diseases and Pulmonary Hypertension Research Group of the Ministry of Health, Labour and Welfare of Japan (JPMH20FC1027, JPMH23FC1031).

References

1. American Academy of Sleep Medicine. International Classification of Sleep Disorders. 3ed ed, text revision. Dairen, IL: American Academy of Sleep Medicine; 2023.
2. Benjafield AV, Ayas NT, Eastwood PR, et al. Estimation of the global prevalence and burden of obstructive sleep apnoea: a literature-based analysis. Lancet Respir Med. 2019;7:687–98.
3. Matsumoto T, Murase K, Tabara Y, et al. Sleep disordered breathing and metabolic comorbidities across sex and menopausal status in East Asians: the Nagahama Study. Eur Respir J. 2020;56:1902251.
4. Matsumoto T, Murase K, Tabara Y, et al. Impact of sleep characteristics and obesity on diabetes and hypertension across genders and menopausal status: the Nagahama study. Sleep. 2018;41:zsy071.
5. Jordan AS, McSharry DG, Malhotra A. Adult obstructive sleep apnoea. Lancet. 2014;383(9918):736–47.
6. Murase K, Minami T, Hamada S, at al. Multimodal Telemonitoring for Weight Reduction in Patients With Sleep Apnea: A Randomized Controlled Trial. Chest. 2022;162(6):1373–1383.
7. Akashiba T, Inoue Y, Uchimura N, et al. Sleep Apnea Syndrome (SAS) Clinical practice guidelines 2020. Respir Investig. 2022;60(1):3–32.
8. Akashiba T, Inoue Y, Uchimura N, et al. Sleep Apnea Syndrome (SAS) Clinical practice guidelines 2020. Sleep Biol Rhythms. 2022;20(1):5–37.

Tokyo, Japan Kazuo Chin

Contents

Part I
Epidemiology and Social Issues

Chapter 1
Epidemiology of Sleep Apnea Syndrome in Adult: What is the Current Prevalence of Obstructive Sleep Apnea in Adults?

Yoshihito Kameda, Yuito Ueda, Hiroo Wada, and Takeshi Tanigawa

Abstract Obstructive sleep apnea (OSA) and sleep-related breathing disorders (SRBDs) are significant health concerns characterized by abnormal breathing during sleep. OSA is typically diagnosed using polysomnography (PSG), with various classifications and monitoring types outlined by the American College of Physicians and the American Academy of Sleep Medicine. Epidemiological studies reveal varying prevalence rates of OSA and SRBD, influenced by diagnostic methods, definitions, and demographic factors. The global prevalence of OSA is notably high in populous countries, with a marked increase in recent years due to aging populations and the obesity epidemic.

Epidemiological data show that the prevalence of OSA and SRBD varies by gender, age, and diagnostic criteria, with a generally higher prevalence in men and older age groups. The economic impact of OSA is substantial, with significant costs associated with undiagnosed cases, including lost productivity, motor vehicle accidents, and increased risk of comorbidities.

Risk factors for OSA include anatomical features like micrognathia and enlarged adenoids, as well as lifestyle factors such as obesity and alcohol consumption. Postmenopausal women also show an elevated risk. Central sleep apnea (CSA) is less prevalent but more common in older males and those with heart disease.

In conclusion, the diagnosis and treatment of sleep apnea syndrome (SAS), encompassing OSA and SRBD, are crucial due to the rising global prevalence and significant economic burden. The overlap of the risk factors for SAS with those for lifestyle diseases underscores the need for increased awareness and understanding for SAS across various medical specialties.

Y. Kameda · Y. Ueda · H. Wada · T. Tanigawa (✉)
Department of Public Health, Juntendo University, Tokyo, Japan

K. Chin (ed.), *The Current State of Sleep Disordered Breathing in Japan and Around the World*, Respiratory Disease Series: Diagnostic Tools and Disease Managements, https://doi.org/10.1007/978-981-96-6030-8_1

Keywords Sleep apnea syndrome (SAS) · Sleep-related breathing disorders (SRBDs) · Polysomnography (PSG) · Epidemiology · Risk factor

1 Diagnosis of Obstructive Sleep Apnea or SRBD

Obstructive sleep apnea (OSA) is characterized by episodes of complete collapse of the airway or partial collapse with an associated decrease in oxygen saturation or arousal from sleep [1]. Sleep-related breathing disorders (SRBDs) are characterized by abnormal breathing during sleep [2]. SRBDs are grouped into OSA, central sleep apnea, sleep-related hypoventilation, and sleep-related hypoxemia disorder. The diagnosis of OSA is usually based on the results of polysomnography (PSG) in clinical practice. Some reports have defined OSA as "SRBD plus excessive daytime sleepiness (EDS)" [3, 4] and others as "SRBD plus EDS or hypertension and cardiovascular disorders" [5].

The American College of Physicians (ACP) published a guideline to present the evidence and provide clinical recommendations for the diagnosis of obstructive sleep apnea in adults [6]. In this guideline, the diagnosis of OSA is classified into four types (Table 1.1). Type I monitors are facility-based PSG. Type II monitors are portable, measure most of the same channels (physiologic parameters) as type I monitors (including ≥2 respiratory channels), and can differentiate between sleep and awake states. Type III monitors also measure at least 2 respiratory channels but cannot reliably distinguish between sleep and awake

Table 1.1 Types of monitors for diagnosis of obstructive sleep apnea ([6], Table 1.1)

Type I	Type I monitors mean facility-based testing with 14–16 channels, including EEG, EOG, EMG, ECG/HR, airflow, effort, SaO_2. It has ≥2 airflow/effort channels, identifies sleep and awake states, and measures AHI
Type II	Type II monitors mean portable testing with ≥7 channels, including EEG, EOG, EMG, ECG/HR, airflow, effort, SaO_2. It has ≥2 airflow/effort channels, identifies sleep and awake states, and measures AHI
Type III	Type III monitors mean portable testing with >4 channels, including airflow and/or effort, ECG/HR, SaO_2. It has ≥2 airflow/effort channels, does not identify sleep and awake states, but estimates AHI. Type III monitors estimate the AHI by measuring the total number of episodes of apnea and hypopnea divided by the number of recording hours/time (as opposed to the number of hours of sleep determined by EEG)
Type IV	Type IV monitors mean portable testing with 1–3 channels. They include all monitors that do not fit into type III classification, do not have ≥2 airflow/effort channels, do not identify sleep and awake states, but estimate AHI similarly to type III monitors. Some type IV devices estimate sleep and awake state by peripheral arterial tone and estimate the AHI from the estimated sleep time. Type IV monitors may have more than 3 channels provided that criteria for type III monitors are not met. Type IV monitors may include devices that measure signals that are, in principle, able to identify arousals from sleep

AHI apnea-hypopnea index, *ECG* electrocardiography, *EEG* electroencephalography, *EMG* electromyography, *EOG* electro-oculography, *HR* heart rate

Table 1.2 Definition of hypopnea by the American Academy of Sleep Medicine guidelines ([7], Table 1.1)

1999 guideline	≥50% decrease in flow OR a clear reduction in flow that does not reach ≥50% AND is associated with either an oxygen desaturation of ≥3% or an arousal
2007 guideline	≥30% decrease in flow from baseline with an associated oxygen desaturation of ≥4%
2012 guideline	≥30% decrease in flow from baseline with an associated oxygen desaturation of ≥3% OR an associated arousal

states. Type IV monitors are those that do not fit into type III classification and can vary in the number of channels that they record. Type III monitors and type IV monitors provide estimated AHI. A significant limitation of type IV monitors is that they cannot differentiate between obstructive and central apneas. The American Academy of Sleep Medicine (AASM) guidelines defined hypopnea criteria in 1999, 2007, and 2012. These criteria were used for worldwide survey of OSA [7] (Table 1.2).

In large epidemiological studies, it is difficult to perform PSG examination (type I or type II monitors) on all participants, and therefore, those with impaired breathing and oxygenation during sleep were often examined by flow sensors with monitoring methods such as ECG/heart rate, respiration effort, and oxygen saturation (type III monitors) or by pulse oximetry with a total of 1–3 channels of monitoring methods (type IV monitors) and reported as having SRBD. When sleep events were reported by type III monitors or type IV monitors, they were often reported as estimated AHI or respiratory event index (REI) instead of AHI. Flow sensors and pulse oximetry are more convenient for screening, but pulse oximetry is reported to be less sensitive than flow sensor. For normal weight subjects, the diagnostic sensitivity of flow sensor was 94%, 93%, and 92% at REI cutoff values of 5, 10, and 15 or higher, respectively, compared to 86%, 87%, and 84% for pulse oximetry [8, 9].

2 Number of Patients with Obstructive Sleep Apnea Worldwide

Figure 1.1 shows the top 10 estimated numbers of OSA patients worldwide according to the American Academy of Sleep Medicine 2012 criteria [7]. The most populous countries, India, China, the United States, and Brazil, are ranked high. The cumulative number of affected individuals in the top 10 countries is 516 million for apnea hypopnea index (AHI) ≥5 and 228 million for AHI ≥15. The prevalence of OSA has been reported to have increased in recent years. Increasing age and the global epidemic of obesity have been associated with increased prevalence of OSA [10].

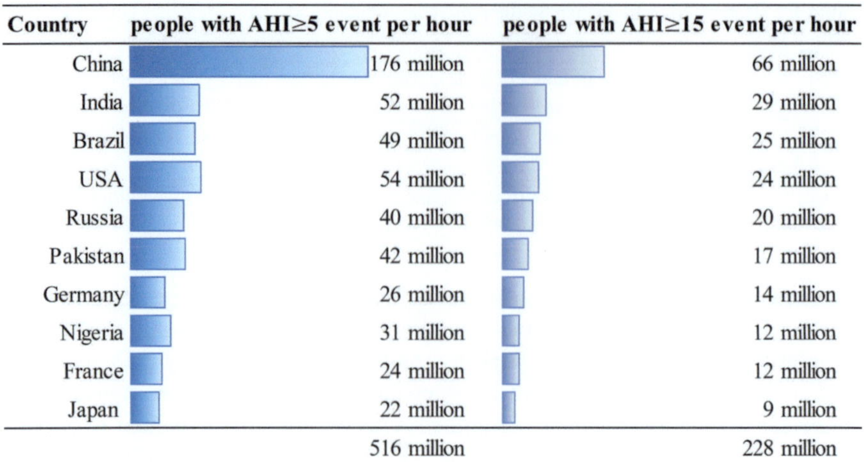

Fig. 1.1 Top ten countries with the highest estimated number of individuals with obstructive sleep apnea based on the American Academy of Sleep Medicine 2012 criteria (Compiled from [7])

3 Summary of Epidemiological Studies That Have Investigated the Prevalence of Obstructive Sleep Apnea

Table 1.3 summarizes epidemiological studies that have investigated the prevalence of OSA [3–5, 11–34]. For studies classified by age, the portion of the study that includes people in their 50 s is excerpted. Results obtained with PSG are indicated as AHI, and results from simple monitors such as flow sensor or pulse oximetry are indicated as REI.

The reported frequency of OSA varies depending on the testing method and definition. When OSA was defined as "SRBD combined with excessive daytime sleepiness (EDS)," most of the reports showed that AHI ≥ 5 combined with EDS was around 5% in men and 2–3% in women [3, 4, 11–14, 22]. AHI ≥ 15 combined with EDS is less reported but is reported to be about 3% in men [3] and 1% in women [4]. Some articles have noted that the correlation between SRBD and EDS is weak [3, 4, 26]. When OSA was defined as "SRBD combined with EDS or hypertension and cardiovascular disorders," its prevalence was higher, around 15%, although the results concerned only to men [5]. In a study using a pulse oximetry, 40.4% of males and 9.0% of females had SRBD with 3% ODI (oxygen desaturation index) ≥ 5 and 3% ODI ≥ 15, respectively, in a community population aged 40–69 years [27]. The prevalence of SRBD among Japanese women aged 30–69 years was 20.2% for those with a 3% ODI ≥5 and 2.8% for those with a 3% ODI ≥15 [24]. In a research using airflow sensors that involved 978 community dwellers, a total of 18.4% of participants had an REI ≥15 as determined by the airflow sensor [28]. One study attempted to diagnose OSA by utilizing a multisensor mattress [34]. This device contains pneumatic and sound sensors to detect body movements, respiratory rate, heart rate, snoring, and episodes of breathing cessation. This study involving 67,278

Table 1.3 Summary of the prevalence of obstructive sleep apnea

Author	Year	Age	Country	Examination	Gender		Population	AHI ≥ 5	AHI ≥ 10	AHI ≥ 15	AHI ≥ 20	AHI ≥ 30
					Male	Female						
Young et al. [11]	1993	30–60	United States	PSG	1670	1843	Workplace	M:31.0% F:16.0%	M:14.0% F:5.9%	M:9.1% F:4.0%		
Bixler et al. [12]	2001	20–100	United States	PSG		1000	Community			F:2.0%		
Duran et al. [13]	2001	30–70	Spain	PSG	255	135	Community	M:27.9% F:31.0%	M:24.1% F:16.2%	M:19.4% F:8.6%	M:14.7% F:8.3%	M:11.4% F:4.3%
Kim et al. [14]	2004	40–70	South Korea	PSG	309	148	Community	M:33.7% F:25.2%	M:21.6% F:10.0%	M:11.9% F:2.9%		
Ip et al. [3]	2001	30–60	Hong Kong	PSG	153		Workplace	M:17.2%				
Ip et al. [4]	2004	30–60	Hong Kong	PSG		106	Workplace	F:10.1%				
Baldw et al. [15]	2004	40≤	United States	PSG	3042	3398	Community	M:57.7% F:30.1%		M:25.0% F:11.5%		M:9.3% F:3.5%
Frankl et al. [16]	2013	20–70	Sweden	PSG		398	Community	F:56.0%		F:17.0%		F:4.6%
Bixler et al. [5]	1998	0–100	United States	PSG	741		Community	M:19.7%	M:11.8%		M:6.4%	
Heinzer et al. [17]	2015	35–75	Switzerland	PSG	1024	1097	Cardiovascular/ psychiatric cohort	M:83.8% F:60.8%		M:49.7% F:23.4%		
Tufik et al. [18]	2010	20–80	Brazil	PSG	466	576	Community	M:46.5% F:30.6%		M:24.8% F:9.6%		
Fietze et al. [19]	2019	20–81	Germany	PSG	649	559	Community	M:53.6% F:24.1%		M:23.4% F:8.3%		M:8.0% F:2.5%
McArdle et al. [20]	2022	45–65	Australia	PSG	366	537	Parents of children cohort	M:86.2% F:58.2%		M:42.4% F:20.3%		

(continued)

Table 1.3 (continued)

Author	Year	Age	Country	Examination	Gender		Population	REI ≥ 5	REI ≥ 10	REI ≥ 15	REI ≥ 20	REI ≥ 30
					Male	Female						
Cunningham et al. [21]	2021	46–69	Australia	Flow sensor, pulse oximetry	1191	1495	Community	M:57.7% F:40.7%		M:20.2% F:10.0%		M:5.1% F:2.0%
Udwadia et al. [22]	2004	35–65	India	PSG without EEG	200		Community	M:21.9%	M:14.0%	M:11.7%		
Nakayama-Ashida et al. [23]	2008	20–59	Japan	Pulse oximetry	476		Workplace	M:74.1%		M:30.6%		M:11.8%
Cui et al. [24]	2008	30–69	Japan	Pulse oximetry		3626	Community	F:20.2%	F:6.4%	F:2.8%		
Sakurai et al. [25]	2007	20–69	Japan	Pulse oximetry	1465		Workplace (truck driver)	M:25.4%	M:11.1%	M:6.6%		
Sakamoto et al. [26]	2014	30–79	Japan	Pulse oximetry	314	452	Community	M:44.9% F:24.6%		M:17.8% F:5.1%		
Tanigawa et al. [27]	2004	40–69	Japan	Pulse oximetry	1424		Community	M:40.4%		M:9.0%		
Yamagishi et al. [28]	2010	30≤	Japan	Flow sensor	446	532	Community			M:18.4% F:11.4%		
Matsuo et al. [31]	2020	30–80	Japan	Flow sensor	380	667	Community		M:67.6% F:41.4%			

Miyachi, H. et al. [32]	2022	18–67	Japan	Flow sensor		688	Workplace		F:23.0%			
Wada et al. [33]	2024	20–69	Japan	Flow sensor	19,699		Workplace (truck driver)	M:38.2%		M:12.8%		M:2.8%
Lechat et al. [34]	2022	18–90	Europe: 62%, North America :30%, Asia:6%	Under-mattress sleep sensor	52,533	14,745	Community (Customer user)	M:32.8% F:29.4%		M:16.1% F:10.4%		M:9.6% F:4.1%
Matsumoto, T et al. [37]	2018	34-80	Japan	Pulse oximetry with actigraph	2274	Pre-menopausal(pre) 1585, Post menopausal(post) 3160	Community	M:81.0% F(pre): 25.1% F(post): 60.2%	M:23.7% F(pre):1.5% F(post):9.5%			M:4.4% F(pre):0% F(post):1.2%

AHI apnea-hypopnea index, *REI* respiratory event index, *PSG* polysomnography, *M* male, *F* female, *EEG* electroencephalography
Males with an AHI of 5 or higher as measured by PSG testing ranged from 17.2% to 86.2% and males with an AHI of 15 or higher ranged from 9.1% to 49.7%; females with an AHI of 5 or higher ranged from 10.1% to 60.8% and females with an AHI of 15 or higher ranged from 2.0% to 23.4%
Males with REI of 5 or greater, as measured by pulse oximetry or flow sensor, ranged from 21.9% to 74.1%, and males with REI of 15 or greater ranged from 6.6% to 30.6%. 20.2% to 40.7% of females with REI of 5 or greater, and 2.8% to 11.4% of females with REI of 15 or greater ranged from 2.8% to 11.4%

subjects who underwent multinight in-home monitoring using noninvasive under-mattress sensor technology found a global prevalence of moderate-to-severe OSA at approximately 20%.

The prevalence of SRBDs has been examined using criteria such as an AHI of 5, 10, 15, 20, or 30 or higher by full polysomnography, with many reports adopting the criterion of an AHI ≥15. An analysis of sex- and age-stratified data revealed that the prevalence of sleep-related breathing disorders, when defined as AHI ≥5, varies widely; however, when defined as AHI ≥15, the data exhibit more uniformity.

The prevalence of men with AHI ≥5 ranged from 17.2% to 86.2% and those with AHI ≥15 ranged from 9.1% to 49.7%, while the percentages of women with AHI ≥5 ranged from 10.1% to 60.8% and those with AHI ≥15 ranged from 2.0% to 23.4%. The percentage of men with REI ≥5 ranged from 21.9% to 74.1% and 6.6% to 30.6% with REI ≥15, while the percentage of women with REI ≥5 ranged from 20.2% to 40.7% and 2.8% to 11.4% with REI ≥15. Although few studies showed AHI and REI ≥ 30, the percentages of REI ≥30 ranged from 5.1% to 11.8% for men and 2% to 4.6% for women. Although there is a large variation among the study subjects, for both AHI and REI, the prevalence is higher in men than in women, and AHI ≥ 15 shows less variation in results than AHI ≥ 5. Studies in the community-dwelling population show that the percentage of AHI and REI ≥15 is approximately 10–20% for men in their 50s, compared to less than 10% for women in their 50s. Comparing age groups, in the younger age group (30–40 years old), 10% of men and 5% of women have SRBD. Therefore, the prevalence is higher in older age groups and in males.

4 The Prevalence of Adult Patients with Sleep Apnea at Present

Focusing on recent trends, reports from 2019 to 2024 provide the following insights into the prevalence of OSA and SRDB: In two studies evaluated using polysomnography, the prevalence of AHI ≥5 ranged from 53.6% to 86.2% in men and 24.1% to 58.2% in women, while the prevalence of AHI ≥15 ranged from 23.4% to 42.4% in men and 8.3% to 20.3% in women [19, 20]. An Australian study utilizing flow sensors reported that the prevalence of REI ≥5 was 57.7% in men and 40.7% in women, and the prevalence of REI ≥15 was 20.2% in men and 10.0% in women [21]. Japanese studies using flow sensors found a prevalence of REI ≥10 at 67.6% in men and 23.0% to 41.4% in women [31, 32]. Additionally, a 2024 study of truck drivers reported a prevalence of REI ≥5 at 38.2% and REI ≥15 at 12.8% [33]. In contrast, a 2007 study conducted under similar conditions found that REI ≥5 was 25.4% and REI ≥15 was 6.6% [25]. These findings, consistent with other previous studies, suggest that the prevalence of SDB has been increasing.

5 The Economic Impact of Obstructive Sleep Apnea and the Cost-Effectiveness for Diagnosis and Treatment of OSA

An analysis of the economic impact of OSA was conducted by the AASM [10]. OSA affects approximately 12% of the U.S. population, or 29.4 million adults. Of these, 20% were diagnosed, while 80% were undiagnosed. The estimated economic burden of undiagnosed OSA in the U.S. adults was $149.6 billion in 2015. This includes $86.9 billion from lost productivity and absenteeism, $30 billion from the increased risk of comorbidities, $26.2 billion attributed to motor vehicle accidents, and $6.5 billion due to workplace injuries. Reports from Italy, Australia, and the UK also assess the cost-effectiveness of diagnosing and treating OSA.

6 Risk Factors for Obstructive Sleep Apnea

OSA was characterized by the collapse of the upper airway during sleep, which is a multifaceted occurrence under influence of various factors including reduced ventilatory drive, neuromuscular, and anatomical factors. Predominant anatomical risk factors for OSA include micrognathia, retrognathia, enlarged adenoids, and tonsillar hypertrophy [35, 36]. Other risk factors encompass gender (with males being more susceptible), advanced age, and obesity [18]. Notably, postmenopausal women are at an elevated risk for OSA. A study, adjusted for objective sleep duration measured via sleep diary and actigraphy, analyzed 7051 Japanese participants. Using a 3% ODI as a metric, it was found that 23.7% of men, 1.5% of premenopausal women, and 9.5% of postmenopausal women presented with moderate to severe SRBD (3% ODI ≥15) [37]. Alcohol consumption has been consistently linked with a heightened risk for OSA [29]. A meta-analysis incorporating 21 studies primarily from Europe and the United States demonstrated a 25% increased relative risk for OSA in individuals who consume alcohol as compared to those who do not drink [38]. The risk exacerbates if alcohol is consumed immediately before bedtime [39]. Even results from a survey on daily alcohol consumption, rather than a survey on drinking just before bedtime, increase the probability of developing OSA by about two-fold [30, 40, 41]. Epidemiological research in Japan, examining both community dwellers [42, 43] and male professional drivers [44], has identified a positive association between alcohol intake and OSA prevalence across genders [25, 42, 43]. Moreover, even after adjusting for age, a significant association between alcohol consumption and the prevalence of SRDB is observed.

7 Prevalence of Central Sleep Apnea

Most studies define central sleep apnea (CSA) as a condition where the central apnea index (CAI) is ≥5 and greater than the obstructive apnea index (OAI) [44–50]. In an epidemiological study involving 5804 healthy participants, when CSA's prevalence was determined using these criteria, the prevalence was around 0.1% in women aged about 50 years and 1.0% in men [46]. For women aged 70 and above, the prevalence rose to 0.3%, and for men aged 70 and above, it increased to approximately 2.7%. These findings, in line with other studies [5, 44–51], suggest that being older and male are associated with a higher prevalence of CSA.

8 Risk Factors for Central Sleep Apnea

In patients diagnosed with heart failure and an ejection fraction (EF) of less than 45%, the prevalence of CSA ranged from 11.7% to 49% based on the aforementioned criteria [44, 49, 50]. It is important to note that these studies have limitations, including varying definitions of heart failure. Nonetheless, in general, the prevalence of CSA in heart failure patients is notably higher than in the general healthy population [52–58]. Additionally, associations between CSA and conditions such as stroke [59–62], atrial fibrillation [63, 64], chronic kidney disease [65, 66], and opioid use [67] have been reported.

9 Conclusion

Sleep apnea syndrome (SAS) is assessed using various methods, including polysomnography, flow sensors, and pulse oximetry. Therefore, the prevalence of SAS varies depending on the diagnostic method and cutoff values set; however, there is a global increase in prevalence due to aging populations and the rise in obesity. This increase is particularly notable in countries with particularly large populations. SAS leads to significant economic burdens, including decreased productivity, increased risk of complications, and a higher incidence of car crashes. The diagnosis and treatment of SAS have been shown to be cost-effective, highlighting the importance of addressing SAS. In addition to anatomical factors like micrognathia and adenoids, risk factors for lifestyle diseases such as age, male gender, obesity, and alcohol consumption also overlap with the risk factors for SAS. Given these overlaps, it may be crucial for various medical specialties to enhance their understanding of SAS.

References

1. Slowik JM SA, Collen JF. Obstructive Sleep Apnea StatPearls Publishing2022 [updated Updated 2022 Dec 11. Available from: https://www.ncbi.nlm.nih.gov/books/NBK459252/.
2. Burman D. Sleep Disorders: Sleep-Related Breathing Disorders. FP Essent. 2017;460:11–21.
3. Ip MS, Lam B, Lauder IJ, Tsang KW, Chung KF, Mok YW, et al. A community study of sleep-disordered breathing in middle-aged Chinese men in Hong Kong. Chest. 2001;119(1):62–9.
4. Ip MS, Lam B, Tang LC, Lauder IJ, Ip TY, Lam WK. A community study of sleep-disordered breathing in middle-aged Chinese women in Hong Kong: prevalence and gender differences. Chest. 2004;125(1):127–34.
5. Bixler EO, Vgontzas AN, Ten Have T, Tyson K, Kales A. Effects of age on sleep apnea in men: I. Prevalence and severity. Am J Respir Crit Care Med. 1998;157(1):144–8.
6. Qaseem A, Dallas P, Owens DK, Starkey M, Holty JE, Shekelle P, et al. Diagnosis of obstructive sleep apnea in adults: a clinical practice guideline from theAmerican College of Physicians. Ann Intern Med. 2014;161(3):210–20.
7. Benjafield AV, Ayas NT, Eastwood PR, Heinzer R, Ip MSM, Morrell MJ, et al. Estimation of the global prevalence and burden of obstructive sleep apnoea: a literature-based analysis. Lancet Respir Med. 2019;7(8):687–98.
8. Nakano H, Tanigawa T, Furukawa T, Nishima S. Automatic detection of sleep-disordered breathing from a single-channel airflow record. Eur Respir J. 2007;29(4):728–36.
9. Nakano H, Tanigawa T, Ohnishi Y, Uemori H, Senzaki K, Furukawa T, et al. Validation of a single-channel airflow monitor for screening of sleep-disordered breathing. Eur Respir J. 2008;32(4):1060–7.
10. Lyons MM, Bhatt NY, Pack AI, Magalang UJ. Global burden of sleep-disordered breathing and its implications. Respirology. 2020;25(7):690–702.
11. Young T, Palta M, Dempsey J, Skatrud J, Weber S, Badr S. The Occurrence of Sleep-Disordered Breathing among Middle-Aged Adults. New Engl J Med. 1993;328(17):1230–5.
12. Bixler EO, Vgontzas AN, Lin HM, Ten Have T, Rein J, Vela-Bueno A, et al. Prevalence of sleep-disordered breathing in women: effects of gender. Am J Respir Crit Care Med. 2001;163(3 Pt 1):608–13.
13. Duran J, Esnaola S, Rubio R, Iztueta A. Obstructive sleep apnea-hypopnea and related clinical features in a population-based sample of subjects aged 30 to 70 yr. Am J Resp Crit Care. 2001;163(3):685–9.
14. Kim J, In K, Kim J, You S, Kang K, Shim J, et al. Prevalence of sleep-disordered breathing in middle-aged Korean men and women. Am J Respir Crit Care Med. 2004;170(10):1108–13.
15. Baldwin CM, Kapur VK, Holberg CJ, Rosen C, Nieto FJ, Grp SHHS. Associations between gender and measures of daytime somnolence in the Sleep Heart Health Study. Sleep. 2004;27(2):305–11.
16. Franklin KA, Sahlin C, Stenlund H, Lindberg E. Sleep apnoea is a common occurrence in females. Eur Respir J. 2013;41(3):610–5.
17. Heinzer R, Vat S, Marques-Vidal P, Marti-Soler H, Andries D, Tobback N, et al. Prevalence of sleep-disordered breathing in the general population: the HypnoLaus study. Lancet Respir Med. 2015;3(4):310–8.
18. Tufik S, Santos-Silva R, Taddei JA, Bittencourt LR. Obstructive sleep apnea syndrome in the Sao Paulo Epidemiologic Sleep Study. Sleep Med. 2010;11(5):441–6.
19. Fietze I, Laharnar N, Obst A, Ewert R, Felix SB, Garcia C, et al. Prevalence and association analysis of obstructive sleep apnea with gender and age differences – Results of SHIP-Trend. J Sleep Res. 2019;28(5):e12770.
20. McArdle N, Reynolds AC, Hillman D, Moses E, Maddison K, Melton P, et al. Prevalence of common sleep disorders in a middle-aged community sample. J Clin Sleep Med. 2022;18(6):1503–14.

21. Cunningham J, Hunter M, Budgeon C, Murray K, Knuiman M, Hui J, et al. The prevalence and comorbidities of obstructive sleep apnea in middle-aged men and women: the Busselton Healthy Ageing Study. J Clin Sleep Med. 2021;17(10):2029–39.
22. Udwadia ZF, Doshi AV, Lonkar SG, Singh CI. Prevalence of sleep-disordered breathing and sleep apnea in middle-aged urban Indian men. Am J Respir Crit Care Med. 2004;169(2):168–73.
23. Nakayama-Ashida Y, Takegami M, Chin K, Sumi K, Nakamura T, Takahashi K, et al. Sleep-disordered breathing in the usual lifestyle setting as detected with home monitoring in a population of working men in Japan. Sleep. 2008;31(3):419–25.
24. Cui R, Tanigawa T, Sakurai S, Yamagishi K, Imano H, Ohira T, et al. Associations of sleep-disordered breathing with excessive daytime sleepiness and blood pressure in Japanese women. Hypertens Res. 2008;31(3):501–6.
25. Sakurai S, Cui R, Tanigawa T, Yamagishi K, Iso H. Alcohol consumption before sleep is associated with severity of sleep-disordered breathing among professional Japanese truck drivers. Alcohol Clin Exp Res. 2007;31(12):2053–8.
26. Sakamoto Y, Kokubo Y, Toyoda K, Watanabe M, Tanigawa T, Miyamoto Y. Sleep-disordered breathing is associated with elevated human atrial natriuretic peptide levels in a Japanese urban population: The Suita study. Int J Cardiol. 2014;173(2):334–5.
27. Tanigawa T, Tachibana N, Yamagishi K, Muraki I, Kudo M, Ohira T, et al. Relationship between sleep-disordered breathing and blood pressure levels in community-based samples of Japanese men. Hypertens Res. 2004;27(7):479–84.
28. Yamagishi K, Ohira T, Nakano H, Bielinski SJ, Sakurai S, Imano H, et al. Cross-cultural comparison of the sleep-disordered breathing prevalence among Americans and Japanese. Eur Respir J. 2010;36(2):379–84.
29. Bearpark H, Elliott L, Grunstein R, Cullen S, Schneider H, Althaus W, et al. Snoring and Sleep-Apnea – a Population Study in Australian Men. Am J Resp Crit Care. 1995;151(5):1459–65.
30. Peppard PE, Austin D, Brown RL. Association of Alcohol Consumption and Sleep Disordered Breathing In Men And Women. J Clin Sleep Med. 2007;3(3):265–70.
31. Matsuo R, Tanigawa T, Tomooka K, Ikeda A, Wada H, Maruyama K, et al. Sleep disordered breathing and subjective excessive daytime sleepiness in relation to the risk of motor vehicle crash: the Toon Health Study. Sci Rep-Uk. 2020;10(1)
32. Miyachi N, Ikeda A, Filomeno R, Wada H, Maruyama K, Suzuki Y, et al. Impaired psychomotor vigilance associated with sleep-disordered breathing in women working in the care of older adults in Japan. Sleep Breathing. 2022;26(1):259–67.
33. Wada H, Nakano H, Sakurai S, Tanigawa T. Self-reported sleep tendency poorly predicts the presence of obstructive sleep apnea in commercial truck drivers. Sleep Med. 2024;115:109–13.
34. Lechat B, Naik G, Reynolds A, Aishah A, Scott H, Loffler KA, et al. Multinight Prevalence, Variability, and Diagnostic Misclassification of Obstructive Sleep Apnea. Am J Respir Crit Care Med. 2022;205(5):563–9.
35. Schwab RJ, Gupta KB, Gefter WB, Metzger LJ, Hoffman EA, Pack AI. Upper airway and soft tissue anatomy in normal subjects and patients with sleep-disordered breathing. Significance of the lateral pharyngeal walls. Am J Respir Crit Care Med. 1995;152(5 Pt 1):1673–89.
36. Sankri-Tarbichi AG. Obstructive sleep apnea-hypopnea syndrome: Etiology and diagnosis. Avicenna J Med. 2012;2(1):3–8.
37. Matsumoto T, Murase K, Tabara Y, Gozal D, Smith D, Minami T, et al. Impact of sleep characteristics and obesity on diabetes and hypertension across genders and menopausal status: the Nagahama study. Sleep. 2018;41(7)
38. Simou E, Britton J, Leonardi-Bee J. Alcohol and the risk of sleep apnoea: a systematic review and meta-analysis. Sleep Med. 2018;42:38–46.
39. Kolla BP, Foroughi M, Saeidifard F, Chakravorty S, Wang Z, Mansukhani MP. The impact of alcohol on breathing parameters during sleep: a systematic review and meta-analysis. Sleep Med Rev. 2018;42:59–67.
40. Yang SS, Guo XH, Liu W, Li YH, Liu YX. Alcohol as an independent risk factor for obstructive sleep apnea. Irish J Med Sci. 2022;191(3):1325–30.

41. Huang Z, Aarab G, Chattrattrai T, Su N, Volgenant CMC, Hilgevoord AAJ, et al. Associated factors of primary snoring and obstructive sleep apnoea in patients with sleep bruxism: A questionnaire study. J Oral Rehabil. 2022;49(10):970–9.
42. Tanigawa T, Tachibana N, Yamagishi K, Shimamoto T, Iso H. Usual alcohol consumption and arterial oxygen desaturation during sleep. JAMA. 2004;292(8):923–5.
43. Cui RZ, Tanigawa T, Sakurai S, Yamagishi K, Muraki I, Imano H, et al. Associations between alcohol consumption and sleep-disordered breathing among Japanese women. Respir Med. 2011;105(5):796–800.
44. Bitter T, Westerheide N, Hossain SM, Prinz C, Horstkotte D, Oldenburg O. Symptoms of sleep apnoea in chronic heart failure--results from a prospective cohort study in 1,500 patients. Sleep Breath 2012;16(3):781–791.
45. Javaheri S, Blackwell T, Ancoli-Israel S, Ensrud KE, Stone KL, Redline S, et al. Sleep-disordered Breathing and Incident Heart Failure in Older Men. Am J Respir Crit Care Med. 2016;193(5):561–8.
46. Donovan LM, Kapur VK. Prevalence and Characteristics of Central Compared to Obstructive Sleep Apnea: Analyses from the Sleep Heart Health Study Cohort. Sleep. 2016;39(7):1353–9.
47. Johansson P, Alehagen U, Svanborg E, Dahlstrom U, Brostrom A. Sleep disordered breathing in an elderly community-living population: Relationship to cardiac function, insomnia symptoms and daytime sleepiness. Sleep Med. 2009;10(9):1005–11.
48. Stone KL, Blackwell TL, Ancoli-Israel S, Barrett-Connor E, Bauer DC, Cauley JA, et al. Sleep Disordered Breathing and Risk of Stroke in Older Community-Dwelling Men. Sleep. 2016;39(3):531–40.
49. Ward NR, Roldao V, Cowie MR, Rosen SD, McDonagh TA, Simonds AK, et al. The effect of respiratory scoring on the diagnosis and classification of sleep disordered breathing in chronic heart failure. Sleep. 2013;36(9):1341–8.
50. Redeker NS, Muench U, Zucker MJ, Walsleben J, Gilbert M, Freudenberger R, et al. Sleep disordered breathing, daytime symptoms, and functional performance in stable heart failure. Sleep. 2010;33(4):551–60.
51. Mehra R, Stone KL, Blackwell T, Ancoli Israel S, Dam TT, Stefanick ML, et al. Prevalence and correlates of sleep-disordered breathing in older men: osteoporotic fractures in men sleep study. J Am Geriatr Soc. 2007;55(9):1356–64.
52. Wang H, Parker JD, Newton GE, Floras JS, Mak S, Chiu KL, et al. Influence of obstructive sleep apnea on mortality in patients with heart failure. J Am Coll Cardiol. 2007;49(15):1625–31.
53. Javaheri S, Parker TJ, Liming JD, Corbett WS, Nishiyama H, Wexler L, et al. Sleep apnea in 81 ambulatory male patients with stable heart failure. Types and their prevalences, consequences, and presentations. Circulation. 1998;97(21):2154–9.
54. Sin DD, Fitzgerald F, Parker JD, Newton G, Floras JS, Bradley TD. Risk factors for central and obstructive sleep apnea in 450 men and women with congestive heart failure. Am J Respir Crit Care Med. 1999;160(4):1101–6.
55. Javaheri S, Shukla R, Zeigler H, Wexler L. Central sleep apnea, right ventricular dysfunction, and low diastolic blood pressure are predictors of mortality in systolic heart failure. J Am Coll Cardiol. 2007;49(20):2028–34.
56. Sin DD, Logan AG, Fitzgerald FS, Liu PP, Bradley TD. Effects of continuous positive airway pressure on cardiovascular outcomes in heart failure patients with and without Cheyne-Stokes respiration. Circulation. 2000;102(1):61–6.
57. Brack T, Thuer I, Clarenbach CF, Senn O, Noll G, Russi EW, et al. Daytime Cheyne-Stokes respiration in ambulatory patients with severe congestive heart failure is associated with increased mortality. Chest. 2007;132(5):1463–71.
58. Giannoni A, Gentile F, Sciarrone P, Borrelli C, Pasero G, Mirizzi G, et al. Upright Cheyne-Stokes Respiration in Patients With Heart Failure. J Am Coll Cardiol. 2020;75(23):2934–46.
59. Seiler A, Camilo M, Korostovtseva L, Haynes AG, Brill AK, Horvath T, et al. Prevalence of sleep-disordered breathing after stroke and TIA: A meta-analysis. Neurology. 2019;92(7):e648–e54.

60. Schutz SG, Lisabeth LD, Hsu CW, Kim S, Chervin RD, Brown DL. Central sleep apnea is uncommon after stroke. Sleep Med. 2021;77:304–6.
61. Bonnin-Vilaplana M, Arboix A, Parra O, Garcia-Eroles L, Montserrat JM, Massons J. Cheyne-stokes respiration in patients with first-ever lacunar stroke. Sleep Disord. 2012;2012:257890.
62. Parra O, Arboix A, Bechich S, Garcia-Eroles L, Montserrat JM, Lopez JA, et al. Time course of sleep-related breathing disorders in first-ever stroke or transient ischemic attack. Am J Respir Crit Care Med. 2000;161(2 Pt 1):375–80.
63. Leung RST, Huber MA, Rogge T, Maimon N, Chiu KL, Bradley TD. Association between atrial fibrillation and central sleep apnea. Sleep. 2005;28(12):1543–6.
64. May AM, Blackwell T, Stone PH, Stone KL, Cawthon PM, Sauer WH, et al. Central Sleep-disordered Breathing Predicts Incident Atrial Fibrillation in Older Men. Am J Resp Crit Care. 2016;193(7):783–91.
65. Hanly PJ, Pierratos A. Improvement of sleep apnea in patients with chronic renal failure who undergo nocturnal hemodialysis. New Engl J Med. 2001;344(2):102–7.
66. Nigam G, Pathak C, Riaz M. A systematic review of central sleep apnea in adult patients with chronic kidney disease. Sleep Breath. 2016;20(3):957–64.
67. Wang D, Teichtahl H, Drummer O, Goodman C, Cherry G, Cunnington D, et al. Central sleep apnea in stable methadone maintenance treatment patients. Chest. 2005;128(3):1348–56.

Chapter 2
Epidemiology of SAS in Children: What Should We Understand About the Current Prevalence of Pediatric Sleep Apnea?

Yuito Ueda, Yoshihito Kameda, Hiroo Wada, and Takeshi Tanigawa

Abstract Pediatric sleep-disordered breathing (SDB) is a significant public health problem that affects the health, growth, and development of children. Key risk factors include obesity, enlarged tonsils and adenoids, allergic rhinitis, and asthma, while the consequences can include neurobehavioral problems, growth delays, and developmental delays. SDB also impacts healthcare utilization and contributes to socioeconomic disparities, with its prevalence ranging from 1% to 5% in children. Public health strategies to address SDB should focus on raising awareness, early detection, and timely intervention. Continued research is essential to improve health outcomes for children affected by SDB.

Keyword Prevalence

1 Introduction

Since sleeping plays a crucial role in growth and health, children with sleep-disordered breathing (SDB) may experience growth retardation and impaired development, as well as neurobehavioral problems [1]. Since children with neurobehavioral manifestations may claim restlessness and attention deficits, and they might be sometimes even diagnosed with attention deficit hyperactivity disorder (ADHD).

Y. Ueda · Y. Kameda · H. Wada · T. Tanigawa (✉)
Department of Public Health, Juntendo University Graduate, School of Medicine, Hongo, Bunkyo-Ku, Tokyo, Japan
e-mail: tataniga@juntendo.ac.jp

K. Chin (ed.), *The Current State of Sleep Disordered Breathing in Japan and Around the World*, Respiratory Disease Series: Diagnostic Tools and Disease Managements, https://doi.org/10.1007/978-981-96-6030-8_2

In case SDB is the underlying cause, those symptoms may be treatable or alleviated [2]. Furthermore, it is believed that SDB can have persistent impacts on a future life of children. Therefore, early identification of case children and their appropriate treatment are crucial for positively influencing their future. This chapter focuses on and discusses the current status and evidence from epidemiological studies of SDB. There is accumulated evidence on pediatric OSA and SDB to date, both of which are presented as SDB in this manuscript.

Their therapeutic approaches may be discussed in Part II.

2 Pediatric Sleep-Disordered Breathing

Generally speaking, SDB is characterized by recurrent upper airway obstruction during sleep in both adults and children, often accompanied by snoring and increased upper airway resistance [3, 4]. Diagnosis is typically based on the apnea-hypopnea index (AHI) obtained from overnight polysomnography (PSG) and associated sleep apnea symptoms [5, 6, 7]. SDB is defined as a syndrome of upper airway dysfunction during sleep, characterized by snoring and/or increased respiratory effort due to heightened upper airway resistance and pharyngeal collapsibility. Obstructive SDB can be further categorized into several clinical entities. Primary snoring is defined as "habitual snoring (more than three nights per week) without apneas, hypopneas, frequent arousals from sleep, or gas exchange abnormalities." Upper airway resistance syndrome is characterized by "snoring, increased work of breathing, and frequent arousals, but without recognizable obstructive events or gas exchange abnormalities." Obstructive hypoventilation involves "snoring and abnormally elevated partial pressure of carbon dioxide in the absence of recognizable obstructive events." Finally, obstructive sleep apnea syndrome is characterized by "recurrent events of partial or complete upper airway obstruction (hypopneas, obstructive or mixed apneas) with disruptions in normal oxygenation, ventilation, and sleep patterns" [7]. These symptoms include sleep fragmentation, hypoxemia, hypercapnia, and daytime sleepiness. Utilizing overnight PSG in pediatric clinical practice and epidemiological studies is challenging due to the need for a well-equipped sleep lab, hospitalization, and the reluctance of children to undergo the procedure. Therefore, in epidemiological studies, questionnaires and portable devices, such as pulse oximeters and airflow sensors, are frequently used. These devices provide measures like the 3% oxygen desaturation index (3% ODI) and the respiratory event index (REI). A recently published guideline by the British Thoracic Society discussed the identification of pediatric SDB cases using various AHI thresholds, questionnaires, and new devices [8].

The classification of snoring during sleep generally depends on the auditory perception of the sounds produced by the individual [9]. Primary snoring is specifically defined as snoring that is not accompanied by apneas, hypopneas, hypoxemia, hypercapnia, or sleep fragmentation [10].

3 Prevalence of Pediatric Sleep-Disordered Breathing

The prevalence of sleep-disordered breathing (SDB) in children varies depending on the indicators used and their threshold values. As summarized in Fig. 2.1, two systematic reviews have reported on the prevalence rates of obstructive sleep apnea (OSA) in pediatric populations. A review by the American Academy of Pediatrics (AAP), incorporating data from ten studies summarized by Marcus et al., found that the prevalence of SDB based on polysomnography (PSG) in the general pediatric population ranged from 0% to 5.7% [11].

A recent systematic review by Magnusdottir and Hill determined the prevalence of OSA in preschool-aged children by reviewing 30 studies. This review highlighted significant variation in reported OSA prevalence, ranging from 0.7% to 13.0%, depending on the methods and criteria used. Higher rates were observed in studies using subjective measures, such as questionnaires, compared to those employing objective measures such as PSG. Notably, only two studies in this review utilized PSG, reporting OSA prevalence of 1.8% and 6.4%. Additionally, studies published between 2016 and 2023 reported higher OSA prevalence, ranging from 12.8% to 20.4%, suggesting a possible increase over the past decade [12]. Similarly, the prevalence of habitual snoring (HS), a primary symptom of SDB, has been reported in various studies. As summarized in Fig. 2.2, the prevalence of HS shows wide variation. In the AAP review summarized by Marcus et al., HS prevalence based on parent-reported questionnaires ranged from 1.5% to 27.6%. The criteria for defining HS differed among studies, contributing to the broad range in prevalence estimates [11].

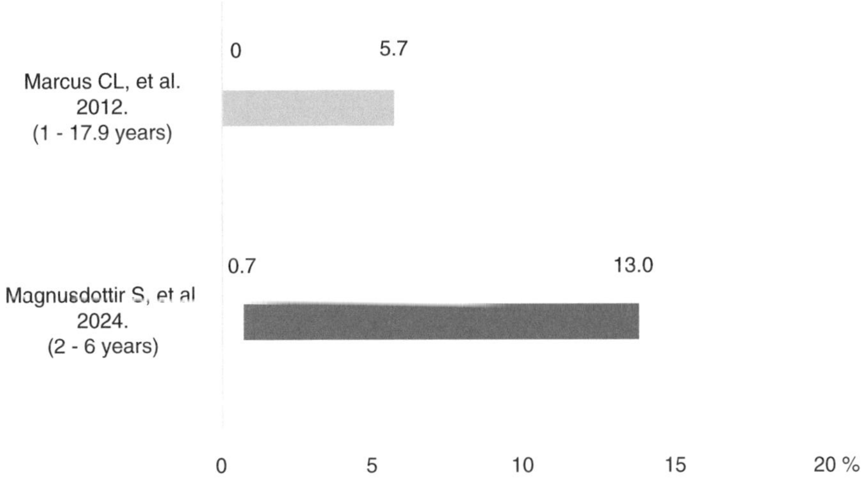

Fig. 2.1 Prevalence of sleep disordered breathing (Based on Marcus et al. [11] and Magnusdottir and Hill [12])

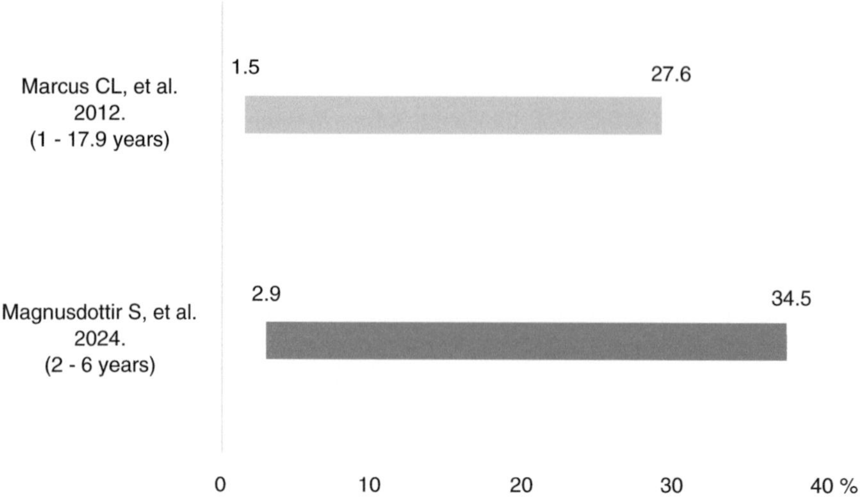

Fig. 2.2 Prevalence of habitual snoring (Based on Marcus et al. [11] and Magnusdottir and Hill [12])

In the systematic review by Magnusdottir and Hill, HS prevalence ranged from 2.9% to 34.5% across several studies. This variation was largely due to differences in the methods used to define and assess HS, with most studies relying on parent-reported questionnaires. For instance, one study using non-validated questionnaires reported an HS prevalence of 12.1%, while another using a validated sleep questionnaire reported a prevalence of 35.6%. The review emphasized that the inconsistency in criteria for defining HS, such as the frequency of snoring, contributed to the wide range in prevalence estimates [12]. Although these prevalence estimates are based on subjective responses rather than objective evaluations, they suggest that HS, and by extension of SDB, is relatively common in pediatric populations. The variability in prevalence underscores the importance of using standardized and validated questionnaires in future research [11]. Despite the high prevalence of pediatric SDB and its significant impact on children's physical and mental health, awareness remains comparatively low, representing a substantial public health concern.

4 Risk Factors and Associated Health Problems of Pediatric Sleep-Disordered Breathing

Understanding the risk factors and comorbidities of pediatric sleep-disordered breathing is essential for early screening, prevention of progression, effective intervention, and preventive strategies.

4.1 Obesity

Obesity is a significant independent risk factor for pediatric SDB. With the increasing prevalence of childhood obesity, particularly central obesity, the incidence of SDB has also risen, because obesity contributes to the accumulation of fat around the neck and the throat, increasing the vulnerability of airway obstruction during sleep [13]. This was confirmed by strong correlations between body mass index (BMI), waist size, and the severity of SDB, suggesting that metabolic factors play a crucial role in the etiology of SDB in children [14]. The relationship between BMI and respiratory event index in children older than 7 years is noteworthy, highlighting the increasing impact of obesity on the severity of SDB with age [15].

4.2 Adenotonsillar Hypertrophy

Adenotonsillar hypertrophy is one of the common causes of SDB in children. This enlargement can narrow the upper airway, especially when muscle tone decreases during sleep, leading to breathing difficulties [16]. This condition is most prevalent in children aged 2–6 years, coinciding with the peak incidence of pediatric SDB [17]. Traditionally, many children with tonsillar hypertrophy and SDB were underweight [18], but with the rise in childhood obesity, this clinical picture has changed.

4.3 Allergic Rhinitis and Upper Airway Abnormalities

Allergic rhinitis (AR) is another significant risk factor for developing pediatric SDB. Nasal congestion secondary to the inflammatory process associated with AR increases airway resistance [19]. A meta-analysis by Cao et al. showed that children with AR are more likely to have habitual snoring and an increased risk of SDB [20], and the incidence of AR in children with SDB was higher than those without SDB by 2.12 times [20].

4.4 Asthma

Asthma and other respiratory diseases are closely associated with pediatric SDB. Children with asthma are more likely to suffer from habitual snoring and SDB compared to those without asthma [21]. The prevalence of SDB is higher in children with asthma, and the severity of SDB increases with the severity of asthma [21]. Ross et al. also showed that children with SDB are 3.62 times more likely to have severe asthma after a year of asthma treatment, suggesting that SDB may exacerbate the severity of asthma [22].

4.5 Neurobehavioral and Cognitive Abnormalities

Children with SDB may experience difficulties in attention, learning, and memory and exhibit neurocognitive and behavioral problems such as hyperactivity and aggressiveness [23, 24]. These issues are thought to be caused by multiple factors including nocturnal intermittent hypoxemia, sleep fragmentation, and overall reduced sleep quality. Such neurocognitive deficits can have long-term effects on academic performance and social interactions.

4.6 Growth and Developmental Issues

Pediatric SDB is not just a disorder of sleep disturbance but is associated with significant health problems affecting the growth and development of children. Additionally, sleep fragmentation and reduced sleep quality can further exacerbate these growth issues by interfering with normal developmental processes. Impaired secretion of growth hormone has been shown in children with SDB, and improvements in SDB by adenotonsillectomy have been associated with recovery of growth hormone secretion and weight gain [25]. Pediatric SDB is a multifaceted condition with widespread impacts on the health of children. The associations of impaired sleep quality with cardiovascular diseases, growth retardation, neurobehavioral, metabolic, and respiratory disorders indicated the need for comprehensive management strategies. Understanding these associations is crucial in providing holistic care to children with SDB.

4.7 Evidence for Children in Japan

Although there are accumulated data on pediatric SDB, their evidence is still scarce. Therefore, we conducted several epidemiological studies. We first developed a Japanese version of the severity hierarchy score (SHS) [26]. The original version of SHS was developed by Spruyt and Gozal [27] and was translated into French [28], Chinese [29], and Thailand [30] and had a cut-off value of ≥2.72–1.9. However, our validation study indicated that an SHS score ≥ 1.88 identifies those children in Japan at high risk for SDB [26].

In an epidemiological study of all elementary school students in Matsuyama city (N ≥ 20,000), when SDB was defined as SHS ≥2.72, the prevalence of SDB is 0.6%, but that prevalence will be greater with the definition of SHS ≥1.88. High

SHS scores were associated with obesity and problematic behaviors including restlessness, fidgeting, and inattentiveness [31]. It has also been shown that SDB-related symptoms derived from the parent-reported questionnaire were associated with nocturnal enuresis [32], pectus excavatum [33], and common cold [34]. Collectively, SDB has a significant impact on the physical and mental health of children.

5 Pediatric Sleep-Disordered Breathing from a Public Health Perspective

Pediatric SDB raises a significant public health issue due to its high prevalence, its association with health risks, and its impact on the healthcare system. From surveys based on questionnaires to those on PSG and PVT, the challenges in pediatric epidemiology lie in the fact that while the British Thoracic Society (BTS) guidelines consider AHI as a major indicator (BTS GL 2024), a study has shown that even snoring frequency as infrequent as once a week can alter neurological and behavioral parameters, and those indices are more sensitive than AHI [35].

From experimental studies on adult participants, Van Dongen showed that self-reported sleepiness is not sufficiently reliable, however, the psychomotor vigilance test (PVT) provides more accurate data on physical and mental conditions following chronic sleep deprivation [36]. PVT measures your response time between red digits appearing on a small window, and your pressing button, and this process is repeated many times for 10 minutes or 3 minutes of the test time. After evaluating your responsiveness during the test period, your vigilance is objectively indicated, as lapses or mean reaction time. We also found that PVT may identify individuals at-risk for psychological health crises, such as burnout and depression in adults [37], and anxiety and hyperactiveness in children, and believe that PVT is promising to assess the psychological condition of children.

5.1 Burden on the Healthcare System and Socioeconomic Disparities

SDB in children imposes a substantial burden on the healthcare system. Children with untreated SDB often have increased healthcare utilization, including hospital visits and medical interventions [38]. This increase in healthcare usage is not only due to the direct impacts of SDB but also related comorbidities, such as cardiovascular disorders, diabetes, neurobehavioral abnormalities, and metabolic disorders [23]. Consequently, there is an increase in healthcare costs for families and the healthcare system. These costs include not only social costs but also the loss derived from impaired longer-term health and development from untreated or inadequately managed SDB among children at their levels.

Children from disadvantaged socioeconomic backgrounds, such as impoverished households or single-parent homes, are more likely to be diagnosed with SDB [39]. Then, those with SDB, when they grow to be adults, are more likely to have social disadvantages and suffer from economic damages [40]. Therefore, SDB and social disadvantages form a vicious cycle, and thus, social disparities may become broader.

The focus should be on ensuring that all children, regardless of socioeconomic status, have access to necessary diagnostic and treatment services. Addressing socioeconomic disparities in the context of pediatric SDB is essential for achieving health equity, and the screening, diagnosis, and treatment of SDB in children is one of the measures to address these issues.

Key strategies to address pediatric SDB from a public health perspective include raising awareness among healthcare professionals, schoolteachers, and parents. Public health campaigns and educational programs can play a key role in raising awareness of the signs of SDB, the importance of early diagnosis, and the treatment options available. Regular screening for symptoms of SDB can also lead to earlier diagnosis and treatment. For example, simple questionnaires on SDB administered to parents during routine pediatric visits can be an effective tool for identifying children at risk of SDB. Early intervention can improve individual health outcomes and reduce the long-term public health burden by preventing the progression of associated conditions.

6 Summary

Pediatric SDB is a significant public health issue due to its high prevalence, impact on health and development, and the burden it places on the healthcare system. Public health strategies focusing on awareness, early detection, intervention, and addressing socioeconomic disparities are crucial. Continued research can further improve our understanding and management of pediatric SDB, ultimately benefiting children's health worldwide.

References

1. Simola P, Liukkonen K, Pitkäranta A, Pirinen T, Aronen ET. Psychosocial and somatic outcomes of sleep problems in children: a 4-year follow-up study. Child Care Health Dev. 2014 Jan;40(1):60–7.
2. Dillon JE, Blunden S, Ruzicka DL, Guire KE, Champine D, Weatherly RA, Hodges EK, Giordani BJ, Chervin RD. DSM-IV diagnoses and obstructive sleep apnea in children before and 1 year after adenotonsillectomy. J Am Acad Child Adolesc Psychiatry. 2007;46(11):1425–36.
3. Kaditis A, Kheirandish-Gozal L, Gozal D. Algorithm for the diagnosis and treatment of pediatric OSA: a proposal of two pediatric sleep centers. Sleep Med. 2012;13:217–27.

4. Carroll JL. Obstructive sleep-disordered breathing in children: new controversies, new directions. Clin Chest Med. 2003 Jun;24(2):261–82.
5. American Thoracic Society. Standards and indications for cardiopulmonary sleep studies in children. Am J Respir Crit Care Med. 1996;153:866–78.
6. Dayyat E, Kheirandish-Gozal L, Gozal D. Childhood obstructive sleep apnea: one or two distinct disease entities? Sleep Med Clin. 2007;2:433–44.
7. Kaditis AG, Alonso Alvarez ML, Boudewyns A, Alexopoulos EI, Ersu R, Joosten K, Larramona H, Miano S, Narang I, Trang H, Tsaoussoglou M, Vandenbussche N, Villa MP, Van Waardenburg D, Weber S, Verhulst S. Obstructive sleep disordered breathing in 2- to 18-year-old children: diagnosis and management. Eur Respir J. 2016 Jan;47(1):69–94.
8. Evans HJ, Gibson NA, Bennett J, Chan SY, Gavlak J, Harman K, Ismail-Koch H, Kingshott RN, Langley R, Morley A, Opstad KS, Russo K, Samuels MP, Tan HL, Tweedie D, Yanney M, Whitney A. BTS paediatric sleep disorders guideline development group. British Thoracic Society guideline for diagnosing and monitoring paediatric sleep-disordered breathing. Thorax. 2023;78(Suppl 2):s1–s27.
9. Strollo PJ Jr, Sanders MH. Significance and treatment of nonapneic snoring. Sleep. 1993;16(5):403–8.
10. American Academy of Pediatrics. Section on Pediatric Pulmonology, Subcommittee on Obstructive Sleep Apnea Syndrome. American Academy of Pediatrics. Clinical practice guideline: diagnosis and management of childhood obstructive sleep apnea syndrome. Pediatrics. 2002;109(4):704–12.
11. Marcus CL, Brooks LJ, Draper KA, Gozal D, Halbower AC, Jones J, Schechter MS, Ward SD, Sheldon SH, Shiffman RN, Lehmann C, Spruyt K, American Academy of Pediatrics. Diagnosis and management of childhood obstructive sleep apnea syndrome. Pediatrics. 2012;130(3):e714–55.
12. Magnusdottir S, Hill EA. Prevalence of obstructive sleep apnea (OSA) among preschool aged children in the general population: a systematic review. Sleep Med Rev. 2024;73:101871.
13. Newman AB, Foster G, Givelber R, Nieto FJ, Redline S, Young T. Progression and regression of sleep-disordered breathing with changes in weight: the sleep heart health study. Arch Intern Med. 2005;165(20):2408–13.
14. Bixler EO, Vgontzas AN, Lin HM, Liao D, Calhoun S, Vela-Bueno A, Fedok F, Vlasic V, Graff G. Sleep-disordered breathing in children in a general population sample: prevalence and risk factors. Sleep. 2009;32(6):731–6.
15. Kaditis AG, Alexopoulos EI, Hatzi F, Karadonta I, Chaidas K, Gourgoulianis K, Zintzaras E, Syrogiannopoulos GA. Adiposity in relation to age as predictor of severity of sleep apnea in children with snoring. Sleep Breath. 2008;12(1):25–31.
16. Marcus CL, McColley SA, Carroll JL, Loughlin GM, Smith PL, Schwartz AR. Upper airway collapsibility in children with obstructive sleep apnea syndrome. J Appl Physiol. 1985). 1994;77(2):918–24.
17. Arens R, McDonough JM, Costarino AT, Mahboubi S, Tayag-Kier CE, Maislin G, Schwab RJ, Pack AI. Magnetic resonance imaging of the upper airway structure of children with obstructive sleep apnea syndrome. Am J Respir Crit Care Med. 2001;164(4):698–703.
18. Kelly A, Marcus CL. Childhood obesity, inflammation, and apnea: what is the future for our children? Am J Respir Crit Care Med. 2005;171(3):202–3.
19. Kimple AJ, Ishman SL. Allergy and sleep-disordered breathing. Curr Opin Otolaryngol Head Neck Surg. 2013;21(3):277–81.
20. Cao Y, Wu S, Zhang L, Yang Y, Cao S, Li Q. Association of allergic rhinitis with obstructive sleep apnea: a meta-analysis. Medicine (Baltimore). 2018;97(51):e13783.
21. Goldstein NA, Aronin C, Kantrowitz B, Hershcopf R, Fishkin S, Lee H, Weaver DE, Yip C, Liaw C, Saadia TA, Abramowitz J, Weedon J. The prevalence of sleep-disordered breathing in children with asthma and its behavioral effects. Pediatr Pulmonol. 2015;50(11):1128–36.

22. Ross KR, Storfer-Isser A, Hart MA, Kibler AM, Rueschman M, Rosen CL, Kercsmar CM, Redline S. Sleep-disordered breathing is associated with asthma severity in children. J Pediatr. 2012;160(5):736–42.
23. Kheirandish-Gozal L, Gozal D. Pediatric OSA syndrome morbidity biomarkers: the hunt is finally on! Chest. 2017;151(2):500–6.
24. Horne RSC, Ong C, Weichard A, Nixon GM, Davey MJ. Are there gender differences in the severity and consequences of sleep disordered in children? Sleep Med. 2020;67:147–55.
25. Nieminen P, Löppönen T, Tolonen U, Lanning P, Knip M, Löppönen H. Growth and biochemical markers of growth in children with snoring and obstructive sleep apnea. Pediatrics. 2002;109(4):e55.
26. Zhu Q, Wada H, Onuki K, Kitazawa T, Furuya R, Miyakawa M, Sato S, Yonemoto N, Ueda Y, Nakano H, Gozal D, Tanigawa T. Validity and reliability of the Japanese version of the severity hierarchy score for pediatric obstructive sleep apnea screening. Sleep Med. 2023;101:357–64. Epub 2022 Nov 22. Erratum in: Sleep Med. 2023 May;105:36
27. Spruyt K, Gozal D. Screening of pediatric sleep-disordered breathing: a proposed unbiased discriminative set of questions using clinical severity scales. Chest. 2012;142(6):1508–15.
28. Nguyên XL, Lévy P, Beydon N, Gozal D, Fleury B. Performance characteristics of the French version of the severity hierarchy score for paediatric sleep apnoea screening in clinical settings. Sleep Med. 2017;30:24–8.
29. Zhang J, Tang MY, Jiang F. The reliability and validity of Chinese version of a short pediatric obstructive sleep apnea syndrome screening scale. Chinese J Evidence - Based Pediatric. 2017;12:17–21.
30. Tanphaichitr A, Chuenchod P, Ungkanont K, Banhiran W, Vathanophas V, Gozal D. Validity and reliability of the Thai version of the pediatric obstructive sleep apnea screening tool. Pediatr Pulmonol. 2021;56(9):2979–86.
31. Sakamoto N, Gozal D, Smith DL, Yang L, Morimoto N, Wada H, Maruyama K, Ikeda A, Suzuki Y, Nakayama M, Horiguchi I, Tanigawa T. Sleep duration, snoring prevalence, obesity, and behavioral problems in a large cohort of primary school students in Japan. Sleep. 2017;40(3)
32. Wada H, Kimura M, Tajima T, Shirahama R, Suzuki Y, Suzuki Y, Hayashi T, Maruyama K, Endo M, Sakamoto N, Ikeda A, Gozal D, Tanigawa T. Nocturnal enuresis and sleep disordered breathing in primary school children: potential implications. Pediatr Pulmonol. 2018;53(11):1541–8.
33. Wada H, Kimura M, Shirahama R, Ikeda A, Gozal D, Tanigawa T. Pectus excavatum is associated with sleep-related breathing disorders in children. Eur Respir J. 2019;54(4):1900524.
34. Kitazawa T, Wada H, Onuki K, Furuya R, Miyakawa M, Zhu Q, Ueda Y, Sato S, Kameda Y, Nakano H, Gozal D, Tanigawa T. Snoring, obstructive sleep apnea, and upper respiratory tract infection in elementary school children in Japan. Sleep Breath. 2023.
35. Smith DL, Gozal D, Hunter SJ, Kheirandish-Gozal L. Frequency of snoring, rather than apnea-hypopnea index, predicts both cognitive and behavioral problems in young children. Sleep Med 2017 J34:170–178.
36. Van Dongen HP, Maislin G, Mullington JM, Dinges DF. The cumulative cost of additional wakefulness: dose-response effects on neurobehavioral functions and sleep physiology from chronic sleep restriction and total sleep deprivation. Sleep. 2003;26(2):117–26.
37. Wada H, Basner M, Cordoza M, Dinges D, Tanigawa T. Objective alertness, rather than sleep duration, is associated with burnout and depression: a national survey of Japanese physicians. J Sleep Res. 2025;34(1):e14304.
38. Tarasiuk A, Greenberg-Dotan S, Simon-Tuval T, Freidman B, Goldbart AD, Tal A, Reuveni H. Elevated morbidity and health care use in children with obstructive sleep apnea syndrome. Am J Respir Crit Care Med. 2007;175(1):55–61.

39. Wang R, Dong Y, Weng J, Kontos EZ, Chervin RD, Rosen CL, Marcus CL, Redline S. Associations among neighborhood, race, and sleep apnea severity in children. A Six-City analysis. Ann Am Thorac Soc. 2017;14(1):76–84.
40. Borsoi L, Armeni P, Donin G, Costa F, Ferini-Strambi L. The invisible costs of obstructive sleep apnea (OSA): systematic review and cost-of-illness analysis. PLoS One. 2022;17(5):e0268677.

Chapter 3
OSA, Morphology, and Pathophysiology: Why is the Morphology so Important in the Pathophysiology of Obstructive Sleep Apnea?

Shiroh Isono

Abstract Some specific morphological differences between obstructive sleep apnea (OSA) and non-OSA persons account for mechanisms for development of pharyngeal airway obstruction during sleep. The pharyngeal airway is analogous to a collapsible tube within a rigid box which can demonstrate three key mechanisms of pharyngeal closure: increase of respiratory efforts during OSA; increase of tissue pressure surrounding the pharynx caused upper airway anatomical imbalance by the excessive amount of soft tissue (obesity) and small maxillomandibular enclosure; reduction of longitudinal tension of the pharyngeal airway particularly in central obese patients with reduced lung volume. Contribution of craniofacial abnormalities to OSA differs among the countries and races with larger influence in the Asian people. The anatomical imbalance can be detected by lower hyoid bone in the lateral cephalogram. There are, however, OSA mechanisms unexplained by the simple collapsible tube model. For example, mechanical disadvantage of fat deposition at the tongue base, mechanical interaction between the tongue base and soft palate through the gravitational impact on the soft tissue, valve-like behavior of the soft palate and epiglottis, and surface tension of pharyngeal airway mucosa. Clearly, it is necessary to develop a more comprehensive clinically useful morphological model in understanding the OSA pathophysiology.

Keywords Pharynx · Collapsible tube · Obstruction · Flow dynamics

---

S. Isono (✉)
Department of Anesthesiology, Graduate School of Medicine, Chiba University, Chuo-Ku, Chiba, Japan

K. Chin (ed.), *The Current State of Sleep Disordered Breathing in Japan and Around the World*, Respiratory Disease Series: Diagnostic Tools and Disease Managements, https://doi.org/10.1007/978-981-96-6030-8_3

1 A Collapsible Tube Within a Rigid Box: Can It Mimic Pharyngeal Obstruction in OSA?

The pharyngeal airway, where OSA occurs, is structurally surrounded by soft tissue such as the tongue, soft palate, tonsils, and pharyngeal fat pads. The soft tissue is enclosed by bony structures such as the mandible, maxilla, and cervical spines [1]. The pharynx is inherently collapsible during sleep when upper airway (UA) dilating muscle activity decreases [2] and is mechanically analogous to an artificial collapsible tube in a rigid box (Fig. 3.1). The behavior of an atonic or hypotonic pharyngeal airway (passive pharynx) is demonstrable by a collapsible tube within a rigid box [3, 4].

In this mechanical model, the luminal size (airway size) is determined by the pressure difference between the inside (P_{lumen}) and outside (P_{tissue}) of the tube (transmural pressure: $P_{tm} = P_{lumen}—P_{tissue}$) and mechanical properties of the tube ("tube law") [5]. Three distinct but mutually interactive mechanisms result in luminal

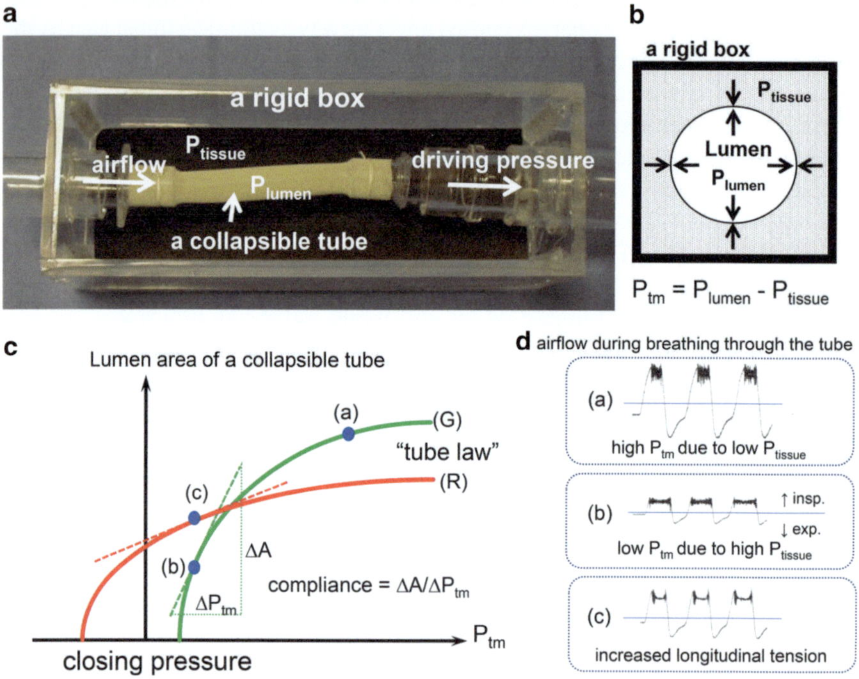

Fig. 3.1 (**a**) An artificial collapsible tube in a rigid box. Pressure differences across the collapsible tube (driving pressure) introduce airflow through the tube. (**b**) Definition of transmural pressure (P_{tm}). P_{tm} is defined as intraluminal pressure (P_{lumen}) minus surrounding tissue pressure (P_{tissue}). (**c**) "tube law" of the collapsible tube. Cross-sectional area of the tube changes in accordance with the "tube law." Compliance of the tube varies with Ptm and is determined as slope of the "tube law." Two different "tube law" (G and R) are presented. (**d**) Typical airflow patterns produced during breathing starting from three different points on the "tube law"

narrowing or closure: decrease of P_{lumen}, increase of P_{tissue}, and reduction of longitudinal tension of the collapsible tube. Even without airflow through the tube, any mechanisms increasing P_{tissue} can narrow the lumen area. In the human pharyngeal airway, P_{tissue} can be increased by UA anatomical imbalance and gravitational impact on the pharyngeal airway as discussed below. Longitudinal traction of the pharyngeal airway can be decreased by lung volume reduction particularly in obese patients, as also discussed below. Airflow through the collapsible tube (inspiration) decreases P_{lumen} with different pressure distributions along the tube due to dissipative energy loss and/or conversion of kinetic energy to potential energy (Bernoulli's law) [5, 6]. When the reduction of P_{lumen} results in a critical luminal narrowing (choking point), the tube wall starts vibrating (snoring) with a flattened airflow signal (inspiratory flow limitation) in accordance with the fluid dynamics. For the points (a), (b), and (c) on the tube law curves (Fig. 3.1), P_{tm} progressively decreases due to progressive decrease of P_{lumen} during inspiration and luminal area progressively decreases in accordance with the tube law curves. However, the maximum airflow values significantly differ between the points (a > c > b) because different P_{tissue} results in different lumen area at the beginning of inspiration and different longitudinal tension of the tube leads to different lumen area change during inspiration. Using the tube law concept, Isono et al. first evidenced anatomically more collapsible pharyngeal airway in OSA patients than non-OSA subjects [7]. UA Starling resistor model, an extremely collapsible tube, is widely applied for measurements of UA P_{crit} (critical closing pressure) in OSA patients [8].

In this way, the collapsible tube model is useful for understanding mechanisms of pharyngeal narrowing and closure during OSA. Based on the behavior of the mechanical model, we need to explain the sources of the P_{tissue} and changes of longitudinal forces of the airway in addition to changes of the luminal pressure during breathing. Furthermore, the actual pharyngeal airway and surrounding structures are not as simple as the collapsible tube within a rigid box. In fact, some types of obstructive apnea and hypopnea are not explainable by the model. Part of the answer can be obtained by considering specific structural aspects of the pharyngeal airway and the human body as well as the neural control system interacting with the structures as is summarized in Fig. 3.2 and discussed below.

2 UA Anatomical Imbalance

In the pharynx analogous to a collapsible tube within a rigid box, the balance between the size of the maxillomandibular bony enclosure and the amount of soft tissue within the enclosure may determine the airway space and P_{tissue} [1, 9]. Excessive soft tissue within the bony enclosure or a small maxilla and/or mandible would result in limited space available for the airway and, consequently, a pharyngeal airway narrowing and increase of P_{tissue} (Fig. 3.2). This UA anatomical balance theory was first proposed by Watanabe et al. who found association between sites of positive closing pressure (P_{close}) and morphological differences: smaller maxilla and

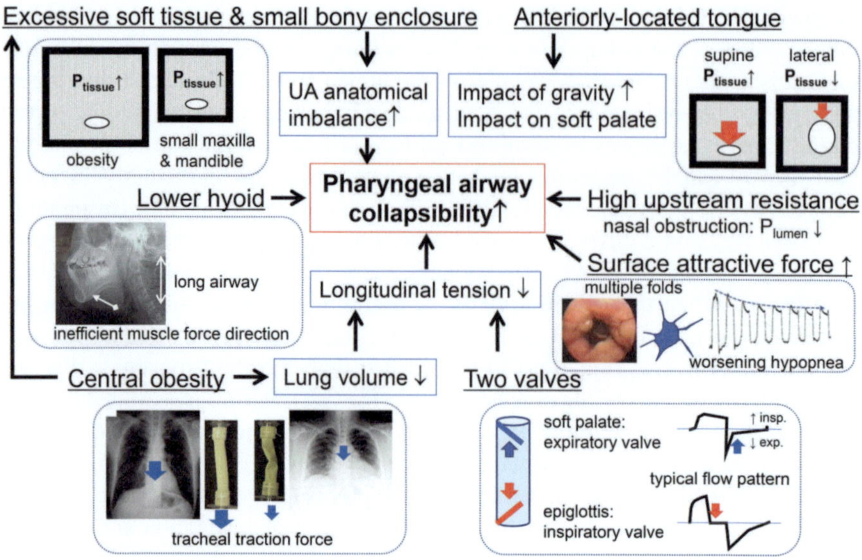

Fig. 3.2 Key morphologies possibly leading to pharyngeal airway obstruction. Refer this figure for each of the section in this chapter

mandible in OSA patients with positive P_{close} at the retropalatal and retroglossal airways, and obesity in OSA patients with positive P_{close} exclusively at the retropalatal airway [1]. Furthermore, Tsuiki et al. evidenced the UA anatomical imbalance by demonstrating significantly larger tongues for any given maxillomandibular size in OSA patients than BMI-matched non-OSA controls [10]. Kairaitis et al. confirmed that an increase of mass surrounding the pharyngeal airway resulted in increases of both P_{tissue} and UA resistance in anesthetized rabbits [11]. Tongue volume is not always larger in OSA patients [12, 13]. It should be noted that sole measurements of soft tissue volume without craniofacial dimension control do not reflect UA anatomical balance and P_{tissue}. In fact, UA anatomical balance assessed by relative soft tissue volume to maxillomandibular dimensions have differed between OSA patients and non-OSA controls in two studies that did not detect larger tongue volumes in OSA patients [12, 13].

3 Excessive Soft Tissue Surrounding the Pharynx

Any causes of increased amount of soft tissue within the maxillomandibular enclosure can influence the UA anatomical balance. Schwab et al. identified tongue volume and lateral pharyngeal wall volume as independent risk factors for OSA [14]. More fat deposition surrounding the pharynx in OSA patients is documented compared with BMI-matched non-OSA subjects [15, 16]. The pharyngeal fat volume was significantly associated with AHI, but not BMI [17] and appeared to contribute to the collapsibility of retropalatal and retroglossal airway [18].

It remains unclear how much increase in soft tissue volume is necessary for OSA to develop. Schwab et al. reported 30 cm^3 larger soft tissue volume in obese OSA than non-obese controls without controlling BMI (36 versus 26 kg/m^2) and craniofacial dimensions [14]. In contrast to the study in primarily Caucasian and African-American, study performed in Japanese males found that the difference of UA soft tissue volume between OSA and craniofacial size-matched non-OSA controls was approximately 20 cm^3 [13]. Sutherland et al. found a reduction of the UA fat volume by approximately 17 cm^3 after 8 kg weight reduction resulted a 31% AHI reduction in Caucasian OSA patients [19]. These upper airway imaging studies in adults suggest that OSA would presumably develop following a 20–30 cm^3 increase in UA soft tissue volume depending on the maxillomandibular enclosure size.

4 Contribution of Pharyngeal Fat Deposition to OSA Pathophysiology

In addition to the mass effect, fat deposition alters soft tissue elasticity which is a significant determinant of soft tissue movement and deformation. Interestingly, fat content in the posterior tongue (30%) was significantly higher than in the anterior tongue (11%) or other somatic muscles (3%) and correlated with BMI in autopsy specimens from the general population [20]. In general, Young's elastic modulus of muscle (0.0675 MPa) is half of that of fat (0.182 MPa), suggesting that the tongue base is less mobile than other part of the tongue during the genioglossus muscle contraction and/or other extrinsic forces on the tongue. In fact, this prediction is in agreement with the movements of the tongue musculature during hypoglossal nerve stimulation analyzed by a tagged MRI technique in rats [21]. Kato et al. demonstrated more effectiveness of submental negative pressure application in non-obese than obese OSA patients with significant improvement of stiffness and P_{close} at the retroglossal airway [22].

An animal study demonstrated increase of oil droplet areas together with increase in muscle fiber diameter in the genioglossus and geniohyoid muscles, but not in the masseter muscle after high-fat diet feeding [23]. Furthermore, intermittent hypoxemia appeared to induce a transition from endurant type IIa fibers to the more fatigable type IIb fibers [24]. In patients with OSA, this transition has been shown to be reversible with CPAP treatment [25].

5 Small Maxillomandibular Bony Enclosure

Any persons even without obesity can develop OSA due to increase of P_{tissue} when soft tissue surrounding the pharynx is excess for the individual maxillomandibular bony enclosure size. Therefore, small maxilla and/or mandible are significant risk factors for development of OSA without obesity (Fig. 3.2). However, small maxilla and/or mandible in most of non-obese adult OSA patients are rarely recognized as abnormal in the routine clinical assessments and are detected by imaging techniques such as lateral cephalogram [26, 27]. Various cephalogram parameters can be used to assess maxillomandibular bony enclosure size; however, caution is required since UA anatomical balance is capable of assessment by both soft tissue and bony enclosure. In this context, detection of excess sub-mandible soft tissue, high Mallampati class, and lowered hyoid bone are considered to reflect the UA anatomical balance in non-obese OSA patients [28].

In contrast to western countries where obesity is predominant in OSA patients, most Japanese OSA patients are non-obese [29]. Reginal and/or racial differences of the morphologic features of OSA patients appear to be explained by the UA anatomical concept [30, 31]. Lee et al. reported that Chinese patients had more craniofacial bony restriction (a shorter cranial base, maxilla and mandible length) and Caucasian patients had greater BMI and large neck circumference [30]. Notably, the ratios of BMI to the maxilla or mandible size were similar when OSA severity was matched between Chinese and Caucasian OSA patients.

Although rare, it is well-known that syndromes with craniofacial abnormalities (Pierre Robin sequence, Treacher Collins syndrome, Crouzon syndrome, Apert syndrome, etc.) are accompanied by obstructive sleep apnea and some suffer from airway obstruction during wakefulness requiring tracheostomy in the early period of life. Surgical correction of craniofacial bony restriction is effective for improving OSA both in adults and children [32, 33]. In particular, small children with the syndromic craniosynostosis can avoid tracheostomy by early midfacial and/or mandibular distraction surgery [34].

6 Central Obesity: Reduction of Longitudinal Tracheal Traction Force and P_{tissue} Increase

The trachea mechanically connects the lung and pharyngeal airway. Static and dynamic inflation of the lung produces sustained and inspiratory longitudinal tracheal traction forces, respectively (Fig. 3.2). The static force may be reduced in obese patients with lower functional residual capacity by changing the tube law of the pharynx. The dynamic tracheal traction force serves to stabilize the pharyngeal airway and airflow during inspiration as predicted by the behavior of an artificial collapsible tube.

In response to either static tracheal traction or lung inflation, reduction of UA resistance and collapsibility was reported in both animal and human studies [35–39]. Kairaitis et al. found small but significant reductions in P_{tissue} in response to tracheal traction in anesthetized rabbits [36]. The genioglossus activity decreased during lung inflation in sleeping OSA patients suggesting structural mechanisms [38, 39]. In fact, in anesthetized and paralyzed OSA patients, Tagaito et al. found a significant reduction in retropalatal P_{close} during lung inflation and a direct association between changes in retropalatal P_{close} and BMI [37]. Kohno et al. further evidenced the stronger lung volume dependence of longitudinal tracheal traction particularly in OSA patients with central obesity [40].

Tracheal traction forces dynamically change in accordance with respiratory cycles during spontaneous breathing. Negative intra-thoracic pressure regardless of lung inflation appears to produce the phasic tracheal traction forces [35]. Maximum tracheal displacement was directly associated with peak inspiratory efforts and greater in patients with severe OSA [41]. Therefore, tracheal tug during OSA without lung volume increase could serve to improve pharyngeal collapsibility while it also serves to maintain obstruction by increasing the negative P_{lumen}. Because of the increased diaphragmatic curvature in reduced lung volume, this mechanism should operate more efficiently in obese patients with reduced lung volume central obesity than non-obese subjects.

7 Morphological Changes as Compensatory Mechanisms for Anatomical Imbalance

As discussed above, specific morphologies are associated with development of OSA. In contrast, some morphological changes are considered to play roles as compensatory mechanisms in particular for UA anatomical imbalance. Unlike the rigid box shown in Fig. 3.1, the human maxillomandibular bony enclosure is not a closed space. Therefore, the excessive soft tissue within the bony enclosure can be displaced outside it through the submandible space, possibly partly improving the UA anatomical imbalance and decreasing the P_{tissue}. The displaced excessive submandible soft tissue can be detected in OSA patients as increased neck circumference, a "double chin," or reduced cricomental space [28]. Furthermore, the excessive soft tissue displaces the mobile hyoid bone caudally and elongates the pharyngeal airway length by 15–30%. The lowered hyoid bone is a common finding in the lateral cephalogram in OSA patients [10, 26, 27] and may be an indicator of UA anatomical imbalance rather than a cause of OSA [10] (Fig. 3.2). Elongation of the pharyngeal airway could have different impacts on OSA: an increase in UA resistance, worsening OSA, and an increase of longitudinal tension, improving OSA. The hyoid bone serves as an anker for supra- and infra-hyoid bone muscles including pharyngeal airway dilators. Caudal displacement of hyoid bone decreases anteriorly oriented muscle force leading to airway narrowing and increases upward muscle force decreasing longitudinal tension. The inefficient muscle force may contribute to increase of pharyngeal airway collapsibility, although it is speculative at present.

8 Anteriorly Located Tongue: Impacts of Gravity and Its Impact on the Soft Palate

Soft tissues surrounding the pharyngeal airway are not uniformly distributed within the bony enclosure (Fig. 3.2). The larger mass of the soft tissues, such as the tongue, anteriorly overrides on the pharyngeal airway, producing greater P_{tissue} derived from the gravity onto the anterior soft tissues [42]. The impact of gravity can be altered by position change from the supine to other positions such as the lateral, sitting, and prone positions [42, 43].

When the relatively smaller amount of the soft tissues locates laterally in OSA patients, lateral position reduces impact of gravity on the lateral wall soft tissue decreasing P_{tissue} and passive P_{close} [42]. Sleep in the lateral position significantly decreased AHI particularly in non-obese OSA patients [44]. Notably, the position-dependent OSA patients presented smaller lateral soft tissue volume compared with BMI-, age-, and AHI-matched non-positional OSA patients [13]. Sitting position also decreases the impact of gravity on the anteriorly located soft tissue and, in fact, decreased the passive P_{close} [43] and AHI [45].

Furthermore, because of the unique structural arrangements of the tongue and soft palate, the tongue base can push the soft palate posteriorly. By measuring the contact pressure between them, Isono et al. evidenced significant dynamic interactions between them during both obstructive apnea and each inspiratory effort, possibly maintaining closure at the retropalatal airway only in anesthetized OSA patients with positive P_{close} at retroglossal airway [46].

9 Valve-Like Behavior of Two Peninsulas in the Pharynx: The Soft Palate and Epiglottis

Morphologically, the soft palate and epiglottis resemble peninsulas protruding from the pharyngeal wall (Fig. 3.2). Both the epiglottis and soft palate function as valves for prevention of food from entering the trachea and nose, respectively, during swallowing. Similarly, the expiratory and inspiratory airflows through the pharyngeal airway hit the valves, consequently narrowing or closing the airway when they are not stabilized by contraction of the surrounding UA muscles. Opening or closing of the swing valve is mainly determined by the pressure difference between anterior and posterior valve surfaces, valve mass, and valve angle for the airflow [47].

Safar was the first to document the possibility that expiratory obstruction during positive pressure intranasal ventilation is caused by the valve-like behavior of the soft palate [48]. A sudden reduction of expiratory flow was reported in both spontaneously breathing, as well as mechanically ventilated OSA patients [49–51]. Recently, Okuyama et al. endoscopically confirmed that expiratory obstruction of the soft palate causes an expiratory flow limitation [52]. Very interestingly, the dynamic airway P_{close} during the expiratory obstruction at the soft palate was much greater than the static P_{close} at the soft palate indicating that the valve-like behavior is not explainable by the simple tube law theory.

Zarbarzin et al. endoscopically observed the valve-like epiglottic collapse covering the vocal cords together with a sudden fall of the airflow signal during inspiration in sleeping OSA patients (Fig. 3.2) [53]. This type of epiglottic closure is considered to occasionally occur in 20–30% of OSA patients. Notably, despite the dynamic mid-inspiratory closure at the atmospheric upstream pressure, there was unstable but relatively normal inspiratory flow indicating the negative epiglottis P_{crit}. Accordingly, neither the Starling resistor model nor the collapsible tube with variable compliance adequately describes the sudden mid-inspiratory flow reduction.

Clearly, the more advanced and comprehensive theory, hopefully uncomplicated, for explaining dynamic closure of the pharyngeal airway needs to be developed to describe and understand the upper airway behavior during sleep in OSA patients. Due to the strong associations of features of airflow signals and the site of airway closure, establishment of a pharyngeal mechanical model closer to its anatomical structure would lead to automatic determination of the responsible site of OSA development and serve to accelerate the formulation of individualized OSA treatment strategies.

10 Nose: An Upstream Resistance for the Pharyngeal Airway During Inspiration

The nose has important physiological functions such as humidification, heating, filtration, and olfaction and accounts for more than 50% of the total resistance of the upper airway [54]. The nose locates upstream to the pharynx and consists of nasal wings and nasal cavity which have different mechanical properties. The nasal wings are collapsible particularly when inspiratory drive increases. The ala nasi muscles dilate and stiffen the wings. In contrast, mechanical properties of nasal cavity change little during breathing while its cross-sectional area changes in accordance with the nasal cycle of mucosal blood flow and body position. Therefore, the nose has two different aspects: a collapsible as well as fixed upstream resistance decreasing P_{lumen} during inspiration, but it is not the responsible site for OSA. The amount of P_{lumen} decrease depends on the airflow and resistive properties of the nasal cavity (collapsibility, cross-sectional area, shape, and curvature of the lumen, smoothness of the nasal mucosa, respiratory drive). While P_{lumen} decreases by less than 1–2 cm H_2O during quiet breathing in normal subjects without nasal symptoms, it significantly decreases by more than twice that amount in patients with nasal congestion.

Even in patients with sub-atmospheric P_{close}, P_{lumen} at the most collapsible site within the pharyngeal airway reaches it leading to complete airway closure at the site.

Normal subjects without nasal symptoms predominantly breathe more frequently through the nose during wakefulness and sleep (92% and 96%, respectively) [55]. Although the fraction of oral breathing is much higher in OSA patients [56], OSA patients start breathing through the nose during sleep and switch to mouth breathing with cortical arousal when the nasal resistance exceeds to a certain level. High nasal resistance in supine position was an independent risk factor for OSA [57]. However, effectiveness of nasal surgery on decrease in AHI is not evidenced and limited if exists despite significant improvement of daytime clinical symptoms and patients' satisfaction [54]. Effective CPAP pressure is higher by the amount of P_{lumen} reduction within the nose in patients with nasal congestion. Accordingly, nasal surgery is to be considered for OSA patients with nasal symptoms, not for OSA treatment, but for improvement of CPAP compliance. A nasal strip is helpful for preventing inspiratory collapse and flow limitation at the nasal wings [58].

11 Surface Attractive Forces: Multiple Folds in the Pharynx During OSA and Snoring

Pharyngeal endoscopy often reveals multiple folds, particularly in a narrowed pharynx similar to an artificial collapsible tube [59, 60] (Fig. 3.2). In this multi-folding condition, cohesive and adhesive forces (attractive forces) appear to contribute to difficulty in reopening of the completely closed airway and progressive worsening of hypopnea. At termination of OSA, pharyngeal muscle activity is much greater than that in quiet breathing during wakefulness. This well-known phenomenon can be explained by the fact that a pressure required to reopen the completely closed pharyngeal airway (opening pressure) is greater by approximately 5 cm H_2O than the pressure at which the airway completely closes (closing pressure) [61]. The pressure hysteresis strongly suggests a role of surface attractive forces between the opposed luminal surfaces. The role of surface attractive forces in the partially collapsed airway is considered to be negligible since the pressure produced by surface cohesive forces calculated by Laplace's law does not exceed 1 cm H_2O until the radius of the airway decreases to 1 mm assuming a single circular shape and pharyngeal mucosal lining liquid surface tension of 60 mN m^{-1}. However, in the multi-folding condition shown in Fig. 3.2, the sum of the surface cohesive forces at each fold may resist reopening of the airway. During inspiratory flow limitation, pharyngeal airway progressively narrows and does not return to the original airway size at the beginning of the subsequent breath producing progressive reduction of airflow within a breath (negative effort dependence) and worsening of hypopneas [6, 59]. This phenomenon is not observed in a collapsible tube within a rigid box, but it is produced when adhesive material is applied inside the collapsible tube (Fig. 3.2). This multi-folding hypothesis is supported by the observations that injection of a surfactant into the canine pharyngeal airway decreased intensity of snoring sound [62], and that injection of surfactant into the pharynx of OSA patients significantly decreased frequency of hypopneas but not apneas [63]. Surface attractive forces possibly modulate the pharyngeal behavior even in the partially collapsed airway.

12 Conclusions

Some specific morphological differences between OSA and non-OSA persons account for mechanisms for development of pharyngeal airway obstruction during sleep. Both structural mechanisms surrounding the pharyngeal airway, as well as those in a distance from the airway operate to increase the pharyngeal airway collapsibility. Although most of these can be explained by behavior of a collapsible tube inside a rigid box, it is necessary to develop more comprehensive clinically useful morphological model to understand the overview of the OSA pathophysiology.

Acknowledgments We would like to thank Dr. Sara Shimizu (Shimizu Orthopedic Plastic Surgery Clinic, Tokyo, Japan) for her assistance with improving this manuscript.

References

1. Watanabe T, Isono S, Tanaka A, Tanzawa H, Nishino T. Contribution of body habitus and craniofacial characteristics to segmental closing pressures of the passive pharynx in patients with sleep-disordered breathing. Am J Respir Crit Care Med. 2002;165(2):260–5.
2. Remmers JE, deGroot WJ, Sauerland EK, Anch AM. Pathogenesis of upper airway occlusion during sleep. J Appl Physiol. 1978;44:931–8.
3. Isono S. Obesity and obstructive sleep apnea: mechanisms for increased collapsibility of passive pharyngeal airway. Respirology. 2012;17:32–42.
4. Isono S. Physiology and dynamics of the pharyngeal airway. In: Kushida CA, Lane L, editors. Encyclopedia of sleep. 2nd ed. Oxford: Elsevier Ltd; 2023. p. 220–37.
5. Isono S, Remmers JE (1994) Anatomy and physiology of upper airway obstruction. In: Principles and practice of sleep medicine (2nd edition), ed M.H. Kryger, T. Roth, and W.C. Dement, Philadelphia: WB Saunders Inc., 642–656.
6. Isono S, Feroah TR, Hajduk EA, Brant R, Whitelaw WA, Remmers JE. Interaction of cross-sectional area, driving pressure, and airflow of passive velopharynx. J Appl Physiol. 1997;83(3):851–9.
7. Isono S, Remmers JE, Tanaka A, Sho Y, Sato J, Nishino T. Anatomy of pharynx in patients with obstructive sleep apnea and in normal subjects. J Appl Physiol. 1997;82(4):1319–26.
8. Gold AR, Schwartz AR. The pharyngeal critical pressure. The whys and hows of using nasal continuous positive airway pressure diagnostically. Chest. 1996;110(4):1077–88.
9. Shelton KE, Gay SB, Hollowell DE, Woodson H, Suratt PM. Mandible enclosure of upper airway and weight in obstructive sleep apnea. Am Rev Respir Dis. 1993;148:195–200.
10. Tsuiki S, Isono S, Ishikawa T, Yamashiro Y, Tatsumi K, Nishino T. Anatomical balance of the upper airway and obstructive sleep apnea. Anesthesiology. 2008;108:1009–15.

11. Kairaitis K, Howitt L, Wheatley JR, Amis TC. Mass loading of the upper airway extraluminal tissue space in rabbits: effects on tissue pressure and pharyngeal airway lumen geometry. J Appl Physiol. 1985). 2009;106(3):887–92.
12. Iida-Kondo C, Yoshino N, Kurabayashi T, Mataki S, Hasegawa M, Kurosaki N. Comparison of tongue volume/oral cavity volume ratio between obstructive sleep apnea syndrome patients and normal adults using magnetic resonance imaging. J Med Dent Sci. 2006;53:119–26.
13. Saigusa H, Suzuki M, Higurashi N, Kodera K. Three-dimensional morphological analyses of positional dependence in patients with obstructive sleep apnea syndrome. Anesthesiology. 2009;110:885–90.
14. Schwab RJ, Pasirstein M, Pierson R, Mackley A, Hachadoorian R, Arens R, Maislin G, Pack AI. Identification of upper airway anatomic risk factors for obstructive sleep apnea with volumetric magnetic resonance imaging. Am J Respir Crit Care Med. 2003;168:522–30.
15. Horner RL, Mohiaddin RH, Lowell DG, Shea SA, Burman ED, Longmore DB, Guz A. Sites and sizes of fat deposits around the pharynx in obese patients with obstructive sleep apnoea and weight matched controls. Eur Respir J. 1989;2:613–22.
16. Mortimore IL, Marshall I, Wraith PK, Sellar RJ, Douglas NJ. Neck and total body fat deposition in nonobese and obese patients with sleep apnea compared with that in control subjects. Am J Respir Crit Care Med. 1998;157:280–3.
17. Shelton KE, Woodson H, Gay S, Suratt PM. Pharyngeal fat in obstructive sleep apnea. Am Rev Respir Dis. 1993;148:462–6.
18. Li Y, Lin N, Ye J, Chang Q, Han D, Sperry A. Upper airway fat tissue distribution in subjects with obstructive sleep apnea and its effect on retropalatal mechanical loads. Respir Care. 2012;57:1098–105.
19. Sutherland K, Lee RW, Phillips CL, Dungan G, Yee BJ, Magnussen JS, Grunstein RR, Cistulli PA. Effect of weight loss on upper airway size and facial fat in men with obstructive sleep apnoea. Thorax. 2011;66:797–803.
20. Nashi N, Kang S, Barkdull GC, Lucas J, Davidson TM. Lingual fat at autopsy. Laryngoscope. 2007;117:1467–73.
21. Brennick MJ, Pickup S, Dougherty L, Cater JR, Kuna ST. Pharyngeal airway wall mechanics using tagged magnetic resonance imaging during medial hypoglossal nerve stimulation in rats. J Physiol. 2004;561:597–610.
22. Kato S, Isono S, Amemiya M, Sato S, Ikeda A, Okazaki J, Sato Y, Ishikawa T. Submental negative pressure application decreases collapsibility of the passive pharyngeal airway in nonobese women. J Appl Physiol (1985). 2015;118(7):912–20.
23. Saito T, Yamane A, Kaneko S, Ogawa T, Ikawa T, Saito K, Sugisaki M. Changes in the lingual muscles of obese rats induced by high-fat diet feeding. Arch Oral Biol. 2010;55:803–8.
24. Pae EK, Wu J, Nguyen D, Monti R, Harper RM. Geniohyoid muscle properties and myosin heavy chain composition are altered after short-term intermittent hypoxic exposure. J Appl Physiol. 2005;98:889–94.
25. Carrera M, Barbé F, Sauleda J, Tomás M, Gómez C, Santos C, Agustí AG. Effects of obesity upon genioglossus structure and function in obstructive sleep apnoea. Eur Respir J. 2004;23:425–9.
26. Ferguson KA, Ono T, Lowe AA, Ryan CF, Fleetham JA. The relationship between obesity and craniofacial structure in obstructive sleep apnea. Chest. 1995;108(2):375–81.
27. Sakakibara H, Tong M, Matsushita K, Hirata M, Konishi Y, Suetsugu S. Cephalometric abnormalities in non-obese and obese patients with obstructive sleep apnoea. Eur Respir J. 1999;13(2):403–10.
28. Tsai WH, Remmers JE, Brant R, Flemons WW, Davies J, Macarthur C. A decision rule for diagnostic testing in obstructive sleep apnea. Am J Respir Crit Care Med. 2003;167(10):1427–32.
29. Noda A, Okada T, Yasuma F, Sobue T, Nakashima N, Yokota M. Prognosis of the middle-aged and aged patients with obstructive sleep apnea syndrome. Psychiatry Clin Neurosci. 1998;52(1):79–85.

30. Lee RW, Vasudavan S, Hui DS, Prvan T, Petocz P, Darendeliler MA, Cistulli PA. Differences in craniofacial structures and obesity in Caucasian and Chinese patients with obstructive sleep apnea. Sleep. 2010;33(8):1075–80.
31. Xu L, Keenan BT, Wiemken AS, Chi L, Staley B, Wang Z, Wang J, Benedikstdottir B, Juliusson S, Pack AI, Gislason T, Schwab RJ. Differences in three-dimensional upper airway anatomy between Asian and European patients with obstructive sleep apnea. Sleep. 2020;43(5):zsz273.
32. Ogisawa S, Nishikubo S, Nakajima J, Azaki H, Mayahara K, Shinozuka K, Tonogi M. The changes in oral volume and hyoid bone position after maxillomandibular advancement and genioglossus advancement for patients with obstructive sleep apnea. Sleep Breath. 2023;27(1):239–44.
33. Mitsukawa N, Kaneko T, Saiga A, Akita S, Satoh K. Early midfacial distraction for syndromic craniosynostotic patients with obstructive sleep apnoea. J Plast Reconstr Aesthet Surg. 2013;66(9):1206–11.
34. Mitsukawa N, Satoh K, Suse T, Hosaka Y. Clinical success of mandibular distraction for obstructive sleep apnea resulting from micrognathia in 10 consecutive Japanese young children. J Craniofac Surg. 2007;18(4):948–53.
35. Van de Graaff WB. Thoracic traction on the trachea: mechanisms and magnitude. J Appl Physiol. 1991;70:1328–36.
36. Kairaitis K, Byth K, Parikh R, Stavrinou R, Wheatley JR, Amis TC. Tracheal traction effects on upper airway patency in rabbits: the role of tissue pressure. Sleep. 2007;30:179–86.
37. Tagaito Y, Isono S, Remmers JE, Tanaka A, Nishino T. Lung volume and collapsibility of the passive pharynx in patients with sleep-disordered breathing. J Appl Physiol. 2007;103:1379–85.
38. Stanchina ML, Malhotra A, Fogel RB, Trinder J, Edwards JK, Schory K, White DP. The influence of lung volume on pharyngeal mechanics, collapsibility, and genioglossus muscle activation during sleep. Sleep. 2003;26:851–6.
39. Begle RL, Badr S, Skatrud JB, Dempsey JA. Effect of lung inflation on pulmonary resistance during NREM sleep. Am Rev Respir Dis. 1990;141:854–60.
40. Kohno A, Kitamura Y, Kato S, Imai H, Masuda Y, Sato Y, Isono S. Displacement of the hyoid bone by muscle paralysis and lung volume increase: the effects of obesity and obstructive sleep apnea. Sleep. 2019;42(1):zsy198.
41. Tong J, Jugé L, Burke PG, Knapman F, Eckert DJ, Bilston LE, Amatoury J. Respiratory-related displacement of the trachea in obstructive sleep apnea. J Appl Physiol. 1985). 2019 Nov 1;127(5):1307–16.
42. Isono S, Tanaka A, Nishino T. Lateral position decreases collapsibility of the passive pharynx in patients with obstructive sleep apnea. Anesthesiology. 2002;97(4):780–5.
43. Tagaito Y, Isono S, Tanaka A, Ishikawa T, Nishino T. Sitting posture decreases collapsibility of the passive pharynx in anesthetized paralyzed patients with obstructive sleep apnea. Anesthesiology. 2010;113(4):812–8.
44. Cartwright RD, Lloyd S, Lilie J, Kravitz H. Sleep position training as treatment for sleep apnea syndrome: a preliminary study. Sleep. 1985;8(2):87–94.
45. McEvoy RD, Sharp DJ, Thornton AT. The effects of posture on obstructive sleep apnea. Am Rev Respir Dis. 1986;133(4):662–6.
46. Isono S, Tanaka A, Nishino T. Dynamic interaction between the tongue and soft palate during obstructive apnea in anesthetized patients with sleep-disordered breathing. J Appl Physiol (1985). 2003;95(6):2257–64.
47. Isono S. Two valves in the pharynx. Eur Respir J. 2017;50(3):1701496.
48. Safar P. Ventilatory efficacy of mouth-to-mouth artificial respiration; airway obstruction during manual and mouth-to-mouth artificial respiration. JAMA J Am Med Assoc. 1958;167:335–41.
49. Sato S, Hasegawa M, Okuyama M, Okazaki J, Kitamura Y, Sato Y, Ishikawa T, Sato Y, Isono S. Mask ventilation during induction of general anesthesia: influences of obstructive sleep apnea. Anesthesiology. 2017;126(1):28–38.
50. Stănescu D, Kostianev S, Sanna A, Liistro G, Veriter C. Expiratory flow limitation during sleep in heavy snorers and obstructive sleep apnoea patients. Eur Respir J. 1996;9:2116–21.

51. Azarbarzin A, Sands SA, Marques M, Genta PR, Taranto-Montemurro L, Messineo L, White DP, Wellman A. Palatal prolapse as a signature of expiratory flow limitation and inspiratory palatal collapse in patients with obstructive sleep apnoea. Eur Respir J. 2018;51(2):1701419.
52. Okuyama M, Kato S, Sato S, Okazaki J, Kitamura Y, Ishikawa T, Sato Y, Isono S. Dynamic behaviour of the soft palate during nasal positive pressure ventilation under anaesthesia and paralysis: comparison between patients with and without obstructive sleep-disordered breathing. Br J Anaesth. 2018;120(1):181–7.
53. Azarbarzin A, Marques M, Sands SA, Op de Beeck S, Genta PR, Taranto-Montemurro L, de Melo CM, Messineo L, Vanderveken OM, White DP, Wellman A. Predicting epiglottic collapse in patients with obstructive sleep apnoea. Eur Respir J. 2017;50(3):1700345.
54. Georgalas C. The role of the nose in snoring and obstructive sleep apnoea: an update. Eur Arch Otorrinolaringol. 2011;268(9):1365–73.
55. Fitzpatrick MF, Driver HS, Chatha N, Voduc N, Girard AM. Partitioning of inhaled ventilation between the nasal and oral routes during sleep in normal subjects. J Appl Physiol. 1985;94(3):883–90.
56. Gleeson K, Zwillich CW, Braier K, White DP. Breathing route during sleep. Am Rev Respir Dis. 1986;134(1):115–20.
57. Lofaso F, Coste A, d'Ortho MP, Zerah-Lancner F, Delclaux C, Goldenberg F, Harf A. Nasal obstruction as a risk factor for sleep apnoea syndrome. Eur Respir J. 2000;16(4):639–43.
58. Höijer U, Ejnell H, Hedner J, Petruson B, Eng LB. The effects of nasal dilation on snoring and obstructive sleep apnea. Arch Otolaryngol Head Neck Surg. 1992;118(3):281–4.
59. Isono S. Upper airway muscle function during sleep. In: Loughlin GM, Marcus CL, Carroll JL, editors. Sleep and breathing in children: a developmental approach. New York: Marcel Dekker Inc; 2000. p. 261–91.
60. Kairaitis K, Foster S, Amatoury J, Verma M, Wheatley JR, Amis TC. Pharyngeal mucosal wall folds in subjects with obstructive sleep apnea. J Appl Physiol. 1985). 2015 Mar 15;118(6):707–15.
61. Wilson SL, Thach BT, Brouillette RT, Abu-Osba YK. Upper airway patency in the human infant: influence of airway pressure and posture. J Appl Physiol Respir Environ Exerc Physiol. 1980;48(3):500–4.
62. Widdicombe JG, Davies A. The effects of a mixture of surface-active agents (Sonarex) on upper airways resistance and snoring in anaesthetized dogs. Eur Respir J. 1988;1(9):785–91.
63. Kirkness JP, Madronio M, Stavrinou R, Wheatley JR, Amis TC. Relationship between surface tension of upper airway lining liquid and upper airway collapsibility during sleep in obstructive sleep apnea hypopnea syndrome. J Appl Physiol. 1985). 2003 Nov;95(5):1761–6.

Chapter 4
Obstructive Sleep Apnea and Lifestyle Diseases: Clinical Question Is There a Correlation Between Sleep Apnea and Lifestyle Diseases?

Takeshi Matsumoto and Kazuo Chin

Abstract In the relationship between obstructive sleep apnea (OSA) and hypertension, the presence of moderate-to-severe OSA is significantly associated with the presence of hypertension, as well as the development of hypertension. Continuous positive airway pressure (CPAP) therapy has shown a significant antihypertensive effect, especially when CPAP is used for ≥4 h per day. In the relationship between OSA and diabetes, the presence of moderate-to-severe OSA is significantly associated with the presence of diabetes, as well as the development of diabetes. The effect of CPAP therapy on the improvement of insulin resistance in OSA patients has been indicated in meta-analyses, although the result of each study is not consistent. In the relationship between OSA and dyslipidemia, some cross-sectional studies have shown a significant association, and the effects of CPAP therapy on dyslipidemia are inconclusive. There is a certain association between lifestyle diseases and OSA, but evidence for the improvement of these conditions with CPAP therapy is not robust.

Keywords Obstructive sleep apnea · Lifestyle diseases · Hypertension · Diabetes · Dyslipidemia · Continuous positive airway pressure

The original version of the chapter has been revised. A correction to this chapter can be found at https://doi.org/10.1007/978-981-96-6030-8_17

T. Matsumoto (✉)
Department of Respiratory Medicine, Saiseikai-Noe Hospital, Osaka, Japan

Department of Respiratory Medicine, Graduate School of Medicine, Kyoto University, Kyoto, Japan
e-mail: mtakeshi@kuhp.kyoto-u.ac.jp

K. Chin
Department of Sleep Medicine and Respiratory Care, Division of Sleep Medicine, Nihon University of Medicine, Itabashi-ku, Tokyo, Japan

Center for Genomic Medicine, Graduate School of Medicine, Kyoto University, Kyoto, Japan

K. Chin (ed.), *The Current State of Sleep Disordered Breathing in Japan and Around the World*, Respiratory Disease Series: Diagnostic Tools and Disease Managements, https://doi.org/10.1007/978-981-96-6030-8_4

1 Introduction

The importance of sleep in maintaining good health is widely recognized, and the relationship between sleep and health has been particularly emphasized and studied in recent years [1]. Among the various disorders that compromise sleep in different ways, one of the most significant conditions is sleep-related breathing disorders, or sleep-disordered breathing (SDB). Among SDB, obstructive sleep apnea (OSA) is a main disorder where sleep disruptions occur due to episodes of apnea or hypopnea during sleep, leading to impaired restful sleep, excessive daytime sleepiness, and significant impact on daily life. Furthermore, it is known to contribute to conditions such as hypertension, insulin resistance, and cardiovascular diseases [2]. Treatment, mainly continuous positive airway pressure (CPAP) therapy, has been recognized as crucial for managing this condition. In this chapter, we will introduce the relationship between OSA and lifestyle diseases (hypertension, diabetes, and dyslipidemia).

2 OSA and Hypertension

The mechanisms through which OSA affects hypertension involve intermittent hypoxia and sleep fragmentation, both of which trigger the activation of the sympathetic nervous system, leading to neurogenic hypertension and elevated nocturnal blood pressure [3]. Furthermore, OSA not only causes sympathetic activation during periods of apnea but also during wakefulness, and if nocturnal hypertension due to OSA persists until the early morning, it can result in morning hypertension. Additionally, the impact of oxidative stress and systemic inflammation due to OSA is suggested [2].

The main observational studies investigating the relationship between OSA and hypertension are summarized in Table 4.1. In the Wisconsin Sleep Cohort Study (WSCS), a significant positive correlation was observed between the rise in blood pressure and the increase in apnea-hypopnea index (AHI). The odds ratio for hypertension was 1.8 times higher for AHI ≥15/h compared to AHI 0/h [4]. In the Sleep Heart Health Study (SHHS), the odds ratio for hypertension was 1.37 times higher for AHI ≥30/h compared to AHI <1.5/h [5].

Taking an overview of longitudinal studies, in the WSCS, the odds ratios for developing hypertension were as follows when compared to AHI 0/h: AHI 0.1–4.9/h had an odds ratio of 1.42, AHI 5–14.9/h had an odds ratio of 2.03, and AHI ≥15/h had an odds ratio of 2.89 [6]. However, in the SHHS, when adjusted for body mass index (BMI), the significant association between high AHI values and the onset of hypertension disappeared [7]. However, the subjects in WSCS had an average age of 47, while the subjects in SHHS had an average age of 60, which may have influenced the differences in the results.

In a meta-analysis that included 26 studies, the association between OSA and treatment-resistant hypertension was reported to have an odds ratio of 2.84. When

Table 4.1 Reports on the association between obstructive sleep apnea and hypertension

Reference	Sample size	Follow-up period	Characteristics	Main results
Cross-sectional or observational study				
Young et al. 1997 [4]	1060	Cross-sectional	Report from WSCS	Significant positive correlation between blood pressure elevation and AHI was noted, where the OR for hypertension was 1.8 when comparing AHI ≥15/h to AHI of 0/h
Nieto et al. 2000 [5]	6132	Cross-sectional	Report from SHHS	OR for hypertension was 1.37 when comparing AHI ≥30/h to AHI <1.5/h
Peppard et al. 2000 [6]	709	4 years	Report from WSCS, mean value of BMI was 29 kg/m^2	OR for developing hypertension, when compared to an AHI of 0/h, was 1.42 for an AHI of 0.1–4.9/h, 2.03 for an AHI of 5–14.9/h, and 2.89 for an AHI ≥15/h
O'Connor et al. 2009 [7]	2470	2 years	Report from SHHS, mean value of BMI was 27.9 kg/m^2	When adjusting for BMI, the significant association between high AHI values and the development of hypertension disappeared
Interventional study (CPAP treatment)				
Norman et al. 2006 [11]	46	2 weeks	Comparison among CPAP, sham CPAP, and oxygen therapy	CPAP therapy led to a reduction in both daytime and nighttime blood pressure, whereas oxygen therapy alone did not show a decrease in blood pressure
Barbe et al. 2012 [13]	723	4 years	Comparison between CPAP and control, both groups received dietary and sleep environment guidance	No significant difference in the incidence of new-onset hypertension between the two groups; however, a significant difference was observed when considering only the group that used CPAP for an average ≥ 4 h per day
Gottlieb et al. 2014 [12]	281	12 weeks	Comparison among CPAP, oxygen therapy, and education-only in patients at high cardiovascular risk	24-hour average blood pressure-lowering effect observed only in the CPAP group
Chirinos et al. 2014 [10]	181	24 weeks	Comparison among weight loss, CPAP and combination	Blood pressure reduction was observed in all groups, but the combination of CPAP and weight loss was the most effective
Sapina-Beltran E et al. 2019 [14]	272	12 weeks	Comparison between CPAP and sham CPAP in two groups divided into dippers and non-dippers	The antihypertensive effect of CPAP was observed only in the non-dipper group
Lui MM et al. 2021 [15]	92	8 weeks	Comparison between CPAP and control, targeting patients using ≥3 antihypertensive medications	The antihypertensive effect of CPAP was observed, but subanalysis did not show a significant antihypertensive effect in the dipper group

SHHS Sleep Heart Health Study, *WSCS* Wisconsin Sleep Cohort Study, *AHI* apnea-hypopnea index, *BMI* body mass index, *OR* odds ratio, *CPAP* continuous positive airway pressure

OSA was categorized as mild/moderate/severe, the odds ratios for the association with hypertension were reported as 1.18/1.32/1.56, respectively (AHI of less than 5/h is considered normal, 5–15/h is categorized as mild, 15–30/h as moderate, and ≥ 30/h as severe) [8]. In a recent meta-analysis that included ten studies, the association between OSA and hypertension was reported with an odds ratio of 1.8 [9].

Next, Table 4.1 illustrates the main randomized controlled trials (RCTs) investigating whether CPAP therapy improves hypertension. A study focused on OSA patients with obesity and C-reactive protein levels ≥1 mg/L examined the effects of CPAP therapy alone, weight loss alone, and a combination of CPAP therapy and weight loss. The results showed that each group had a positive effect on blood pressure improvement, with the combined CPAP therapy and weight loss group showing the highest efficacy [10]. In another study comparing three groups—CPAP, sham CPAP, and oxygen therapy—it was found that CPAP lowered both daytime and nocturnal blood pressure, whereas oxygen therapy alone did not lead to blood pressure reduction [11]. Similarly, another study divided OSA patients at high cardiovascular risk into three groups: CPAP, oxygen therapy, and education-only. This study also revealed a blood pressure-lowering effect in only the CPAP group for 24-hour average blood pressure, suggesting the presence of mechanisms not dependent on hypoxia [12]. However, contrasting findings exist as well. In a study comparing two groups—CPAP with dietary and sleep environment guidance, and a control group without intervention—no significant difference was observed in the incidence of new-onset hypertension between the two groups, leading to differing opinions [13]. Nonetheless, this study found a significant difference when analyzing a subgroup that used CPAP for an average of ≥4 h per day. Furthermore, recent RCTs have focused on the patterns of nocturnal blood pressure, suggesting that the antihypertensive effects of CPAP may be limited in individuals classified as dippers [14, 15].

Looking into this matter further with the results of meta-analyses, a meta-analysis of 29 RCTs comprising 1820 individuals found that CPAP had a blood pressure-lowering effect; however, the change was mild, with a decrease of 2.6 mmHg in systolic blood pressure and 2.0 mmHg in diastolic blood pressure [16]. Another meta-analysis involving 4 RCTs comprising 1206 individuals found that in patients without daytime sleepiness, a blood pressure-lowering effect was not observed when CPAP usage averaged less than 4 h per day [17]. In a recent meta-analysis that included 19 studies and 1904 participants, the observed reductions in systolic and diastolic blood pressure of 5.0 mmHg and 3.3 mmHg, respectively, were reported. However, there was no significant effect in studies with follow-up periods of <3 months [18]. From these results, it can be said that maintaining good adherence, such as using CPAP for more than 4 h per day and for more than 3 months, has a significant impact on the antihypertensive effect. In the meanwhile, CPAP is not able to completely correct all factors contributing to blood pressure elevation, such as fluid retention or excess sodium intake. Although an additional effect of CPAP is noted, antihypertensive medications appear to yield better blood pressure-lowering effects [19, 20]. Therefore, the impact of SDB on hypertension might be more significant in exacerbating existing hypertension rather than contributing to its onset.

3 OSA and Diabetes

SDB has been known to be a risk factor for impaired glucose tolerance. However, the global recognition of its association significantly expanded after the International Diabetes Federation released a report on epidemiology and prevention for SDB and type 2 diabetes in 2008 [21].

The mechanisms underlying the impact of OSA on glucose metabolism involve intermittent hypoxia and sleep fragmentation, each of which is thought to independently contribute to insulin resistance. Specific mechanisms include activation of the sympathetic nervous system, increased oxidative stress, elevation of cortisol due to activation of the hypothalamus-pituitary-adrenal axis, activation of transcription factors like nuclear factor κB, Interleukin-6, Tumor Necrosis Factor-α, and inflammatory cytokines [2, 22]. Moreover, a bidirectional relationship is also suggested, as elevated blood glucose levels can exacerbate OSA by decreasing the reactivity of carotid bodies and the genioglossus muscle [23, 24].

The main observational studies investigating the relationship between OSA and diabetes are summarized in Table 4.2. Numerous studies highlight the higher prevalence of diabetes in individuals with OSA. SHHS reported an AHI of ≥15/h as an independent risk factor for abnormal glucose metabolism [25]. More recent findings from a large-scale European trial, the European Sleep Apnea Database, reported odds ratios for the co-occurrence of type 2 diabetes as 1.33/1.73/1.87 for mild/moderate/severe OSA, respectively [26].

Taking an overview of longitudinal studies, findings from WSCS reported that after adjusting for the prevalence of diabetes, the odds ratio for AHI ≥15/h compared to AHI <5/h was 2.3 times, and the diabetes incidence rate over a 4-year period was 1.62 times higher. However, these differences did not reach statistical significance [27]. Findings from a cohort study in the United States reported a 1.43 times higher risk of diabetes incidence with an AHI ≥8/h [28]. A Canadian cohort study indicated that the risk of diabetes incidence was 1.23 times higher for moderate OSA and 1.31 times higher for severe OSA [29]. Recently, findings from a cohort study in China, which had a median follow-up of 7.3 years, reported a diabetes incidence risk of 2.01 times for moderate OSA and 2.62 times for severe OSA [30]. In a meta-analysis that included 16 studies, a positive correlation has been reported, indicating that the risk of diabetes increases by 1.08 times for each increment of AHI by 5/h [31]. In another meta-analysis that included 25 studies, both cross-sectional and longitudinal studies consistently showed an association between OSA and impaired glucose metabolism or diabetes [32].

Next, Table 4.2 presents the main RCTs investigating whether CPAP therapy improves diabetes. Previously, the prevailing reports indicated that CPAP therapy did not result in the improvement of diabetes [33–35]. In studies that investigated the effects of CPAP therapy, weight loss, and a combination of CPAP therapy and weight loss on insulin sensitivity in three RCT groups, CPAP therapy alone group did not improve insulin sensitivity, suggesting that weight loss was necessary [10]. Overall, the prevailing reports have been somewhat negative. Insulin resistance may

Table 4.2 Reports on the association between obstructive sleep apnea and diabetes

Reference	Sample size	Follow-up period	Characteristics	Main results
Cross-sectional or observational study				
Punjabi et al. 2004 [25]	2656	Cross-sectional	Report from SHHS, fasting and 2-h post-75 g glucose load blood glucose levels were measured	Moderate-to-severe OSA was associated with glucose metabolism abnormalities (OR 1.46)
Reichmuth et al. 2005 [27]	1387	4 years	Report from WSCS	The adjusted OR for the incidence of diabetes was 1.62, but it was not statistically significant
Botros et al. 2009 [28]	544	2.7 years	The analysis was conducted by dividing the AHI into quartiles, with males making up 93% of the sample	An AHI ≥8/h was associated with a 1.43-fold increased risk of developing diabetes
Lam et al. 2010 [59]	165	Cross-sectional	Report from China, the average BMI of 26.9 kg/m^2 (relatively low compared to other studies)	OSA was not significantly associated with blood glucose or HbA1c levels
Heffner et al. 2012 [60]	16,066	Cross-sectional	Primary care was the focus of the study	18% of diabetes cases were diagnosed with OSA
Kendzerska et al. 2014 [29]	8678	67 months	A longitudinal study with a large sample size	The risk of developing diabetes increased with an HR of 1.23 for moderate and 1.31 for severe OSA
Kent et al. 2014 [26]	6616	Cross-sectional	Report from ESADA study	OR for the comorbidity of diabetes with mild, moderate, and severe OSA is 1.33, 1.73, and 1.87, respectively
Xu et al. 2019 [30]	1206	7.3 years	Long-term follow-up data	The risk of developing diabetes increased with an HR of 2.01 for moderate and 2.62 for severe OSA
Interventional study (CPAP treatment)				
West et al. 2007 [33]	42	3 months	The average CPAP usage time was slightly short at 3.6 h	CPAP therapy showed no significant differences in HbA1c and insulin resistance

Weinstock et al. 2012 [34]	50	8 weeks	A crossover design was used for participants with an AHI ≥15/h	CPAP therapy showed no significant difference in the normalization of blood glucose levels and insulin sensitivity after the glucose tolerance test, except for those with an AHI ≥30/h, where insulin sensitivity improved
Chirinos et al. 2014 [10]	181	24 weeks	Comparison among weight loss, CPAP, and combination	CPAP therapy showed no significant differences in insulin resistance
Pamidi et al. 2015 [36]	39	2 weeks	The average CPAP usage time was 8 h	CPAP therapy showed improvements in insulin sensitivity and post-meal blood glucose levels
Shaw et al. 2016 [35]	298	24 weeks	A large sample size, focused on a group with HbA1c levels 6.5–8.5%	CPAP therapy showed no significant differences in HbA1c
Salord et al. 2016 [61]	80	12 weeks	This study targeted obese patients with a BMI ≥40 kg/m^2, or those with a BMI ≥35 kg/m^2 with comorbidities	CPAP therapy showed no significant difference in HOMA-IR, but improvements were observed in glucose tolerance and post-glucose load blood glucose levels
Martinez-Ceron et al 2016 [37]	50	6 months	The follow-up period was long	HbA1c levels decreased, and insulin resistance improved
Banghoj et al. 2020 [62]	58	12 weeks	The average CPAP usage time was relatively long at 5.6 h	There was no significant difference in average blood glucose levels, and even when limited to the group with good CPAP compliance, there was an improvement trend but no significant difference
Zamarron et al. 2023 [33]	185	52 weeks	The primary endpoint was the change in the urine albumin-to-creatinine ratio with CPAP	Significant change in the urine albumin-to-creatinine ratio was not observed with CPAP treatment, but improvements were noted in blood glucose and insulin resistance

SHHS Sleep Heart Health Study, *WSCS* Wisconsin Sleep Cohort Study, *ESADA* European Sleep Apnea Database, *OR* odds ratio, *HR* hazard ratio, *CPAP* continuous positive airway pressure, *HOMA-IR* homeostatic model assessment for insulin resistance, *HbA1c* hemoglobin A1c, *AHI* apnea-hypopnea index, *BMI* body mass index be more strongly determined by factors such as obesity and lifestyle habits; however, there have also been RCTs that suggest the potential for improvement through CPAP therapy [36–38], leading to a lack of consensus in the conclusions. This lack of consensus could be attributed to variations in CPAP usage time and follow-up periods among different studies.

To shed further light on this matter, exploring the results of meta-analyses reveals a diverse perspective. In a recent meta-analysis that included 31 studies up to February 2022, it was reported that CPAP therapy improved homeostatic model assessment for insulin resistance (HOMA-IR), but it did not lead to improvements in hemoglobin A1c (HbA1c) levels [39]. However, another meta-analysis that focused on 11 studies up to December 2022 reported that CPAP therapy led to improvements in HbA1c levels, and the degree of improvement was correlated with the CPAP usage time [40]. While slight differences may arise due to variations in the studies included, it seems plausible that CPAP therapy might indeed hold the potential to ameliorate insulin resistance.

4 OSA and Dyslipidemia

The mechanism underlying the impact of OSA on lipid metabolism involves intermittent hypoxia triggered by OSA. This hypoxia-induced effect operates through hypoxia-inducible factor 1, upregulating sterol regulatory element binding protein 1 and stearoyl coenzyme A desaturase 1. These factors lead to the migration of lipids from adipose tissue to the liver, thereby increasing the synthesis of cholesterol esters and triglycerides. Additionally, the elevation of oxidative stress and activation of sympathetic nervous activity are believed to induce lipid peroxidation reactions and increase lipoprotein production, leading to dyslipidemia [41, 42].

The main observational studies investigating the relationship between OSA and dyslipidemia are summarized in Table 4.3. These are all cross-sectional study results. Among them, the study with the largest sample size to date is the one involving 4991 participants from SHHS. In individuals under the age of 65, this study found that the severity of OSA was associated with higher levels of total cholesterol and triglycerides, while high-density lipoprotein (HDL) cholesterol levels were decreased [43]. There is an intriguing study that examined the ex vivo inhibition of low-density lipoprotein (LDL) oxidation, a measure of HDL function, in 210 participants. This study found that impaired HDL function was associated with AHI [44]. From studies conducted in Japan, a study involving 275 male workers revealed a correlation between respiratory disturbance index and triglycerides [45]. In the same study, short sleep duration was independently associated with total cholesterol, suggesting that sleep duration is an important factor in lipid metabolism. While several reports indicate a link between OSA severity and lipid metabolism abnormalities, there is variation in the findings. Some reports did not find an association when adjusting for BMI [46], while others found associations only with

Table 4.3 Reports on the association between obstructive sleep apnea and dyslipidemia

Reference	Sample size	Follow-up period	Characteristics	Main results
Cross-sectional or observational study				
Newman et al. 2001 [43]	4991	Cross-sectional	Report from SHHS, the sample size was large	In individuals aged <65, total cholesterol and triglycerides increased, while HDL cholesterol decreased
Tan et al. 2006 [44]	210	Cross-sectional	HDL function was the primary evaluation parameter	HDL dysfunction was associated with AHI
Roche et al. 2009 [63]	846	Cross-sectional	Report from SYNAPSE study, this study applied to individuals aged ≥65	HDL cholesterol was associated, but LDL cholesterol was not associated with OSA
Trzepizur et al. 2013 [64]	2081	Cross-sectional	The severity was determined by ODI	The increase in triglycerides and the decrease in HDL cholesterol were related to ODI, while there was no association with total cholesterol and LDL cholesterol
Toyama et al. 2013 [45]	275	Cross-sectional	The severity was determined by RDI	Triglycerides were associated with RDI
Silva et al. 2021 [65]	708	Cross-sectional	This group had an average age of 46 years, and various metabolic markers were measured	A positive correlation between OSA and cholesterol was observed only in males
Interventional study (CPAP treatment)				
Robinson et al. 2004 [65]	220	1 month	These data were not from fasting blood samples	Total cholesterol decreased, while triglycerides remained unchanged
Phillips et al. 2011 [48]	38	2 months	A crossover design, and the main outcome measure was postprandial lipids	Total cholesterol, HDL cholesterol, triglycerides, and non-HDL cholesterol decreased
Craig et al. 2012 [49]	391	6 months	The median CPAP usage time was 2.6 h, indicating relatively short usage	Total cholesterol did not change significantly

(continued)

Table 4.3 (continued)

Reference	Sample size	Follow-up period	Characteristics	Main results
Chirinos et al. 2014 [10]	146	24 weeks	Comparison among weight loss, CPAP, and combination	LDL cholesterol, HDL cholesterol, and triglycerides did not change significantly
Campos-Rodriguez et al. 2017 [50]	307	12 weeks	All participants were female	Total cholesterol, LDL cholesterol, HDL cholesterol, and triglycerides remained unchanged
Giampa et al. 2022 [52]	100	6 months	The primary endpoint was the improvement rate of metabolic syndrome	HDL cholesterol and triglycerides did not change significantly

SHHS Sleep Heart Health Study, *SYNAPSE* Autonomic Nervous System Activity, Aging and Sleep Apnea/Hypopnea, *CPAP* continuous positive airway pressure, *HDL* high-density lipoprotein, *LDL* low-density lipoprotein, *AHI* apnea-hypopnea index, *ODI* oxygen desaturation index, *RDI* respiratory disturbance index specific aspects of lipid profiles. This variability in results might stem from both study-specific differences and the substantial variability in lipid profiles themselves.

Exploring meta-analytical findings in this regard, an analysis encompassing 18,116 individuals from 64 studies indicated that AHI was associated with decreased HDL cholesterol and increased triglycerides, but no significant association was found with total cholesterol or LDL cholesterol [47].

Table 4.3 shows main RCTs investigating the improvement of dyslipidemia through CPAP therapy. Lipid outcomes are often not the primary endpoints in many studies; however, studies focusing on postprandial lipids as the primary evaluation found that in a crossover study involving 38 participants, reductions in total cholesterol, HDL cholesterol, triglycerides, and non-HDL cholesterol were observed [48]. However, there are also studies with negative findings. In a large study involving 391 participants, total cholesterol remained unchanged; however, it is important to note that the median CPAP usage time in this study was relatively short at 2.6 hours [49]. Additionally, in a study involving 307 women, while a reduction in blood pressure was observed, there was no significant difference in lipid metabolism abnormalities [50]. In the aforementioned comparison of three groups (CPAP therapy alone, weight loss alone, CPAP therapy combined with weight loss), lipid metabolism improvements were not achieved with CPAP therapy alone; weight loss was necessary [10]. In a recent study from the European Sleep Apnea Database, though it was an observational study, it included a substantial sample of 1564 individuals. They reported improvements in total cholesterol after CPAP therapy for over a year on average, but there was no observed change in triglycerides [51]. Even in a recent RCT involving 100 participants, there was no significant change observed in triglycerides and HDL cholesterol [52].

So, when we look at meta-analytical findings in this area, an analysis involving 1958 individuals from 29 studies indicated that CPAP therapy led to improvements in LDL cholesterol, total cholesterol, and HDL cholesterol, but no significant improvement was observed in triglycerides [53]. However, focusing a recent meta-analysis solely on RCTs, an analysis including 12 studies up until January 2021 reported no improvements in total cholesterol, HDL cholesterol, LDL cholesterol, or triglycerides with CPAP therapy, and no correlation was found with the duration of CPAP therapy [54]. Another meta-analysis that included 31 studies up until February 2022 reported improvements in total cholesterol but no improvements in HDL cholesterol, LDL cholesterol, or triglycerides with CPAP therapy [39]. Although the impact of CPAP usage time was not considered, the effectiveness of CPAP for lipid abnormalities may be limited.

5 Large Population Studies in Japan

Indeed, the exploration of the associations between OSA and hypertension, diabetes, and dyslipidemia has provided valuable insights into these health conditions. However, up until now, there has been a lack of large-scale studies, especially among East Asian populations, that take into account the significant confounding factor of obesity. Such studies are highly anticipated and important to further our understanding of the relationships between OSA and these health issues in this specific population.

In Japan, two large-scale epidemiological studies related to sleep have been conducted: the Circulatory Risk in Communities Study (CIRCS) and the Nagahama cohort study. CIRCS is a prospective cohort study conducted in Japan since 1963, and research related to sleep has been jointly conducted by the Osaka University and the University of Tsukuba since 2000 [55]. Between 2001 and 2005, using a pulse oximeter (PULSOX-3Si; Minolta, Osaka, Japan) to assess nocturnal intermittent hypoxia, a study was conducted to investigate its association with the onset of diabetes. Among 4398 individuals aged 40–69, during a median follow-up of three years, 210 individuals developed new-onset diabetes. With a classification of 3% ODI (oxygen desaturation index) as mild for 5 to <15/h and moderate to severe for ≥15/h, the hazard ratio for diabetes onset was 1.26 (0.91–1.76) for mild intermittent hypoxia and 1.69 (1.04–2.76) for moderate to severe intermittent hypoxia [56]. This study is interesting in that it demonstrated a potential association between nocturnal intermittent hypoxia and the onset of diabetes in a large Japanese cohort.

The Nagahama cohort study is a collaborative effort between Nagahama City in Shiga Prefecture and Kyoto University. Its purpose is to promote community health and advance medical research. The study involves various examinations, including sleep assessments, in addition to general health check-ups. The second phase of the study took place from 2012 to 2016. In this cohort study, we investigated objective sleep duration and the severity of SDB [57]. Specifically, we used wrist-worn accelerometers (Actiwatch 2 or the Actiwatch Spectrum Plus; Philips Respironics, Murrysville, PA, USA) to determine bedtime and wake-up time on a daily basis, based on sleep diaries. Objective sleep duration was then calculated using algorithms. For SDB assessment, we utilized a pulse oximeter (PULSOX-Me300; Konica Minolta, Tokyo, Japan) to calculate the average 3% ODI for 4 days. Notably, to enhance the accuracy of ODI, we incorporated the objectively measured sleep duration obtained from the simultaneous accelerometer recordings and adjusted the values, aiming to align them closer to results obtained through polysomnography (in a preliminary study investigating the correlation, the attended polysomnography-measured AHI = 3% ODI adjusted for objective sleep duration × 1.04 + 1.45, $r = 0.99$, $P < 0.001$) [58]. The corrected 3% ODI was then used to determine the severity of SDB, categorizing individuals with ≥5/h as mild, ≥15/h as moderate, and ≥ 30/h as severe SDB.

From 2013 to 2016, 9850 community residents participated in the study. Among them, we conducted analyses on a total of 7713 individuals (78.3% of the initial sample) who had valid data collected from pulse oximeters and accelerometers for two or more days, ranging from 34 to 80 years of age [58].

Patients were defined as having hypertension if they were under antihypertensive medication or if their systolic blood pressure was ≥140 mmHg, or their diastolic blood pressure was ≥90 mmHg; as having diabetes if they were under antidiabetic medication or if their HbA1c levels were ≥ 6.5%; and as having dyslipidemia if they were under antihyperlipidemic medication or if their fasting LDL cholesterol levels were ≥ 140 mg/dL, HDL cholesterol levels were < 40 mg/dL, or triglyceride levels were ≥ 150 mg/dL. As obesity is a strong risk factor for SDB, the frequency of moderate-to-severe SDB was examined based on the presence or absence of obesity (BMI ≥25 kg/m^2) and the presence or absence of lifestyle diseases (hypertension, diabetes, dyslipidemia). Results showed that even in the absence of obesity, the frequency of moderate-to-severe SDB was higher when there were lifestyle diseases (no obesity, no hypertension: 4.4%, no obesity, hypertension: 16.5%, obesity, no hypertension: 20.7%, obesity, hypertension: 38.8%) (no obesity, no diabetes: 7.4%, no obesity, diabetes: 20.1%, obesity, no diabetes: 28.1%, obesity, diabetes: 47.0%) (no obesity, no dyslipidemia: 5.8%, no obesity, dyslipidemia: 10.5%, obesity, no dyslipidemia: 29.8%, obesity, dyslipidemia: 30.0%).

Even after conducting multivariate analysis, lifestyle diseases were strongly associated with SDB in the absence of obesity (odds ratios were 2.3 for hypertension, 1.5 for diabetes, and 1.5 for dyslipidemia). Moreover, when obesity overlapped with these lifestyle diseases, the strength of their association with SDB further increased (8.2-fold for hypertension, 7.8-fold for diabetes, and 5.8-fold for dyslipidemia). In other words, the degree of association with moderate-to-severe SDB increased in the following order: individuals without obesity or lifestyle diseases < individuals with lifestyle diseases only < individuals with obesity only < individuals with both obesity and lifestyle diseases. Therefore, while obesity has been traditionally emphasized as a significant factor in the increased frequency of SDB, the results of this study suggest that even in the absence of obesity, attention should be given to the frequency of SDB when there are lifestyle diseases. However, we should keep in mind that there was no additive effect of dyslipidemia on obesity. As mentioned earlier, the evidence level for the association between dyslipidemia and SDB is lower compared to other lifestyle diseases, and the impact of obesity is thought to be more pronounced.

6 Conclusion

This section reviews previous researches focusing on the relationship between OSA and lifestyle diseases and also introduces the results from large-scale Japanese cohort studies. Findings from various studies do not always align, and this can be attributed to differences in study participants' characteristics and backgrounds (for instance, studies that focus on severe patients with prominent metabolic abnormalities are more likely to yield positive results; additionally, gender and ethnic differences can also play a role), as well as variations in CPAP intervention studies such as differing CPAP usage times and follow-up periods. Although a certain trend of association between lifestyle diseases and SDB is suggested, clear evidence for improvement through CPAP therapy alone is not firmly established, particularly with regards to dyslipidemia where a strong connection with obesity is emphasized, indicating the importance of weight reduction. However, as evident from the Nagahama study, for diagnosing and treating SDB effectively, it is essential to consider the possibility of SDB coexistence in patients with lifestyle diseases, not solely relying on obesity. This is deemed crucial not only for prognosis improvement but also for the treatment of concurrent lifestyle diseases.

References

1. Matricciani L, Bin YS, Lallukka T, Kronholm E, Wake M, Paquet C, et al. Rethinking the sleep-health link. Sleep Health. 2018;4(4):339–48. https://doi.org/10.1016/j.sleh.2018.05.004.
2. Arnardottir ES, Mackiewicz M, Gislason T, Teff KL, Pack AI. Molecular signatures of obstructive sleep apnea in adults: a review and perspective. Sleep. 2009;32(4):447–70.
3. Kario K. Obstructive sleep apnea syndrome and hypertension: ambulatory blood pressure. Hypertens Res. 2009;32(6):428–32. https://doi.org/10.1038/hr.2009.56.
4. Young T, Peppard P, Palta M, Hla KM, Finn L, Morgan B, et al. Population-based study of sleep-disordered breathing as a risk factor for hypertension. Arch Intern Med. 1997;157(15):1746–52.
5. Nieto FJ, Young TB, Lind BK, Shahar E, Samet JM, Redline S, et al. Association of sleep-disordered breathing, sleep apnea, and hypertension in a large community-based study. Sleep Heart Health Study JAMA. 2000;283(14):1829–36.
6. Peppard PE, Young T, Palta M, Skatrud J. Prospective study of the association between sleep-disordered breathing and hypertension. N Engl J Med. 2000;342(19):1378–84. https://doi.org/10.1056/nejm200005113421901.
7. O'Connor GT, Caffo B, Newman AB, Quan SF, Rapoport DM, Redline S, et al. Prospective study of sleep-disordered breathing and hypertension: the sleep heart health study. Am J Respir Crit Care Med. 2009;179(12):1159–64. https://doi.org/10.1164/rccm.200712-1809OC.
8. Hou H, Zhao Y, Yu W, Dong H, Xue X, Ding J, et al. Association of obstructive sleep apnea with hypertension: a systematic review and meta-analysis. J Glob Health. 2018;8(1):010405. https://doi.org/10.7189/jogh.08.010405.
9. Han B, Chen WZ, Li YC, Chen J, Zeng ZQ. Sleep and hypertension. Sleep Breath. 2020;24(1):351–6. https://doi.org/10.1007/s11325-019-01907-2.
10. Chirinos JA, Gurubhagavatula I, Teff K, Rader DJ, Wadden TA, Townsend R, et al. CPAP, weight loss, or both for obstructive sleep apnea. N Engl J Med. 2014;370(24):2265–75. https://doi.org/10.1056/NEJMoa1306187.
11. Norman D, Loredo JS, Nelesen RA, Ancoli-Israel S, Mills PJ, Ziegler MG, et al. Effects of continuous positive airway pressure versus supplemental oxygen on 24-hour ambulatory blood pressure. Hypertension. 2006;47(5):840–5. https://doi.org/10.1161/01.hyp.0000217128.41284.78.
12. Gottlieb DJ, Punjabi NM, Mehra R, Patel SR, Quan SF, Babineau DC, et al. CPAP versus oxygen in obstructive sleep apnea. N Engl J Med. 2014;370(24):2276–85. https://doi.org/10.1056/NEJMoa1306766.
13. Barbé F, Durán-Cantolla J, Sánchez-de-la-Torre M, Martínez-Alonso M, Carmona C, Barceló A, et al. Effect of continuous positive airway pressure on the incidence of hypertension and cardiovascular events in nonsleepy patients with obstructive sleep apnea: a randomized controlled trial. JAMA. 2012;307(20):2161–8. https://doi.org/10.1001/jama.2012.4366.
14. Sapiña-Beltrán E, Torres G, Benítez I, Santamaría-Martos F, Durán-Cantolla J, Egea C, et al. Differential blood pressure response to continuous positive airway pressure treatment according to the circadian pattern in hypertensive patients with obstructive sleep apnoea. Eur Respir J. 2019;54(1) https://doi.org/10.1183/13993003.00098-2019.
15. Lui MM, Tse HF, Lam DC, Lau KK, Chan CW, Ip MS. Continuous positive airway pressure improves blood pressure and serum cardiovascular biomarkers in obstructive sleep apnoea and hypertension. Eur Respir J. 2021;58(5) https://doi.org/10.1183/13993003.03687-2020.

16. Fava C, Dorigoni S, Dalle Vedove F, Danese E, Montagnana M, Guidi GC, et al. Effect of CPAP on blood pressure in patients with OSA/hypopnea a systematic review and meta-analysis. Chest. 2014;145(4):762–71. https://doi.org/10.1378/chest.13-1115.
17. Bratton DJ, Stradling JR, Barbé F, Kohler M. Effect of CPAP on blood pressure in patients with minimally symptomatic obstructive sleep apnoea: a meta-analysis using individual patient data from four randomised controlled trials. Thorax. 2014;69(12):1128–35. https://doi.org/10.1136/thoraxjnl-2013-204993.
18. Shang W, Zhang Y, Liu L, Chen F, Wang G, Han D. Benefits of continuous positive airway pressure on blood pressure in patients with hypertension and obstructive sleep apnea: a meta-analysis. Hypertens Res. 2022;45(11):1802–13. https://doi.org/10.1038/s41440-022-00954-9.
19. Pépin JL, Tamisier R, Barone-Rochette G, Launois SH, Lévy P, Baguet JP. Comparison of continuous positive airway pressure and valsartan in hypertensive patients with sleep apnea. Am J Respir Crit Care Med. 2010;182(7):954–60. https://doi.org/10.1164/rccm.200912-1803OC.
20. Thunström E, Manhem K, Rosengren A, Peker Y. Blood pressure response to losartan and continuous positive airway pressure in hypertension and obstructive sleep apnea. Am J Respir Crit Care Med. 2016;193(3):310–20. https://doi.org/10.1164/rccm.201505-0998OC.
21. Shaw JE, Punjabi NM, Wilding JP, Alberti KG, Zimmet PZ. Sleep-disordered breathing and type 2 diabetes: a report from the international diabetes federation taskforce on epidemiology and prevention. Diabetes Res Clin Pract. 2008;81(1):2–12. https://doi.org/10.1016/j.diabres.2008.04.025.
22. Tahrani AA, Ali A. Obstructive sleep Apnoea and type 2 diabetes. Eur Endocrinol. 2014;10(1):43–50. https://doi.org/10.17925/ee.2014.10.01.43.
23. Framnes SN, Arble DM. The bidirectional relationship between obstructive sleep apnea and metabolic disease. Front Endocrinol (Lausanne). 2018;9:440. https://doi.org/10.3389/fendo.2018.00440.
24. Song SO, He K, Narla RR, Kang HG, Ryu HU, Boyko EJ. Metabolic consequences of obstructive sleep apnea especially pertaining to diabetes mellitus and insulin sensitivity. Diabetes Metab J. 2019;43(2):144–55. https://doi.org/10.4093/dmj.2018.0256.
25. Punjabi NM, Shahar E, Redline S, Gottlieb DJ, Givelber R, Resnick HE. Sleep-disordered breathing, glucose intolerance, and insulin resistance: the sleep heart health study. Am J Epidemiol. 2004;160(6):521–30. https://doi.org/10.1093/aje/kwh261.
26. Kent BD, Grote L, Ryan S, Pépin JL, Bonsignore MR, Tkacova R, et al. Diabetes mellitus prevalence and control in sleep-disordered breathing: the European sleep apnea cohort (ESADA) study. Chest. 2014;146(4):982–90. https://doi.org/10.1378/chest.13-2403.
27. Reichmuth KJ, Austin D, Skatrud JB, Young T. Association of sleep apnea and type II diabetes: a population-based study. Am J Respir Crit Care Med. 2005;172(12):1590–5. https://doi.org/10.1164/rccm.200504-637OC.
28. Botros N, Concato J, Mohsenin V, Selim B, Doctor K, Yaggi HK. Obstructive sleep apnea as a risk factor for type 2 diabetes. Am J Med. 2009;122(12):1122–7. https://doi.org/10.1016/j.amjmed.2009.04.026.
29. Kendzerska T, Gershon AS, Hawker G, Tomlinson G, Leung RS. Obstructive sleep apnea and incident diabetes. a historical cohort study. Am J Respir Crit Care Med. 2014;190(2):218–25. https://doi.org/10.1164/rccm.201312-2209OC.
30. Xu PH, Hui CKM, Lui MMS, Lam DCL, Fong DYT, Ip MSM. Incident type 2 diabetes in OSA and effect of CPAP treatment: a retrospective clinic cohort study. Chest. 2019;156(4):743–53. https://doi.org/10.1016/j.chest.2019.04.130.
31. Qie R, Zhang D, Liu L, Ren Y, Zhao Y, Liu D, et al. Obstructive sleep apnea and risk of type 2 diabetes mellitus: a systematic review and dose-response meta-analysis of cohort studies. J Diabetes. 2020;12(6):455–64. https://doi.org/10.1111/1753-0407.13017.
32. Wang C, Tan J, Miao Y, Zhang Q. Obstructive sleep apnea, prediabetes and progression of type 2 diabetes: a systematic review and meta-analysis. J Diabetes Investig. 2022;13(8):1396–411. https://doi.org/10.1111/jdi.13793.

33. West SD, Nicoll DJ, Wallace TM, Matthews DR, Stradling JR. Effect of CPAP on insulin resistance and HbA1c in men with obstructive sleep apnoea and type 2 diabetes. Thorax. 2007;62(11):969–74. https://doi.org/10.1136/thx.2006.074351.
34. Weinstock TG, Wang X, Rueschman M, Ismail-Beigi F, Aylor J, Babineau DC, et al. A controlled trial of CPAP therapy on metabolic control in individuals with impaired glucose tolerance and sleep apnea. Sleep. 2012;35(5):617–25b. https://doi.org/10.5665/sleep.1816.
35. Shaw JE, Punjabi NM, Naughton MT, Willes L, Bergenstal RM, Cistulli PA, et al. The effect of treatment of obstructive sleep apnea on glycemic control in type 2 diabetes. Am J Respir Crit Care Med. 2016;194(4):486–92. https://doi.org/10.1164/rccm.201511-2260OC.
36. Pamidi S, Wroblewski K, Stepien M, Sharif-Sidi K, Kilkus J, Whitmore H, et al. Eight hours of nightly continuous positive airway pressure treatment of obstructive sleep apnea improves glucose metabolism in patients with prediabetes. A randomized controlled trial. Am J Respir Crit Care Med. 2015;192(1):96–105. https://doi.org/10.1164/rccm.201408-1564OC.
37. Martínez-Cerón E, Barquiel B, Bezos AM, Casitas R, Galera R, García-Benito C, et al. Effect of continuous positive airway pressure on glycemic control in patients with obstructive sleep apnea and type 2 diabetes. A randomized clinical trial. Am J Respir Crit Care Med. 2016;194(4):476–85. https://doi.org/10.1164/rccm.201510-1942OC.
38. Zamarrón E, Jaureguizar A, García-Sánchez A, Díaz-Cambriles T, Alonso-Fernández A, Lores V, et al. Continuous positive airway pressure effect on albuminuria progression in patients with obstructive sleep apnea and diabetic kidney disease: a randomized clinical trial. Am J Respir Crit Care Med. 2023;207(6):757–67. https://doi.org/10.1164/rccm.202206-1091OC.
39. Cattazzo F, Pengo MF, Giontella A, Soranna D, Bilo G, Zambon A, et al. Effect of continuous positive airway pressure on glucose and lipid profiles in patients with obstructive sleep Apnoea: a systematic review and meta-analysis of randomized controlled trials. Arch Bronconeumol. 2023;59(6):370–6. https://doi.org/10.1016/j.arbres.2023.03.012.
40. Herth J, Sievi NA, Schmidt F, Kohler M. Effects of continuous positive airway pressure therapy on glucose metabolism in patients with obstructive sleep apnoea and type 2 diabetes: a systematic review and meta-analysis. Eur Respir Rev. 2023;32(169) https://doi.org/10.1183/16000617.0083-2023.
41. Adedayo AM, Olafiranye O, Smith D, Hill A, Zizi F, Brown C, et al. Obstructive sleep apnea and dyslipidemia: evidence and underlying mechanism. Sleep Breath. 2014;18(1):13–8. https://doi.org/10.1007/s11325-012-0760-9.
42. Barros D, García-Río F. Obstructive sleep apnea and dyslipidemia: from animal models to clinical evidence. Sleep. 2019;42(3) https://doi.org/10.1093/sleep/zsy236.
43. Newman AB, Nieto FJ, Guidry U, Lind BK, Redline S, Pickering TG, et al. Relation of sleep-disordered breathing to cardiovascular disease risk factors: the sleep heart health study. Am J Epidemiol. 2001;154(1):50–9. https://doi.org/10.1093/aje/154.1.50.
44. Tan KC, Chow WS, Lam JC, Lam B, Wong WK, Tam S, et al. HDL dysfunction in obstructive sleep apnea. Atherosclerosis. 2006;184(2):377–82. https://doi.org/10.1016/j.atherosclerosis.2005.04.024.
45. Toyama Y, Chin K, Chihara Y, Takegami M, Takahashi KI, Sumi K, et al. Association between sleep apnea, sleep duration, and serum lipid profile in an urban, male, working population in Japan. Chest. 2013;143(3):720–8. https://doi.org/10.1378/chest.12-0338.
46. Wakabayashi Y, Oka R, Nakaya M, Karashima S, Kometani M, Sakurai M, et al. Associations between sleep-disordered breathing and metabolic risk factors beyond obesity. J Diabetes Res. 2018;2018:1567683. https://doi.org/10.1155/2018/1567683.
47. Nadeem R, Singh M, Nida M, Waheed I, Khan A, Ahmed S, et al. Effect of obstructive sleep apnea hypopnea syndrome on lipid profile: a meta-regression analysis. J Clin Sleep Med. 2014;10(5):475–89. https://doi.org/10.5664/jcsm.3690.
48. Phillips CL, Yee BJ, Marshall NS, Liu PY, Sullivan DR, Grunstein RR. Continuous positive airway pressure reduces postprandial lipidemia in obstructive sleep apnea: a randomized, placebo-controlled crossover trial. Am J Respir Crit Care Med. 2011;184(3):355–61. https://doi.org/10.1164/rccm.201102-0316OC.

49. Craig SE, Kohler M, Nicoll D, Bratton DJ, Nunn A, Davies R, et al. Continuous positive airway pressure improves sleepiness but not calculated vascular risk in patients with minimally symptomatic obstructive sleep apnoea: the MOSAIC randomised controlled trial. Thorax. 2012;67(12):1090–6. https://doi.org/10.1136/thoraxjnl-2012-202178.
50. Campos-Rodriguez F, Gonzalez-Martinez M, Sanchez-Armengol A, Jurado-Gamez B, Cordero-Guevara J, Reyes-Nuñez N, et al. Effect of continuous positive airway pressure on blood pressure and metabolic profile in women with sleep apnoea. Eur Respir J. 2017;50(2) https://doi.org/10.1183/13993003.00257-2017.
51. Gunduz C, Basoglu OK, Kvamme JA, Verbraecken J, Anttalainen U, Marrone O, et al. Long-term positive airway pressure therapy is associated with reduced total cholesterol levels in patients with obstructive sleep apnea: data from the European sleep apnea database (ESADA). Sleep Med. 2020;75:201–9. https://doi.org/10.1016/j.sleep.2020.02.023.
52. Giampá SQC, Furlan SF, Freitas LS, Macedo TA, Lebkuchen A, Cardozo KHM, et al. Effects of CPAP on metabolic syndrome in patients with OSA: a randomized trial. Chest. 2022;161(5):1370–81. https://doi.org/10.1016/j.chest.2021.12.669.
53. Nadeem R, Singh M, Nida M, Kwon S, Sajid H, Witkowski J, et al. Effect of CPAP treatment for obstructive sleep apnea hypopnea syndrome on lipid profile: a meta-regression analysis. J Clin Sleep Med. 2014;10(12):1295–302. https://doi.org/10.5664/jcsm.4282.
54. Xu Y, Wu H, Lu X. Influence of continuous positive airway pressure on lipid profiles of obstructive sleep apnea: a systematic review and meta-analysis. Medicine (Baltimore). 2022;101(42):e31258. https://doi.org/10.1097/md.0000000000031258.
55. Onuki K, Ikeda A, Muraki I, Tanaka M, Yamagishi K, Kiyama M, et al. Nocturnal intermittent hypoxia and the risk of cardiovascular disease among Japanese populations: the circulatory risk in communities study (CIRCS). J Atheroscler Thromb. 2023;30(9):1276–87. https://doi.org/10.5551/jat.63754.
56. Muraki I, Tanigawa T, Yamagishi K, Sakurai S, Ohira T, Imano H, et al. Nocturnal intermittent hypoxia and the development of type 2 diabetes: the circulatory risk in communities study (CIRCS). Diabetologia. 2010;53(3):481–8. https://doi.org/10.1007/s00125-009-1616-0.
57. Matsumoto T, Murase K, Tabara Y, Gozal D, Smith D, Minami T, et al. Impact of sleep characteristics and obesity on diabetes and hypertension across genders and menopausal status: the Nagahama study. Sleep. 2018;41(7) https://doi.org/10.1093/sleep/zsy071.
58. Matsumoto T, Murase K, Tabara Y, Minami T, Kanai O, Takeyama H, et al. Sleep disordered breathing and metabolic comorbidities across sex and menopausal status in east Asians: the Nagahama study. Eur Respir J. 2020;56(2) https://doi.org/10.1183/13993003.02251-2019.
59. Lam DC, Lui MM, Lam JC, Ong LH, Lam KS, Ip MS. Prevalence and recognition of obstructive sleep apnea in Chinese patients with type 2 diabetes mellitus. Chest. 2010;138(5):1101–7. https://doi.org/10.1378/chest.10-0596.
60. Heffner JE, Rozenfeld Y, Kai M, Stephens EA, Brown LK. Prevalence of diagnosed sleep apnea among patients with type 2 diabetes in primary care. Chest. 2012;141(6):1414–21. https://doi.org/10.1378/chest.11-1945.
61. Salord N, Fortuna AM, Monasterio C, Gasa M, Pérez A, Bonsignore MR, et al. A randomized controlled trial of continuous positive airway pressure on glucose tolerance in obese patients with obstructive sleep apnea. Sleep. 2016;39(1):35–41. https://doi.org/10.5665/sleep.5312.
62. Banghøj AM, Krogager C, Kristensen PL, Hansen KW, Laugesen E, Fleischer J, et al. Effect of 12-week continuous positive airway pressure therapy on glucose levels assessed by continuous glucose monitoring in people with type 2 diabetes and obstructive sleep apnoea; a randomized controlled trial. Endocrinol Diabetes Metab. 2021;4(2):e00148. https://doi.org/10.1002/edm2.148.
63. Roche F, Sforza E, Pichot V, Maudoux D, Garcin A, Celle S, et al. Obstructive sleep apnoea/hypopnea influences high-density lipoprotein cholesterol in the elderly. Sleep Med. 2009;10(8):882–6. https://doi.org/10.1016/j.sleep.2008.07.017.

64. Trzepizur W, Le Vaillant M, Meslier N, Pigeanne T, Masson P, Humeau MP, et al. Independent association between nocturnal intermittent hypoxemia and metabolic dyslipidemia. Chest. 2013;143(6):1584–9. https://doi.org/10.1378/chest.12-1652.
65. Silva WA, Almeida-Pititto B, Santos RB, Aielo AN, Giatti S, Parise BK, et al. Obstructive sleep apnea is associated with lower adiponectin and higher cholesterol levels independently of traditional factors and other sleep disorders in middle-aged adults: the ELSA-Brasil cohort. Sleep Breath. 2021;25(4):1935–44. https://doi.org/10.1007/s11325-021-02290-7.
66. Robinson GV, Pepperell JC, Segal HC, Davies RJ, Stradling JR. Circulating cardiovascular risk factors in obstructive sleep apnoea: data from randomised controlled trials. Thorax. 2004;59(9):777–82. https://doi.org/10.1136/thx.2003.018739.

Part II
Treatment and the Related Problems

Chapter 5
Weight Loss and Positional Therapy: For What Type of OSA Patients is Weight Loss Therapy Effective? Is Positional Therapy Effective in Treating OSA Patients?

Misa Takegami

Abstract Obesity is the most important modifiable risk factor for obstructive sleep apnea (OSA). Lifestyle interventions that promote weight loss, including diet and exercise, are not expected to be sufficiently effective to improve apnea hypopnea index-based treatment outcomes in patients with OSA. However, they may be effective in preventing hypertension, lipid abnormalities, and cardiovascular diseases, which typically accompany OSA. Accordingly, lifestyle interventions and patient education are important for weight loss in obese patients with OSA. Additionally, positional therapy is a potential alternative treatment for patients who have difficulty starting and continuously using a continuous positive airway pressure machine. However, there remain no approved medical devices in Japan; moreover, the provided guidelines are only for educational purposes. Future studies are expected to confirm the effectiveness of positional therapy, and approved medical devices are expected to be developed in Japan.

Keywords Obstructive sleep apnea · Lifestyle intervention · Diets · Exercise · Weight loss · Obesity · Positional obstructive sleep apnea · Positional therapy device · Meta-analysis

---

M. Takegami (✉)
Department of Public Health and Health Policy, Graduate School of Medicine, The University of Tokyo, Bunkyo-ku, Tokyo, Japan

Department of Preventive Medicine and Epidemiology, National Cerebral and Cardiovascular Center, Suita, Japan
e-mail: takegami@m.u-tokyo.ac.jp

K. Chin (ed.), *The Current State of Sleep Disordered Breathing in Japan and Around the World*, Respiratory Disease Series: Diagnostic Tools and Disease Managements, https://doi.org/10.1007/978-981-96-6030-8_5

1 Introduction: Weight Loss and Positional Therapy

Obstructive sleep apnea (OSA) is highly prevalent, especially among middle-aged and older adults; further, it increases the risk of cardiovascular disease and metabolic abnormalities. Common risk factors for OSA include older age and male sex, with the most important risk factor being excessive weight gain. The objective of OSA treatment is to relieve airway obstruction during sleep, with the initial treatment option usually being a nasal continuous positive airway pressure (CPAP) machine. Although the use of a CPAP machine can be effective, it is not a definitive treatment; moreover, it has several issues, including discomfort and maladaptation due to skin inflammation, problems with adherence, and treatment interruption. In such cases, behavioral interventions such as lifestyle modifications targeting weight loss and sleep position therapy may be an alternative treatment strategy for patients with mild OSA who have difficulty starting and continuously using a CPAP machine.

This chapter reviews existing literature about OSA and obesity as well as the effectiveness of lifestyle interventions for promoting weight loss and sleep position therapy.

2 Weight Loss and Lifestyle Interventions for Obstructive Sleep Apnea

2.1 Impact of Obesity on Obstructive Sleep Apnea

Risk factors for OSA include sex, age, and craniofacial abnormalities; however, the most important and modifiable risk factor for OSA is obesity. Although the mechanism underlying the relationship between obesity and the onset of OSA remains unclear, obesity-induced upper airway narrowing is a major contributing factor. Weight loss relieves this structural burden on the upper airway, and therefore reduces airway obstruction.

The prevalence of OSA is twice as high in individuals with obesity than in normal-weight individuals; moreover, an estimated 58% of adults with moderate-to-severe OSA have obesity-induced OSA [1]. A 4-year follow-up study reported a dose-response relationship between changes in body mass index (BMI) and apnea-hypopnea index (AHI), which suggests a correlation of OSA severity with body weight [2].

Our previous study on male corporate employees observed a dose-response relationship of BMI with respiratory disturbance index (RDI), with >50% of participants in the fourth quartile of BMI (> 25.9) or higher having an RDI ≥15 [3]. Among Asians, who typically have a lower BMI than Westerners, osteofacial morphology, mainly lower jaw abnormalities, has been suggested to have a greater influence on OSA compared with obesity. Nonetheless, obesity has been established to play a strong role in the onset of OSA in Japanese patients.

2.2 Lifestyle Interventions for Weight Reduction

Weight loss through diet and exercise training can effectively improve primary OSA outcomes (AHI, oxygen desaturation index (ODI), and RDI).

Several randomized control trials (RCTs) on the effectiveness of dietary therapy have used structured diets that replace meals with liquid supplements for 7–16 weeks at the early stages of the intervention [4, 5]. The liquid supplements were prepared meals that contained sufficient amounts of essential amino acids, vitamins, and minerals, which are often lacking during weight loss; moreover, they contained minimal carbohydrates and fats, which served as energy sources. This strategy reduced the daily calorie consumption to 600 kcal/day, did not have adverse health effects, and was more effective than other weight loss methods [6]. The composition of meals consumed after the liquid supplements varies, with some studies following the recommendations by the National Cholesterol Education Program and others limiting fat to <30% of the total caloric intake. All RCTs on the effectiveness of dietary therapy in patients with OSA were conducted in either Europe or the United States; additionally, the average baseline weight of the patients was >100 kg. Therefore, it remains unclear whether dietary therapy using liquid supplements is suitable for Japanese patients with OSA, and further research is warranted. Currently, dietary guidance for the purpose of weight loss is recommended for obese patients with OSA.

Exercise therapy includes both aerobic endurance and muscular resistance training. Usually, aerobic endurance training is considered effective for the prevention and treatment of lifestyle-related diseases, including hypertension and dyslipidemia; however, numerous studies have used a combination of both exercise therapy regimens for patients with OSA [5, 7]. In a study by Tuomilehto et al., in addition to endurance training such as walking, jogging, and swimming, resistance training was performed using a circuit-type machine to improve functional capacity [5]. The study showed that exercise therapy that combines aerobic endurance and resistance training improves AHI outcomes even without weight loss [7]. Resistance training increases lung capacity by strengthening respiratory muscles, which may contribute toward improving OSA symptoms even without weight loss. This suggests it may be effective to combine both aerobic endurance and muscular resistance training as exercise therapy for patients with OSA.

2.3 Effects of Weight Loss and Lifestyle Intervention

There have been meta-analyses on lifestyle interventions for OSA [8–10]. Despite the availability of lifestyle interventions such as sleep hygiene and alcohol avoidance, most RCTs have focused on weight loss though diet and/or exercise. These studies found that diet and/or exercise interventions improved AHI.

Carneiro-Barrera et al. conducted a meta-analyses of 13 RCTs ($n = 840$) and 22 uncontrolled before-and-after studies ($n = 580$) to examine the effects of lifestyle interventions, including diet, exercise-training, sleep hygiene, on OSA outcomes [8]. Both study group showed significant improvements in the AHI, ODI, and EDS. Figure 5.1 shows the effects of the lifestyle interventions on AHI based on the 13 RCTs. All 13 RCTs included diet and/or exercise training.

Araghi et al. conducted a meta-analysis that combined seven RCTs ($n = 519$) and 14 uncontrolled before-and-after studies ($n = 374$) on the effectiveness of lifestyle interventions, including diet and exercise, in weight loss [9]. In an analysis of the RCTs only, the intervention group showed a significant post-intervention improvement in the AHI score compared with the control group. Compared with single-component interventions such as diet therapy or exercise therapy alone, interventions combining diet and exercise therapy allowed greater AHI improvement.

The studies included in these meta-analyses were all conducted abroad; moreover, the average BMI of the included patients was higher than that of Japanese patients, which is a common issue with most meta-analyses. Therefore, caution is required when interpreting the findings given this heterogeneity. However, almost all studies showed that lifestyle interventions, including diet and exercise therapy, for promoting weight loss could effectively improve AHI outcomes [9–14]. Physical exercise has been shown to improve the body composition of patients with OSA; moreover, AHI improvement is not solely attributable to reduced adiposity. Taken together, encouraging exercise among patients with OSA is recommendable [14].

Although lifestyle interventions that promote weight loss can effectively improve OSA symptoms, they cannot easily allow a < 10% reduction in body weight. Therefore, they cannot effectively yield the optimal AHI values [15]. Accordingly, they are recommended to be used in conjunction with a CPAP machine rather than

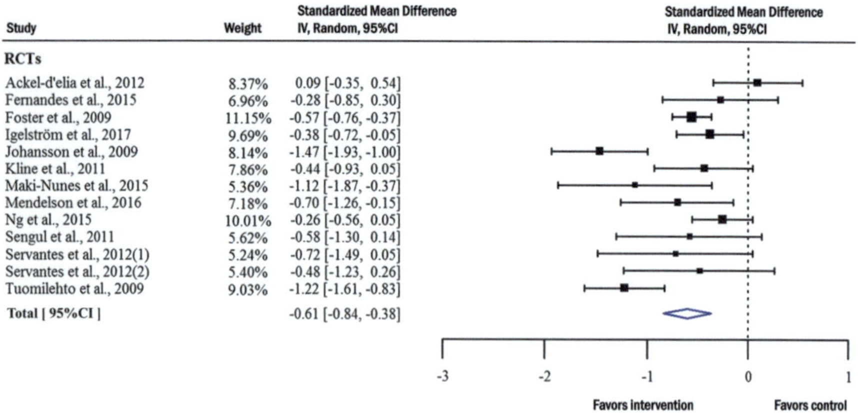

Fig. 5.1 Forest plot of the standardized mean differences for apnea/hypopnea index between lifestyle interventions (diet and/or exercise) and control groups in randomized controlled trials (RCTs). A negative value means a reduction of the outcome after intervention. *IV* inverse variance method, *CI* confidence interval. (Figure is modified with permission received from John Wiley and Sons [8])

as a stand-alone treatment. Weight loss is not only effective against OSA but also can prevent hypertension, lipid abnormalities, and cardiovascular diseases that typically accompany OSA. Additionally, the American College of Physicians' guidelines strongly recommend that patients received education regarding lifestyle habits that promote weight loss [16]. Alternative treatment strategies are necessary, especially for patients not suitable for a CPAP machine [17]. However, there have been no studies on the effects of weight loss on patients with OSA in Japan; therefore, further research is warranted [17].

Key Points

Weight loss reduces apnea in obese patients with OSA. Therefore, in addition to providing standard treatments, such as using a CPAP machine, lifestyle-related guidance for weight loss should be provided.

2.4 *Summary for Weight Loss and Lifestyle Intervention*

Weight loss therapy through lifestyle interventions, including diet and exercise, is not effective as a substitute for standard treatments, such as using a CPAP machine; however, it can contribute to improved AHI scores. Additionally, exercise therapy may have benefits beyond weight loss. Therefore, it is crucial to inform patients that lifestyle changes, including diet and exercise, can help reduce apnea.

3 Positional Therapy for Positional Obstructive Sleep Apnea

3.1 *Positional Obstructive Sleep Apnea (POSA)*

Approximately half of patients with OSA experience worse apnea symptoms due to pharyngeal airway obstruction when sleeping in the supine position [18], which are alleviated when in a non-supine position, such as lying on one's side. Patients whose apnea severity changes depending on their sleep position are considered to have POSA. Overnight polysomnography can confirm whether apnea is exacerbated by the body position during sleep. Although there are varying definitions of POSA [19], it can be defined by the AHI value in the supine position being twice that in a non-supine position, with an overall AHI >5 events/h [20]. Patients with POSA are more likely to be younger, have a lower BMI, and milder apnea severity than patients with non-POSA [21, 22]. In addition, the prevalence of POSA in the Asian population (67%–75%) is higher than in the Caucasian population [22].

Positional therapy (PT) has been proposed as a treatment option for POSA. PT refers to any technique that prevents patients from sleeping in the supine position [23]. This can be achieved through various proprietary devices (Table 5.1) [24].

Table 5.1 Current devices and products used for supine sleep avoidance. (Table is reprinted with permission by CC BY-NC [24])

Method/device/product	Description
Bumpers	
A moderately hard object, usually worn on the back to provide some degree of discomfort in the supine position to encourage avoidance.	
Tennis ball	A tennis ball worn within a tight shirt or secured to chest
iSleepFit™ Posture Belt (iSleepFit System Inc., Michigan, USA)	3 adjustable bumpers/balls secured to chest worn strap
Bolsters	
Bolster pillows (usually inflatable) that are worn close to the body to prevent ability to move into supine sleeping position.	
Sleep Noodle Positional Sleep Aid *(CPAPology, Ontario, Canada)*	Attached to strap worn about chest
WoodyKnows 2021 Side-Sleeping Backpack *(M&M Pure Air Systems LLC, Delaware, USA)*	Attached to backpack worn over chest
Vibrotactile Devices	
Wearable devices that track position and vibrate to warn and condition avoidance of sleeping in the supine position.	
Night Shift™ Sleep Positioner *(Advanced Brain Monitoring Inc., California, USA)*	Worn either neck or chest
Somnibel™ Positional Therapy System *(Sibel, Barcelona, Spain)*	Worn on forehead
Night Balance™ Sleep Positioner Trainer *(Den Haag, The Netherlands)*	Worn on chest
BuzzPOD™ Body Position Orientation Device *(Gorman ProMed Pty Ltd, Victoria, Australia)*	Worn on chest

3.2 Traditional Positional Therapy and Its Effects

Traditional PT techniques apply mechanical avoidance of the supine position and include the use of a bulky object [24]. The most classic technique is the tennis ball technique (TBT) [23]. It involves creation of a pocket in the back of the patient's nightgown, in which a tennis ball is placed. Jackson et al. conducted a 4-week RCT on patients with POSA using a device developed based on TBT [25]. Patients who received PT had significantly lower AHI scores than those who only received typical sleep guidance. In a randomized crossover designed trial, Jokic et al. compared the effectiveness of using a CPAP machine in 13 patients with mild-to-moderate POSA (mean AHI score = 18.0 events/h) [26]. Participants were assigned to either the PT or CPAP group, received treatment for 2 weeks, and then received 2 weeks of treatment that differed from the initial treatment. The AHI scores when using a CPAP machine and during PT decreased by 3.4 events/h and 9.5 events/h, respectively, indicating that sleep apnea did not decrease as much when using a CPAP machine. Other randomized crossover designed trials have reported similar results [27].

There is strong single-night evidence regarding the efficacy of treatments that physically prevent side-to-side movement, including bolsters [28]. A randomized crossover trial on the difference between PT and using a CPAP machine overnight that examined 38 patients with OSA observed no between-intervention difference in AHI improvement, with similar effects on sleep quality and nocturnal oxygenation [28]. However, there are concerns that long-term use of this type of PT device may result in shoulder and hip discomfort given the difficulty in changing sides during sleep[39)]; moreover, patient compliance remains to be established.

3.3 *New Generation Vibrotactile Devices for Positional Therapy and Its Effects*

The vibrotactile PT device was recently developed and is rapidly gaining popularity [23, 29]. It uses a small sensor that detects sleep position; further, it comprises two types: one that is worn on the back of the neck [30] and one that is worn on the chest [31, 32]. Both devices vibrate when the patient is in the supine position during sleep, with the vibrations gradually increasing in intensity until the patient is no longer in this position. Accordingly, the vibrations prevent the patient from sleeping in the supine position. These devices, including the neck-type Night Shift™, the chest-type Night Balance™, and ZZOMA™, have been approved by the US Food and Drug Administration for the treatment of POSA [33]. The chest-type vibrotactile PT device has also been developed in Japan (Fig. 5.2).

In 2011, Bignold et al. conducted a randomized crossover designed trial on the effectiveness of vibrotactile devices in 15 patients with POSA [22]. Participants were randomly assigned to either wear the PT device or receive no treatment for 1 week. They found that the PT device significantly reduced the time spent in the supine position during sleep and the AHI score. Similarly, an RCT that used chest-type vibrotactile devices found a decreased AHI score in the PT device group than

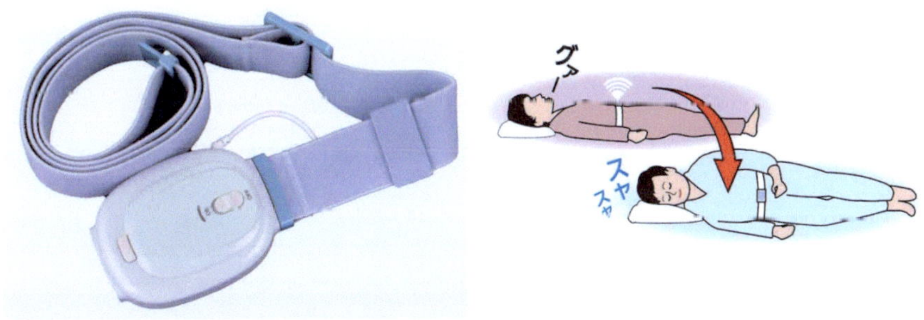

Fig. 5.2 Vibrotactile device, Yokomuki-belt (which means side lying position belt in Japanese) (Baioyakuhin corporation, Tokyo, Japan) Photographic permission granted by Baioyakuhin corporation

in the control group, with this effect persisting for >6 months [33]. In addition, there was improvement in daytime sleepiness.

Several randomized crossover design trials have compared vibrotactile devices with CPAP [34]. Berry et al. conducted a randomized crossover trial in which patients either received a vibrotactile chest worn device or an automatically titrating CPAP device [35]. Among 117 randomized patients, 110 completed 6 weeks of each treatment. Despite being less effective at reducing the AHI compared to CPAP, the PT device met pre-specified non-inferiority margin of five events per hour. The mean AHI difference was 3.58 events/h. Notably, participants indicated that the PT device was more comfortable and easier to use; additionally, 53% of the participants reported a preference for the PT device assuming both devices were equally effective. A similarly designed study conducted by Mok et al. reported that CPAP use allowed a lower AHI value than PT (4.0 ± 3.2 vs. 13.0 ± 13.8 events/hour, respectively, $p = 0.001$). Furthermore, 60% of the patients preferred CPAP, 20% preferred PT, and 20% preferred neither device [36].

3.4 *Effects of Positional Therapy*

There have been several meta-analyses on the effects of PT. Barnes et al. examined four studies on PT and observed a 9.6 reduction in the AHI score when PT was implemented compared with when it was not. This meta-analysis included two TBT-based interventions and two vibrotactile device interventions (Fig. 5.3) [37].

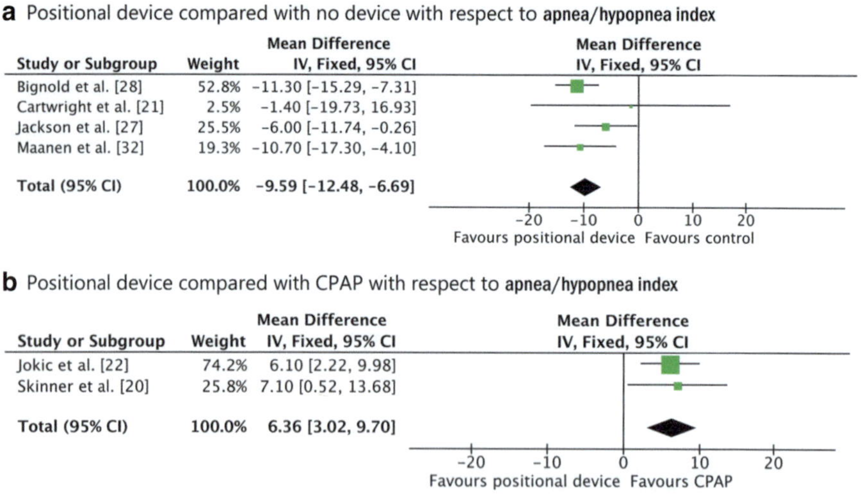

Fig. 5.3 Forest plot of the mean differences for apnea/hypopnea index in Parallel or crossover designed randomized controlled trials. *CPAP* continuous positive airway pressure, *IV* inverse variance method, *CI* confidence interval. (Figure is modified with permission received from Elsevier. [27])

However, compared with using a CPAP machine, PT was not as effective, with the AHI score decreasing by 6.4 with the use of a CPAP machine relative to the value obtained in PT (Fig. 5.3) [37]. Ha et al. also conducted an integrated analysis comparing PT to the use of a CPAP machine and found similar results [38]. However, the included studies did not use a vibrotactile device and only considered TBT therapy.

Al Qarni et al. conducted a meta-analysis of the effect of vibrotactile PT devices that included 18 studies (10 RCTs, 8 cohort studies). PT use reduced the AHI score by an average of −9.19 events/hour at follow-up compared with the baseline value [29].

These meta-analysis results support the efficacy of implementing PT in patients with POSA. However, these meta-analyses included a small number of studies, all RCTs and randomized crossover trials included were small-scale studies, and long-term effects were not verified. Accordingly, the evidence cannot be considered as sufficient. Moreover, all the mentioned studies were conducted outside of Japan and targeted patients with OSA, and the effects of PT remain to be confirmed in all patients with OSA.

Key Points

For patients whose apnea is alleviated when laying on their side, guidance on sleeping position would be effective. In addition, informing patients that adjusting their sleeping position may reduce apnea symptoms, it may be beneficial to also consider using positional therapy devices when necessary.

3.5 *Summary for Positional Therapy*

PT can improve AHI scores in patients with POSA. However, the long-term effects of PT remain unclear and there have been no studies targeting Japanese patients. In Japan, patients with mild symptoms who are not eligible to use a CPAP machine, as well as those who cannot undergo standard treatments, should receive guidance regarding sleeping positions.

4 Conclusion

Weight loss therapy through lifestyle interventions is not effective as a substitute for standard treatments, such as using a CPAP machine; however, it can improve OSA symptoms to a certain extent. Moreover, weight loss can effectively prevent hypertension, lipid abnormalities, and cardiovascular diseases, which are often associated with OSA. Therefore, it is important to provide weight loss-oriented patient education to obese patients with OSA in order to improve their lifestyle habits.

Additionally, although sleep PT may be an alternative treatment for patients who have difficulty starting and continuing using a CPAP machine, there remain no approved medical devices in Japan. Moreover, the only available guidance is for educational use only. Therefore, in the future, it is expected that PT devices will be developed and made available in Japan as well.

References

1. Young T, Skatrud J, Peppard PE. Risk factors for obstructive sleep apnea in adults. JAMA. 2004;291:2013–6.
2. Peppard PE, Young T, Palta M, et al. Longitudinal study of moderate weight change and sleep disordered breathing. JAMA. 2000;284:3015–21.
3. Nakayama-Ashida Y, Takegami M, Chin K, et al. Sleep-disordered breathing in the usual lifestyle setting as detected with home monitoring in a population of working population in Japan. Sleep. 2008;31:419–25.
4. Chirinos JA, Gurubhagavatula I, Teff K, et al. CPAP, weight loss, or both for obstructive sleep apnea. N Engl J Med. 2014;370:2265–75.
5. Tuomilehto HP, Seppa JM, Partinen MM, et al. Lifestyle intervention with weight reduction: first-line treatment in mild obstructive sleep apnea. Am J Respir Crit Care Med. 2009;179:320–7.
6. Flechtner-Mors M, Ditschuneit HH, Johnson TD, et al. Metabolic and weight loss effects of long-term dietary intervention in obese patients: four-year results. Obes Res. 2000;8:399–402.
7. Kline CE, Crowley EP, Ewing GB, et al. The effect of exercise training on obstructive sleep apnea and sleep quality: a randomized controlled trial. Sleep. 2011;34:1631–40.
8. Carneiro-Barrera A, Díaz-Román A, Guillén-Riquelme A, et al. Weight loss and lifestyle interventions for obstructive sleep apnoea in adults: systematic review and meta-analysis. Obes Rev. 2019;20:750–62.
9. Araghi MH, Chen YF, Jagielski A, et al. Effectiveness of lifestyle interventions on obstructive sleep apnea (OSA): systematic review and meta-analysis. Sleep. 2013;36:1553–62.
10. Thomasouli MA, Brady EM, Davies MJ, et al. The impact of diet and lifestyle management strategies for obstructive sleep apnoea in adults: a systematic review and meta-analysis of randomised controlled trials. Sleep Breath. 2013;17:925–35.
11. Anandam A, Akinnusi M, Kufel T, et al. Effects of dietary weight loss on obstructive sleep apnea: a meta-analysis. Sleep Breath. 2013;17:227–34.
12. Aiello KD, Caughey WG, Nelluri B, et al. Effect of exercise training on sleep apnea: a systematic review and meta-analysis. Respir Med. 2016;116:85–92.
13. Mitchell LJ, Davidson ZE, Bonham M, et al. Weight loss from lifestyle interventions and severity of sleep apnoea: a systematic review and meta-analysis. Sleep Med. 2014;15:1173–83.
14. Lins-Filho O, Porto Aguiar JL, Vieira de Almeida JR, et al. Effect of exercise training on body composition in patients with obstructive sleep apnea: a systematic review and meta-analysis. Sleep Med. 2021;87:105–13.
15. Iftikhar IH, Bittencourt L, Youngstedt SD, et al. Comparative efficacy of CPAP, MADs, exercise-training, and dietary weight loss for sleep apnea: a network meta-analysis. Sleep Med. 2017;30:7–14.
16. Qaseem A, Holty JE, Owens DK, et al. Management of obstructive sleep apnea in adults: a clinical practice guideline from the American College of Physicians. Ann Intern Med. 2013;159:471–83.
17. Patil SP, Ayappa IA, Caples SM, et al. Treatment of adult obstructive sleep apnea with positive airway pressure: an American Academy of sleep medicine clinical practice guideline. J Clin Sleep Med. 2019;15:335–43.

18. Oksenberg A, Silverberg DS, Arons E, et al. Positional vs nonpositional obstructive sleep apnea patients: anthropomorphic, nocturnal polysomnographic, and multiple sleep latency test data. Chest. 1997;112:629–39.
19. Omobomi O, Quan SF. Positional therapy in the management of positional obstructive sleep apnea-a review of the current literature. Sleep Breath. 2018;22:297–304.
20. Cartwright RD. Effect of sleep position on sleep apnea severity. Sleep. 1984;7:110–4.
21. Joosten SA, O'Driscoll DM, Berger PJ, et al. Supine position related obstructive sleep apnea in adults: pathogenesis and treatment. Sleep Med Rev. 2014;18:7–17.
22. Mo JH, Lee CH, Rhee CS, et al. Positional dependency in Asian patients with obstructive sleep apnea and its implication for hypertension. Arch Otolaryngol Head Neck Surg. 2011;137:786–90.
23. Yingjuan M, Siang WH, Leong Alvin TK, et al. Positional therapy for positional obstructive sleep apnea. Sleep Med Clin. 2019;14:119–33.
24. Landry SA, Beatty C, Thomson LDJ, et al. A review of supine position related obstructive sleep apnea: classification, epidemiology, pathogenesis and treatment. Sleep Med Rev. 2023;72:101847.
25. Jackson M, Collins A, Berlowitz D, et al. Efficacy of sleep position modification to treat positional obstructive sleep apnea. Sleep Med. 2015;16:545–52.
26. Jokic R, Klimaszewski A, Crossley M, et al. Positional treatment vs continuous positive airway pressure in patients with positional obstructive sleep apnea syndrome. Chest. 1999;115:771–81.
27. Skinner MA, Kingshott RN, Jones DR, et al. Elevated posture for the management of obstructive sleep apnea. Sleep Breath. 2004;8:193–200.
28. Permut I, Diaz-Abad M, Chatila W, et al. Comparison of positional therapy to CPAP in patients with positional obstructive sleep apnea. J Clin Sleep Med. 2010;6:238–43.
29. ALQarni AS, Turnbull CD, Morrell MJ, et al. Efficacy of vibrotactile positional therapy devices on patients with positional obstructive sleep apnoea: a systematic review and meta-analysis. Thorax. 2023;78:1126–34.
30. Levendowski DJ, Seagraves S, Popovic D, et al. Assessment of a neck-based treatment and monitoring device for positional obstructive sleep apnea. J Clin Sleep Med. 2014;10:863–71.
31. van Maanen JP, Meester KA, Dun LN, et al. The sleep position trainer: a new treatment for positional obstructive sleep apnoea. Sleep Breath. 2013;17:771–9.
32. Bignold JJ, Mercer JD, Antic NA, et al. Accurate position monitoring and improved supine-dependent obstructive sleep apnea with a new position recording and supine avoidance device. J Clin Sleep Med. 2011;7:376–83.
33. Laub RR, Tonnesen P, Jennum PJ. A sleep position trainer for positional sleep apnea: a randomized, controlled trial. J Sleep Res. 2017;26:641–50.
34. Positional sleep aids comparison guide. Positional Therapies for Supine Sleep Avoidance. 2021. https://sleepreviewmag.com/sleep-treatments/therapy-devices/positional-therapies-supine/positional-sleep-aids-guide/. Accessed 7th Mar 2024
35. Berry RB, Uhles ML, Abaluck BK, et al. NightBalance sleep position treatment device versus auto-adjusting positive airway pressure for treatment of positional obstructive sleep apnea. J Clin Sleep Med. 2019;15:947–56.
36. Mok Y, Tan A, Hsu PP, et al. Comparing treatment effects of a convenient vibratory positional device to CPAP in positional OSA: a crossover randomised controlled trial. Thorax. 2020;75:331–7.
37. Barnes H, Edwards BA, Joosten SA, et al. Positional modification techniques for supine obstructive sleep apnea: a systematic review and meta-analysis. Sleep Med Rev. 2017;36:107–15.
38. Ha SC, Hirai HW, Tsoi KK. Comparison of positional therapy versus continuous positive airway pressure in patients with positional obstructive sleep apnea: a meta-analysis of randomized trials. Sleep Med Rev. 2014;18:19–24.

Chapter 6
Effect of CPAP Therapy on Weight Changes: How to Understand Weight Changes in Patients with OSA following CPAP Treatment?

Ryo Tachikawa

Abstract Current insights suggest a bidirectional relationship between obesity and obstructive sleep apnea (OSA): obesity can lead to OSA, and conversely, the disrupted energy homeostasis observed in OSA may lead to further weight gain. Similar to the mechanism of weight gain observed in sleep deprivation, it is hypothesized that untreated patients with OSA experience dysregulated energy homeostasis with increased energy intake and expenditure, where intake usually surpasses expenditure. However, existing data indicate that treating OSA with continuous positive airway pressure (CPAP) may also promote weight gain. This paradoxical phenomenon may be attributed to a decrease in basal metabolic rate after initiating CPAP therapy, which might predispose patients with OSA to a positive energy balance. However, it appears that dietary habits and disordered eating behaviors have a more significant impact on actual weight changes compared to alterations in energy expenditure. This underscores the importance of integrating lifestyle modifications into the management of OSA.

Keywords Appetite-related hormone · Basal metabolic rate · Body weight · Continuous positive airway pressure · Eating behavior · Energy homeostasis · Obstructive sleep apnea

R. Tachikawa (✉)
Department of Respiratory Medicine, Kobe City Medical Center General Hospital, Kobe, Japan

K. Chin (ed.), *The Current State of Sleep Disordered Breathing in Japan and Around the World*, Respiratory Disease Series: Diagnostic Tools and Disease Managements, https://doi.org/10.1007/978-981-96-6030-8_6

1 Introduction

Body weight remains stable when there is a balance between energy intake and expenditure. It is widely acknowledged that sleep disturbances can disrupt the intricate regulation of energy, resulting in a positive energy balance, weight gain, and ultimately, obesity. This phenomenon is similarly observed in individuals with obstructive sleep apnea (OSA), as evidenced by a higher risk of weight gain in OSA patients. While one might hypothesize that treating OSA with continuous positive airway pressure (CPAP) would restore energy balance regulation and stabilize weight, evidence suggests that many individuals may still experience an increased risk of weight gain after CPAP therapy. In the following section, we will explore the underlying mechanisms of this paradoxical weight gain trend following CPAP, with a special focus on the dynamics of energy metabolism.

2 Bidirectional Relationship Between OSA and Obesity

It is well established that obesity is the primary risk factor for OSA, with approximately 60–70% of OSA patients being obese. Moreover, current insights suggest a bidirectional relationship between obesity and OSA: not only can obesity lead to OSA, but the existence of OSA might also exacerbate weight gain [1, 2]. In fact, untreated OSA patients have been observed to have a heightened propensity for weight gain compared to those with uncomplicated obesity. A retrospective cohort study comparing weight changes in untreated male OSA patients to those with simple obesity revealed a significant weight gain in the OSA group 1 year prior to the diagnosis of OSA [3]. Data from the Sleep Heart Health Study showed a correlation between the severity of sleep-disordered breathing and an increase in BMI over a 5-year period post-diagnosis [4]. Furthermore, a study comparing the 1-year outcomes of a healthy lifestyle intervention in men with visceral obesity found that those with sleep apnea exhibited lesser reductions in body weight and fewer metabolic improvements than those without, despite equivalent adherence to the program [5]. These studies indicate a bidirectional relationship between obesity and OSA, suggesting that OSA could disrupt energy metabolism and contribute to further weight gain.

3 Putative Mechanisms Behind Sleep Deprivation and Weight Gain

Epidemiological associations between insufficient sleep and various health risks including obesity are well established. A meta-analysis involving approximately 200,000 individuals from 11 prospective cohort studies revealed that short sleep duration (less than 5–6 h) was associated with an increased risk of obesity [6]. In the context of sleep disturbances' impact on energy metabolism, it would be instructive to review the potential underlying mechanisms of obesogenic phenomenon of sleep deprivation.

To understand the mechanisms by which sleep deprivation leads to obesity, one must consider energy metabolism: weight gain results from a sustained positive energy balance, determined by the balance between energy intake and expenditure. Energy expenditure is divided into three main components: basal metabolic rate (BMR), diet-induced thermogenesis, and physical activity energy expenditure, which typically account for 60%, 10%, and 30% of the total expenditure, respectively. During sleep, the BMR is reduced compared to wakeful states, rendering sleep a period of reduced energy consumption.

From the perspective of energy expenditure, a shorter sleep duration can lead to an extended period of wakefulness and activity, thus potentially resulting in stable or slightly increased energy expenditure [7–11]. On the other hand, in terms of energy intake, it has been demonstrated that sleep restriction often leads to overeating when food intake is not controlled [7, 9–14]. This increase in food consumption can be attributed to factors such as more frequent eating opportunities, stress-induced eating, alterations in appetite-regulating hormones, and increased reward-driven eating behaviors, often characterized by increased nighttime intake of fats and carbohydrates. In a systematic review and meta-analysis of 41 studies that implemented sleep restriction interventions, it was shown that sleep deprivation led to an increase in subjective hunger and enhanced brain activity in response to food stimuli, particularly in areas related to cognitive control and reward [15]. As a result, there was an observed increase in caloric intake of approximately 250 kcal/day and a weight gain of 0.34 kg.

Collectively, the primary hypothesized mechanism for weight gain linked to sleep deprivation is the disproportionate increase in caloric intake. Even though there might be an increase in energy expenditure, this is often counteracted or surpassed by a substantial increase in caloric consumption, resulting in a positive energy balance. Experimental evidence further suggests that sleep fragmentation can intensify hunger sensations and amplify caloric consumption [16, 17]. These observations offer a theoretical framework for analogous dynamics in energy metabolism of OSA, where both sleep duration and quality are compromised.

4 Putative Mechanisms Linking OSA and Weight Gain

OSA encompasses not only elements of sleep deprivation but also involves factors directly related to energy metabolism, including increased respiratory effort during apneic events, increased sympathetic nervous system activity, hormonal regulation of hunger/satiety/appetite, and potential reductions in physical activity due to fatigue and sleepiness. This renders the energy metabolism profile in OSA more complex [18].

In terms of energy expenditure, it is plausible that patients with OSA exhibit increased energy consumption. Elevations in BMR have been reported in OSA patients [19–21], with this rise being linked to elevated levels of stress hormones, such as plasma cortisol and urinary norepinephrine [21]. In addition, energy expenditure during sleep also increases not only due to enhanced sympathetic nervous system activity but also due to increased respiratory effort [19]. On the other hand, there is a possibility that physical activity and its associated energy expenditure are reduced in OSA patients, which might offset any increase in basal metabolic rate to some extent [18].

Evidence also suggests that patients with OSA exhibit increased energy intake. A positive correlation exists between the severity of OSA and caloric consumption, with these patients typically showing a preference for fat-rich diets. The inclination toward calorie-dense, high-fat foods remains consistent in OSA patients regardless of their obesity status [22–24]. At the hormonal level, numerous studies have shown elevated serum leptin levels in patients with OSA, a satiety hormone. This elevation is thought to arise from leptin resistance, similar to the hyperleptinemia observed in obese patients. Additionally, increased levels of ghrelin, an appetite-stimulating hormone, have also been suggested in OSA patients. Although these data provide a potential mechanistic basis for the dysregulation of food intake in OSA, more studies are necessary to definitively link hormonal control of hunger and satiety to actual food intake in these patients, given that the levels of appetite-related hormones are influenced by negative feedback mechanisms dependent on dietary and energy intake [18].

In summary, similar to sleep deprivation, it is postulated that both energy expenditure and intake increase in patients with OSA. Considering the observed trend of weight gain in OSA patients, it is theoretically plausible that, in untreated OSA individuals, the increase in energy intake exceeds the rise in energy expenditure. This pattern mirrors the dysregulation of energy balance observed in sleep deprivation.

5 Paradoxical Weight Gain After CPAP

If OSA contributes to weight gain, it would be expected that CPAP would mitigate this obesogenic effect of OSA. However, in a sub-analysis of a randomized controlled trial with 1100 participants in the USA, there was an increase in weight after 6 months in the adherent CPAP group whereas weight decreased in the sham CPAP and non-adherent CPAP groups [25]. A following meta-analysis including 25 RCTs reported an average weight increase of approximately 0.4 kg within several months following CPAP initiation when compared to baseline [26]. A more recent meta-analysis, including 39 RCTs, also indicated a weight gain of 0.148 kg/m^2 in the

CPAP group compared to controls [27]. Additionally, an RCT focused on tonsillectomy in children aged 5–10 showed a postoperative weight gain, with predisposed overweight children trending toward increased obesity [28]. Based on these findings, it is not anticipated that OSA treatment will naturally reduce weight; rather, a short-term increase is more likely. The finding that weight loss does not naturally occur with CPAP therapy alone is clinically relevant, given the high prevalence of overweight and obesity among OSA patients. This highlights the need for a comprehensive risk management strategy in obese individuals, with an emphasis on weight management interventions following CPAP initiation. This was further corroborated by a randomized controlled trial comparing weight loss alone, CPAP therapy alone, and a combination of both in obese patients with OSA [29]. The results clearly demonstrated that for the improvement of cardiovascular risk factors, including blood pressure and insulin sensitivity, weight reduction is crucial, and CPAP therapy by itself is insufficient.

6 Changes in Energy Metabolism After CPAP for OSA

To elucidate the effects of CPAP treatment on energy balance in patients with OSA, it is imperative to concurrently evaluate alterations in energy intake, energy expenditure, and body weight under free-living conditions. Moreover, to understand the mechanisms of changes in energy metabolism, a comprehensive examination of factors related to energy metabolism is required. Elucidating the energy metabolism following CPAP therapy may in turn help understand the underlying mechanisms by which untreated OSA contributes to the dysregulation of energy balance.

In this context, we performed a comprehensive assessment of energy metabolism before and after CPAP [30]. In this study, a comprehensive evaluation of energy metabolism was conducted in 63 newly diagnosed OSA participants (51 males; age 60 ± 10.1 years; apnea–hypopnea index (AHI) > 20/h) at baseline, upon CPAP initiation, and at a 3-month follow-up. Assessments included polysomnography, body weight, body composition, BMR measured by indirect calorimetry, hormone levels (norepinephrine, cortisol, leptin, ghrelin, insulin-like growth factor), dietary intake estimation and eating behavior assessed by questionnaires, and physical activity evaluated using accelerometers. In summarizing the primary measurements pertaining to energy metabolism: BMR notably declined from a mean of 1584 kcal/day prior to CPAP therapy to 1508 kcal/day at the 3-month follow-up. Physical activity levels were consistent over the 3-month duration. Similarly, total caloric intake was unaltered during the same period. Body weight experienced a significant rise from 77.6 kg before CPAP to 78.2 kg after the intervention (Table 6.1).

Table 6.1 Changes in parameters related to energy metabolism before and after CPAP therapy

Variables	Baseline	CPAP initiation[a]	3-month follow-up	*P* value
Indirect calorimetry				
Basal metabolic rate, kcal/day	1584 ± 261	1561 ± 252	1508 ± 258*	<0.001
Physical activity				
Physical activity, activity counts/min	185 ± 80		184 ± 65	0.952
Energy/nutrition intake				
Total caloric intake, kcal/day	2018 ± 509	1906 ± 488	1982 ± 462	0.076
Energy, protein, %	15.8 ± 3.4	15.4 ± 2.9	15.7 ± 3.3	0.525
Energy, fat, %	26.7 ± 6.2	26.2 ± 4.6	27.4 ± 6.3	0.209
Energy, carbohydrate, %	52.7 ± 8.7	53.2 ± 8.1	51.8 ± 8.4	0.245
Anthropometric parameters				
Body weight, kg	77.8 ± 12.6	77.6 ± 12.5	78.2 ± 12.3**	0.010
Fat mass, kg	24.4 ± 7.8	24.3 ± 8.0	24.4 ± 7.9	0.840
Fat-free mass, kg	53.4 ± 8.3	53.3 ± 8.3	53.8 ± 8.6	0.061
Muscle mass, kg	29.7 ± 5.1	29.7 ± 5.1	29.9 ± 5.2	0.253
Hormones				
Cortisol, μg/dL	14.7 ± 3.9	15.3 ± 3.2	14.5 ± 3.4	0.363
Plasma norepinephrine, pg/mL	242 ± 125	230 ± 128	213 ± 101	0.240
Urine norepinephrine, μg/gCr	102 ± 53	107 ± 59	96 ± 41	0.273
IGF-1, ng/mL	130 ± 37	134 ± 33	138 ± 37***	0.004
Leptin, ng/mL	15.0 ± 7.8	16.1 ± 9.6	16.3 ± 10.2	0.078
Acylated ghrelin, fmol/mL	7.1 ± 5.7	7.0 ± 6.3	6.7 ± 6.6	0.766
Sleep parameters				
Total sleep time, min	372 ± 82	383 ± 80	398 ± 66	0.068
Sleep stage 1/2, %	84.4 ± 6.9	78.0 ± 8.1****	77.0 ± 7.5****	<0.001
Sleep stage 3/4, %	1.2 ± 2.3	2.9 ± 4.6***	2.8 ± 5.2*****	0.004
Sleep REM, %	14.6 ± 6.3	19.0 ± 6.5****	20.1 ± 5.7****	<0.001
AHI, events/h	42.2 ± 19.9	5.6 ± 6.2****	3.9 ± 3.7****	<0.001
Time of SpO2 < 90%, %	16.8 ± 20.3	0.6 ± 1.8****	0.7 ± 3.5****	<0.001

Reference [30]. Cite: Tachikawa et al. [30]. The American Journal of Respiratory and Critical Care Medicine is an official journal of the American Thoracic Society

*$p < 0.001$ vs. baseline, $p < 0.01$ vs. CPAP initiation; **$p < 0.05$ vs. CPAP initiation; ***$p < 0.01$ vs. baseline; ****$p < 0.001$ vs. baseline; *****$p < 0.05$ vs. baseline

[a]Values in anthropometric and energy/nutrition intake parameters represent assessments just before CPAP therapy. Other values represent those measured after one night of CPAP therapy

AHI apnea–hypopnea index, *IGF-1* insulin-like growth factor-1, *REM* rapid eye movement

7 Mechanisms Underlying Body Weight Increase After CPAP

The aforementioned study delineated several key mechanisms underlying body weight changes following CPAP therapy [30]. First, in terms of energy expenditure, there was a 5% decline in BMR, while physical activity levels post-CPAP remained unchanged. This reduction in BMR was associated with decreased urine norepinephrine, suggesting a deceased sympathetic nervous system activity following treatment. These findings suggest that the overall energy expenditure following CPAP decreases due to the BMR reduction, predisposing to a positive energy balance.

Second, dietary intake appeared to have a more pronounced effect on weight changes than reduction in BMR. Importantly, the reduction in BMR was consistent between both the weight-increase and weight-decrease groups, indicating that both groups were equally predisposed to a positive energy balance in terms of energy expenditure. In contrast, the estimated caloric intake was higher in the weight-increase group compared to the weight-decrease group at 3-month follow-up (Fig. 6.1). Multivariate analysis further indicated that increased caloric intake was a

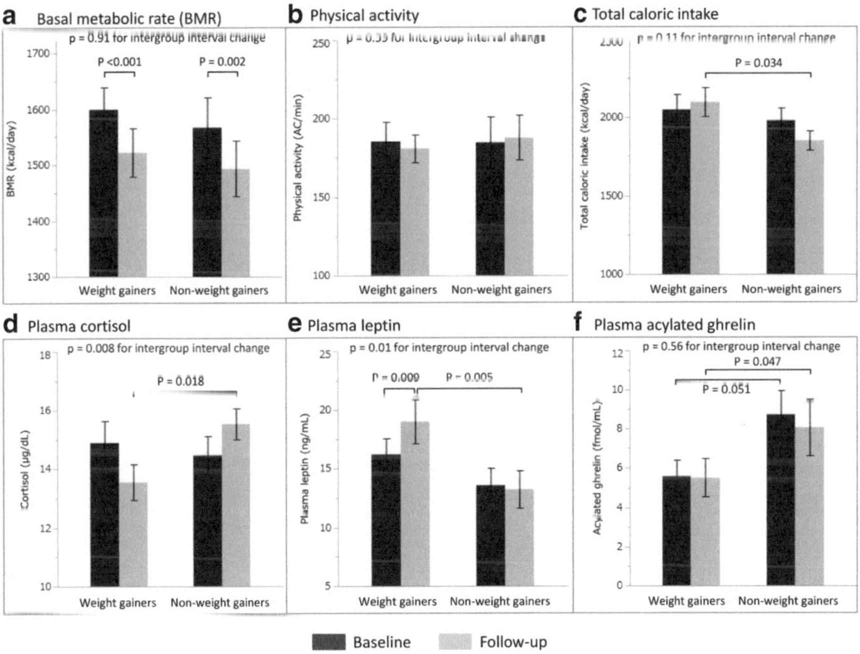

Fig. 6.1 Comparison between weight-increase group (weigh gainers) and weight-decrease group (non-weight gainers). (**a**) Basal metabolic rate, (**b**) physical activity, (**c**) total caloric intake, (**d**) plasma cortisol, (**e**) plasma leptin, and (**f**) plasma acylated ghrelin. Vertical bars represent mean + standard error. *AC* activity counts, *BMR* basal metabolic rate. Reprinted with permission of the American Thoracic Society. Cite: Tachikawa et al. [30]. The American Journal of Respiratory and Critical Care Medicine is an official journal of the American Thoracic Society

particularly significant predictor of weight gain, along with baseline characteristics such as younger age, female gender, non-obesity, and non-smoking status. These insights underscore the primary role of dietary factors in driving individual differences in weight changes beyond the shifts in energy expenditure.

Third, distinct differences were evident in the baseline eating behavior profiles between the weight-increase and weight-decrease groups as assessed by eating behavior questionnaire (Fig. 6.2 and Table 6.2). These differences implicate disordered eating behavior (e.g., misperception of the reasons for gaining weight, disinhibited responsiveness to food cues, and preference for obesogenic foods) as a plausible mechanism that underlies the increased propensity for excessive caloric intake in the weight-increase group. This is in line with previous observations consistently showing that increased caloric intake, rather than the shift in energy expenditure, is the primary cause of weight gain in sleep deprivation, which is in part dependent on disordered eating behaviors [10, 11, 31, 32]. Interestingly, levels of orexigenic hormones, including plasma acylated ghrelin and cortisol, were lower in the weight-increase group at the 3-month follow-up while the plasma leptin level, a satiety hormone, was elevated in the weight-decrease group (Fig. 6.1). While these findings may appear counterintuitive, these associations can be rationalized by assuming that the hormones actually represented the consequence of an energy imbalance rather than a cause of weight change.

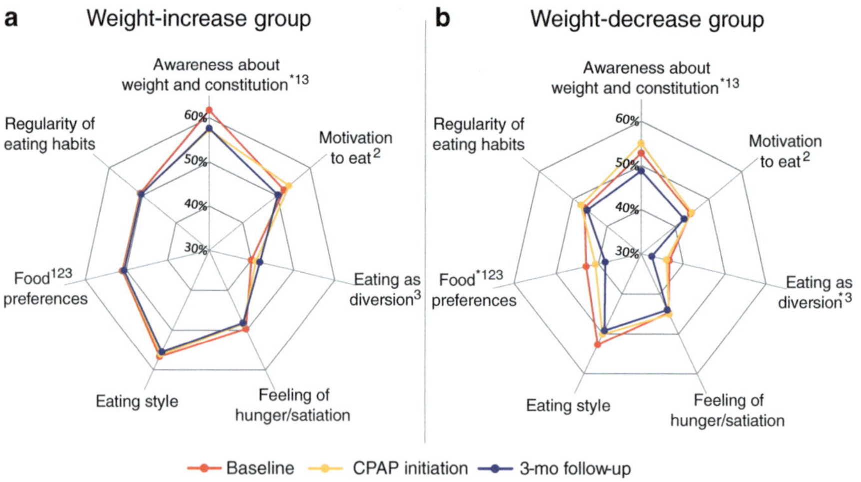

Fig. 6.2 Radar chart for changes in eating behavior scores in the weight-increase group (**a**) and weight-decrease group (**b**). Scores are significantly higher in the weight gainers than the non-weight gainers at baseline, CPAP initiation, and 3-month follow-up ($p < 0.001$, two-way ANOVA). Scores were expressed as a percentage of the maximum possible score for each scale. *$p < 0.05$ for the intra-scale difference during the study period; 1p < 0.05 vs. the other group at baseline; 2p < 0.05 vs. the other group at CPAP initiation; 3p < 0.05 vs. the other group at 3-month follow-up. Reprinted with permission of the American Thoracic Society. Copyright © 2024 American Thoracic Society. All rights reserved. Cite: Tachikawa et al. [30]. The American Journal of Respiratory and Critical Care Medicine is an official journal of the American Thoracic Society

Table 6.2 The eating behavior questionnaire

Answer each question by entering one of the numbers shown below
(1. No, it is not so 2. Yes, occasionally 3. Yes, generally 4. Yes, exactly so)
1. Do you eat fast?
2. Do you think you gain weight because you like sweets?
3. Do you often use convenience stores?
4. Do you often have a fourth meal?
5. Do you feel restless when there is not much food in the refrigerator?
6. Do you think you gain weight because you lie down immediately after eating?
7. Do you often go to dinner parties and drinking parties?
8. Are you often told that you eat too much?
9. Do you feel irritated when hungry?
10. Do you eat well even when you have a cold?
11. Do you snack often?
12. Do you eat more than what you need just to have no leftovers?
13. If your favorite food is offered, do you eat it even immediately after a meal?
14. Do you like heavily seasoned food?
15. Do you feel satiated only when your stomach is full?
16. Do you tend to eat when you feel irritated or anxious?
17. Do you feel unsatisfied with dinner when there are only a few dishes?
18. Are you an evening person?
19. Do you like noodles?
20. Do you tend to gain weight during consecutive holidays, the Bon holidays (Japanese Buddhist holidays in August) and New Year holidays?
21. Do you often eat between meals?
22. Do you really think you gain weight even by drinking water?
23. Do you keep foods readily available?
24. Do you tend to eat when you see others eating?
25. Do you not chew your food well?
26. Do you often eat out or have food delivered?
27. Are your meal times irregular?
28. Do you tend to order more food than needed when you eat out or have food delivered?
29. Do you eat Western dishes more often than Japanese dishes?
30. Do you often go to fast food joints and have burgers and the like?
31. Do you eat something or other when you have nothing else to do?
32. Do you have regrets after eating too much?
33. Do you feel unsatisfied unless you buy more groceries than needed?
34. Do you eat fruit and sweets when they are in front of you because you cannot resist them?
35. Is supper the largest and most sumptuous of your meals?
36. Are you convinced you gain weight because of lack of exercise?
37. Do you have supper late in the evening?
38. Are you not satisfied unless you cook more food than needed?
39. Are you unable to sleep when you are hungry?

(continued)

Table 6.2 (continued)

40. Do you often eat sweet buns?
41. Do you cram food into your mouth when you eat?
42. Do you feel that you are more prone to weight gain than others?
43. Do you like fatty foods?
44. Do you indulge in unplanned buying of food that looks delicious in a supermarket, etc.?
45. Do you think about the next meal even just after finishing one?
46. Do you often drink beer?
47. Do you not have time to enjoy your meals in a leisurely manner?
48. Do you skip breakfast?
49. Do you really not have the feeling of hunger or fullness?
50. Do you often have meals just for social reasons?
51. Do you not lose weight even when you do not eat much?
52. Do you truly have a sweet tooth?
53. Are you often not hungry even just before a meal?
54. Do you eat meat most of the time?
55. During a meal do you stuff food items into your mouth one after another?
Ratings are summed up for each category.
Male
Awareness about weight and constitution: 2, 6, 10, 22, 36, 42, 51
Motivation to eat: 12, 13, 24, 28, 33, 34, 38, 44, 45, 50
Eating as diversion: 5, 16, 23, 31
Feeling of hunger/satiation: 9, 15, 32, 53
Eating style: 1, 8, 25, 41, 55
Food preferences: 11, 14, 26, 29, 30, 40, 43, 52, 54
Regularity of eating habits: 4, 7, 20, 21, 27, 35, 37, 47
Female
Awareness about weight and constitution: 2, 6, 10, 22, 36, 42
Motivation to eat: 12, 13, 17, 24, 28, 33, 38, 44, 50
Eating as diversion: 5, 16, 23, 31
Feeling of hunger/satiation: 9, 15, 32, 39, 49, 53
Eating style: 1, 8, 25, 41, 55
Food preferences: 3, 19, 26, 30, 40, 43, 54
Regularity of eating habits: 4, 18, 20, 21, 27, 35, 37, 48

Reference [30]. Reprinted with permission of the American Thoracic Society.
Cite: Tachikawa et al. [30]. The American Journal of Respiratory and Critical Care Medicine is an official journal of the American Thoracic Society

In summary, a decrease in BMR and excessive energy intake due to disordered eating behaviors are the primary mechanisms contributing to weight gain post-CPAP therapy. It is hypothesized that individuals with disordered eating behaviors are inclined to overeat and may not adjust their energy intake in response to decreased energy expenditure, potentially leading to excessive caloric intake for several months following the initiation of CPAP, beyond the regulation of appetite-related hormone. From another perspective, weight gain following CPAP therapy can be attributed to an inadequate homeostatic regulation of food intake that is overshadowed by non-homeostatic eating behaviors. This mechanism parallels the obesogenic pathways noted in sleep deprivation. Multiple studies have emphasized regulatory processes of food consumption during sleep deprivation that do not rely on energy homeostasis [15, 33–36]. A prominent example is hedonic eating, characterized by eating for pleasure rather than physiological need, mediated by the brain's mesolimbic reward pathways. Sleep deprivation not only amplifies alterations in the reward system, enhancing responsiveness to food stimuli, but also weakens the resistance to high-calorie foods. Investigating the influence of OSA and CPAP therapy on such higher-order central food regulation will be an essential area of study in the future.

8 Conclusion

CPAP therapy may lead to a reduction in BMR, potentially predisposing patients with OSA to a positive energy balance and subsequent weight gain. Nevertheless, dietary habits and disordered eating behaviors exert a more profound influence on weight changes than alterations in energy expenditure. For effective weight management post-CPAP in obese OSA patients, it is imperative to first understand that CPAP is not a treatment for obesity itself. Patients should recognize the possibility that the causes of their weight gain lie within their dysregulated lifestyle habits and dietary behaviors, and addressing these behaviors is considered essential for successful weight management. A pivotal role of healthcare professionals is to motivate patients, provide methods for self-care practices, and encourage continued adherence.

References

1. Romero-Corral A, Caples SM, Lopez-Jimenez F, Somers VK. Interactions between obesity and obstructive sleep apnea: implications for treatment. Chest. 2010;137:711–9.
2. Patel SR. The complex relationship between weight and sleep apnoea. Thorax. 2015;70:205–6.
3. Phillips BG, Kato M, Narkiewicz K, Choe I, Somers VK. Increases in leptin levels, sympathetic drive, and weight gain in obstructive sleep apnea. Am J Phys Heart Circ Phys. 2000;279:H234–7.
4. Brown MA, Goodwin JL, Silva GE, et al. How to understand weight changes in patients with OSA following CPAP treatment? Southwest J Pulm Crit Care. 2011;3:159–68.
5. Borel AL, Leblanc X, Almeras N, et al. Sleep apnoea attenuates the effects of a lifestyle intervention programme in men with visceral obesity. Thorax. 2012;67:735–41.
6. Wu Y, Zhai L, Zhang D. Sleep duration and obesity among adults: a meta-analysis of prospective studies. Sleep Med. 2014;15:1456–62.
7. Bosy-Westphal A, Hinrichs S, Jauch-Chara K, et al. Influence of partial sleep deprivation on energy balance and insulin sensitivity in healthy women. Obes Facts. 2008;1:266–73.

8. Nedeltcheva AV, Kilkus JM, Imperial J, Kasza K, Schoeller DA, Penev PD. Sleep curtailment is accompanied by increased intake of calories from snacks. Am J Clin Nutr. 2009;89:126–33.
9. St-Onge MP, Roberts AL, Chen J, et al. Short sleep duration increases energy intakes but does not change energy expenditure in normal-weight individuals. Am J Clin Nutr. 2011;94:410–6.
10. Calvin AD, Carter RE, Adachi T, et al. Effects of experimental sleep restriction on caloric intake and activity energy expenditure. Chest. 2013;144:79–86.
11. Markwald RR, Melanson EL, Smith MR, et al. Impact of insufficient sleep on total daily energy expenditure, food intake, and weight gain. Proc Natl Acad Sci USA. 2013;110:5695–700.
12. Brondel L, Romer MA, Nougues PM, Touyarou P, Davenne D. Acute partial sleep deprivation increases food intake in healthy men. Am J Clin Nutr. 2010;91:1550–9.
13. Spaeth AM, Dinges DF, Goel N. Effects of experimental sleep restriction on weight gain, caloric intake, and meal timing in healthy adults. Sleep. 2013;36:981–90.
14. Broussard JL, Kilkus JM, Delebecque F, et al. Elevated ghrelin predicts food intake during experimental sleep restriction. Obesity. 2016;24:132–8.
15. Zhu B, Shi C, Park CG, Zhao X, Reutrakul S. Effects of sleep restriction on metabolism-related parameters in healthy adults: a comprehensive review and meta-analysis of randomized controlled trials. Sleep Med Rev. 2019;45:18–30.
16. Gonnissen HK, Hursel R, Rutters F, Martens EA, Westerterp-Plantenga MS. Effects of sleep fragmentation on appetite and related hormone concentrations over 24 h in healthy men. Br J Nutr. 2013;109:748–56.
17. Wang Y, Carreras A, Lee S, et al. Chronic sleep fragmentation promotes obesity in young adult mice. Obesity. 2014;22:758–62.
18. Shechter A. Obstructive sleep apnea and energy balance regulation: a systematic review. Sleep Med Rev. 2017;34:59–69.
19. Stenlof K, Grunstein R, Hedner J, Sjostrom L. Energy expenditure in obstructive sleep apnea: effects of treatment with continuous positive airway pressure. Am J Phys. 1996;271:E1036–43.
20. Ucok K, Aycicek A, Sezer M, et al. Resting metabolic rate and anthropometric measurements in male sleep apnea patients. Intern Med. 2011;50:833–8.
21. de Jonge L, Zhao X, Mattingly MS, et al. Poor sleep quality and sleep apnea are associated with higher resting energy expenditure in obese individuals with short sleep duration. J Clin Endocrinol Metab. 2012;97:2881–9.
22. Vasquez MM, Goodwin JL, Drescher AA, Smith TW, Quan SF. Associations of dietary intake and physical activity with sleep disordered breathing in the apnea positive pressure long-term efficacy study (APPLES). J Clin Sleep Med. 2008;4:411–8.
23. Beebe DW, Miller N, Kirk S, Daniels SR, Amin R. The association between obstructive sleep apnea and dietary choices among obese individuals during middle to late childhood. Sleep Med. 2011;12:797–9.
24. Smith SS, Waight C, Doyle G, Rossa KR, Sullivan KA. Liking for high fat foods in patients with obstructive sleep apnoea. Appetite. 2014;78:185–92.
25. Quan SF, Budhiraja R, Clarke DP, et al. Impact of treatment with continuous positive airway pressure (CPAP) on weight in obstructive sleep apnea. J Clin Sleep Med. 2013;9:989–93.
26. Drager LF, Brunoni AR, Jenner R, Lorenzi-Filho G, Bensenor IM, Lotufo PA. Effects of CPAP on body weight in patients with obstructive sleep apnoea: a meta-analysis of randomised trials. Thorax. 2015;70:258–64.
27. Chen B, Drager LF, Peker Y, et al. Effect of continuous positive airway pressure on weight and local adiposity in adults with obstructive sleep apnea: a meta-analysis. Ann Am Thorac Soc. 2021;18:1717–27.
28. Katz ES, Moore RH, Rosen CL, et al. Growth after adenotonsillectomy for obstructive sleep apnea: an RCT. Pediatrics. 2014;134:282–9.
29. Chirinos JA, Gurubhagavatula I, Teff K, et al. CPAP, weight loss, or both for obstructive sleep apnea. N Engl J Med. 2014;370:2265–75.
30. Tachikawa R, Ikeda K, Minami T, et al. Changes in energy metabolism after continuous positive airway pressure for obstructive sleep apnea. Am J Respir Crit Care Med. 2016;194:729–38.

31. Chaput JP, Despres JP, Bouchard C, Tremblay A. The association between short sleep duration and weight gain is dependent on disinhibited eating behavior in adults. Sleep. 2011;34:1291–7.
32. Garaulet M, Ortega FB, Ruiz JR, et al. Short sleep duration is associated with increased obesity markers in European adolescents: effect of physical activity and dietary habits. The HELENA study. Int J Obes. 2011;35:1308–17.
33. St-Onge MP, McReynolds A, Trivedi ZB, Roberts AL, Sy M, Hirsch J. Sleep restriction leads to increased activation of brain regions sensitive to food stimuli. Am J Clin Nutr. 2012;95:818–24.
34. Benedict C, Brooks SJ, O'Daly OG, et al. Acute sleep deprivation enhances the brain's response to hedonic food stimuli: an fMRI study. J Clin Endocrinol Metab. 2012;97:E443–7.
35. Greer SM, Goldstein AN, Walker MP. The impact of sleep deprivation on food desire in the human brain. Nat Commun. 2013;4:2259.
36. Rihm JS, Menz MM, Schultz H, et al. Sleep deprivation selectively upregulates an amygdala-hypothalamic circuit involved in food reward. J Neurosci. 2019;39:888–99.

Chapter 7
Clinical Considerations and Therapeutic Problems in the Use of Oral Allications Versus CPAP: What is the Position of Oral Appliance for the Treatment of Obstructive Sleep Apnea?

Satoru Tsuiki

Abstract Oral appliances for the treatment of snoring and obstructive sleep apnea (OSA) are defined as devices intended to protrude and stabilize the mandible in order to maintain a patent airway during sleep. Currently, oral appliances are indicated for mild to moderate OSA patients who are not indicated for or cannot tolerate continuous positive airway pressure (CPAP). Although oral appliances are less efficacious in reducing AHI in comparison with CPAP, they are generally well tolerated. The greater efficacy of CPAP is interpreted to offset by inferior adherence relative to oral appliances, suggesting consequently similar effectiveness in comparison with CPAP in OSA treatment. Titration of oral appliance, in which mandibular position is incrementally advanced ventrally until resolution of OSA symptoms and respiratory events, is a key to optimize its efficacy. As oral appliance therapy is a lifelong treatment option for individuals with OSA, every sleep dentist should not overlook short-term side effects that could turn into irreversible long-term adverse consequences. Success in the interdisciplinary management of OSA can be achieved through constant communication and follow-up with the sleep physician and sleep dentist.

Keywords Obstructive sleep apnea · Oral appliance · Mandibular advancement · Titration · Interdisciplinary management

---

S. Tsuiki (✉)
Research Department, Institute of Neuropsychiatry, Shinjuku-ku, Tokyo, Japan

Division of Aging and Geriatric Dentistry, Department of Oral Function and Morphology, Tohoku University Graduate School of Dentistry, Sendai, Miyagi, Japan

Department of Perioperative Medicine, Division of Anesthesiology, Showa Medical University School of Dentistry, Ota-ku, Tokyo, Japan

K. Chin (ed.), *The Current State of Sleep Disordered Breathing in Japan and Around the World*, Respiratory Disease Series: Diagnostic Tools and Disease Managements, https://doi.org/10.1007/978-981-96-6030-8_7

1 Introduction

1.1 Oral Appliances for the Treatment of OSA: Definition and Indication

The Practice Guidelines Committee was charged by the Japanese Respiratory Society in conjunction with the Survey and Research on Refractory Respiratory Diseases and Pulmonary Hypertension Group of the Ministry of Health, Labor and Welfare, Japan to produce clinical guidelines for the treatment of sleep apnea syndrome in Japan [1]. One important aspect of the guidelines is that it intended to increase the clinical availability for the users with the reflection of health insurance system in Japan as well as current trends of related international guidelines. The prevalence of obstructive sleep apnea (OSA) among sleep apnea patients in Japan is higher than previously argued, similar to other developed countries. Patients with moderate-to-severe OSA are estimated approximately 20% of adult males and 10% of postmenopausal women according to a large-scale cohort study [2]. Therefore, clarifying the role and indication of alternative treatment to continuous positive airway pressure (CPAP) for OSA should contribute to improving daytime sleepiness, preventing traffic accidents due to drowsy driving, and decreasing the incident of concomitant diseases.

Oral appliances are now an established treatment option for patients with snoring and OSA [3]. The American Academy of Dental Sleep Medicine has defined oral appliances for the treatment of snoring and OSA as "*devices intended to protrude and stabilize the mandible in order to maintain a patent airway during sleep*" [4]. Traditionally, oral appliances for OSA treatment have fallen into two main categories: those which reposition the mandible forward and those which hold the tongue forward (i.e., tongue retaining device) [5]. However, due to a lack of evidence for their efficacy in OSA, tongue retaining devices are currently distinct from oral appliances [3]. To date, there is still no universally recognized terminology to describe oral appliances for OSA while oral appliances were initially called dental appliances by sleep-related personnel [6]. The most widely used terms for oral appliances are mandibular advancement device (MAD), mandibular repositioning device (MRD), mandibular repositioning appliance (MRA), mandibular advancement splint (MAS), and mandibular advancement appliance (MAA). Although the variety of these similar terms can be confusing, all of these are considered oral appliances based on the above definition by the American Academy of Dental Sleep Medicine. Throughout this chapter, the term "oral appliance" is used to refer to all of these different types of appliance that advance the mandible forward.

In response to a clinical question, "What is the position of oral appliance in the treatment for OSA?", the Guideline Practice Committee has drawn a clearly conclusion and suggested that "oral appliances are indicated for mild to moderate OSA patients who are not indicated for and/or cannot tolerate CPAP." In this chapter, the different types of oral appliances, their adjustment, effects on quality of life, and impact on cardiovascular outcomes, as well as their associated side effects are to be discussed. The details of the guideline can be found and are referred to as Akashiba et al. [1].

2 Types of Oral Appliance

There are currently various oral appliances available, and each differing in design and complexity (Fig. 7.1). Customized, individually fabricated oral appliances can be further classified into either one-piece non-titratable or two-piece titratable designs. Non-titratable oral appliance are generally called "monobloc" where the degree of mandibular advancement is fixed in a certain ventrally advanced mandibular position. In turn, titratable oral appliances allow progressive and gradual adjustment in the degree of mandibular advancement to optimize treatment efficacy. Two-piece titratable oral appliances have become more commonly used and now assumed as standard in the world [3], while monoblocs are rather frequently used in countries including Japan for a considerable reason. Most of OSA patients indicated for an oral appliance after diagnosis select a monobloc in Japan, because this type of oral appliances are partially reimbursable. In principle, patients are responsible for covering 10–30% of the total expenses for medical care for oral appliance therapy, which includes fabrication and adjustment of the appliance, based on factors such as age and income. Selection of oral appliances is likely to be influenced by cost-effectiveness, although evaluating this factor presents a significant challenge.

Whether fabricating a titratable oral appliance or monobloc appliance with subsequent multiple remaking is least inexpensive remains unknown as the cost for appliance fabrication differs between countries and dental laboratories. In addition, the expected lifespan of the appliance varies between patients and is largely associated with materials of appliance. One study from the United Kingdom sophisticatedly compared three different types of monobloc appliance (i.e., thermoplastic device, semi-bespoke (semi-customized) device, custom-made device) in a randomized-controlled crossover manner [7]. Although all three types of oral appliance significantly improved apnea hypopnea index (AHI) and daytime sleepiness compared to baseline, the thermoplastic device was less comfortable and less adherent. On the other hand, the semi-bespoke and custom-made devices were similar in terms of clinical effectiveness; it was then concluded that the most cost-effective

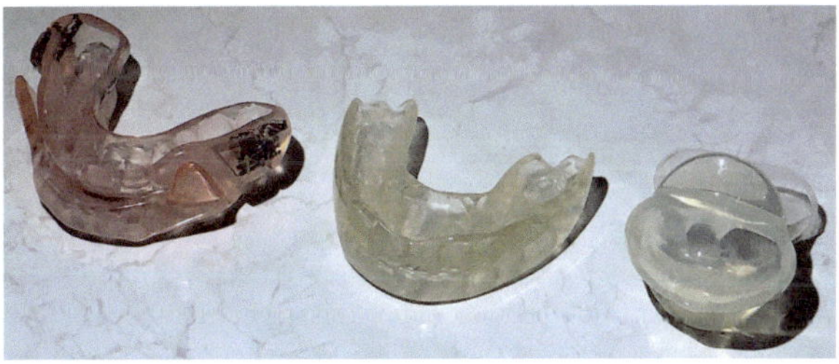

Fig. 7.1 Oral appliances for the treatment of snoring and obstructive sleep apnea. (**left**) A custom-made titratable oral appliance, (**middle**) a monobloc, (**right**) a prefabricated tongue retaining device

option was the less expensive and more accessible semi-bespoke device. Another randomized controlled trial evaluated whether a less expensive, ready-to-use, thermoplastic titratable oral appliance is inferior to a more costly custom-made titratable oral appliance in patients with moderate to severe OSA who were either intolerant to or refused CPAP therapy [8]. The study showed that both appliances had the same effectiveness in reducing OSA severity, symptoms, and blood pressure, as well as improving quality of life. These reports indicate the need for additional studies on the cost-effectiveness of oral appliances. Such complex analyses should encompass not only the differences between monoblocs and titratable appliances, but also within various types of these appliances, as well as between ready-made and custom-made devices. While the majority of current expert recommendations may favor the use of custom-made titratable oral appliances, the lack of sufficient comparative evidence does not necessarily support the use of expensive custom-made titratable devices in countries like Japan, where oral appliance therapy is covered by the national health system. Nevertheless, this situation does not undermine the importance of titration of mandibular position per se in oral appliance therapy.

3 Oral Appliance Titration and CPAP Titration: An Analogy

Understanding of the principles of CPAP titration enhances our knowledge of oral appliance titration in order to maximize appliance efficacy [9] (Table 7.1). When a patient with moderate or severe OSA is indicated for CPAP, a process called CPAP titration is designed for individual patient to manually determine an optimal CPAP by polysomnographic technologists during overnight sleep study [10]. CPAP

Table 7.1 Two different titration in the treatment of OSA

	Oral appliance	CPAP
Indication	Mild to moderate (severe) OSA, primary snoring	Moderate to severe OSA
Target respiratory events	Snoring, obstructive apnea/hypopnea, RERA, etc.	Snoring, obstructive apnea/hypopnea, RERA, etc.
Target of titration	Mandibular advancement	Intraluminal pressure
Upper airway	Enlargement	Enlargement
Initial level	50–70% of maximum mandibular advancement	4 cm H_2O, etc.
Degree of titration	Additional 5–10 mm, etc.	4–20 cm H_2O, etc.
Time or duration to titrate	2–3 weeks to 2–3 months	Single night
Effects on OSA	++	+++

CPAP continuous positive airway pressure, *OSA* obstructive sleep apnea, *RERA* respiratory event related arousal. Plus symbol indicates observation: the both therapies were classified as high (+++), moderate (++)

titration is, for example, started at 4 cm H_2O, with 1 cm H_2O PAP increases for each increment until respiratory events such as apnea, hypopnea, snoring, and respiratory event-related arousals abolished [11]. The optimal PAP is determined as the pressure level that could suppress respiratory events in any sleep position and in any sleep stage.

The concept of titrating oral appliances is based on the idea of this CPAP titration. Instead of application of CPAP, the elimination of targeted respiratory events is performed by mandibular advancement in oral appliance therapy. Patients are usually not able initially to tolerate the degree of mandibular advancement necessary to completely relieve respiratory events. Thus, titration of mandibular position starts from an arbitrary anterior position of the mandible (e.g., 50–75% of the maximum mandibular protrusive position) [12]. Once patients are accustomed to wearing the oral appliance without any trouble at this initial mandibular position, patients are instructed to start advancing the mandible by themselves at home with gradual increments of 0.10–0.25 mm per week beyond initial mandibular position. The use of a titratable oral appliance certainly contribute to saving time during titration without fabricating a new appliance. When the patient or bed partner reports a cessation of snoring and a resolution of OSA symptoms, further advancement will not be performed, and it is considered titrated. Timely follow-up of polysomnography with oral appliance in place would prevent suboptimal treatment outcomes. However, there is not yet a convenient tool for determining whether an oral appliance is adequately titrated or when to perform post-treatment follow-up polysomnographic evaluations. The use of out-of-center sleep testing at patient each visit to dental office is not feasible from the viewpoint of cost and accessibility. A recent report demonstrated that a gradual reduction in the STOP (i.e., snoring, tiredness during daytime, observed apnea, high blood pressure) score, i.e., fewer responses in the STOP questionnaire, in patients undergoing oral appliance therapy could be a simple indicator of a better oral appliance adjustment and best timing for follow-up polysomnography [13]. This evaluation may somewhat ameliorate the existing trial-and-error approach to oral appliance titration and facilitate proper post-treatment assessments.

4 Efficacy of Oral Appliance Versus CPAP

Compared with no treatment, the mean reduction in AHI was 13.6/h with oral appliance in place [3]. In addition, 25 out of 34 randomized controlled studies showed AHI reduction more than 50% of baseline AHI. This evidence further supports the result of a meta-analysis that oral appliances are better than no treatment for patients who are intolerant to CPAP [14]. There have been several reports on the efficacy of oral appliances versus CPAP in the treatment of OSA, suggesting that oral appliances are less efficacious in reducing AHI in comparison with CPAP although both treatments improve in objective measurements including AHI, arousal index, and minimum arterial oxygen saturation [3, 15]. Alternatively, considering that this effect may be related to a higher baseline AHI in CPAP patients (i.e., moderate to severe OSA), oral appliances are first-line treatment option for mild OSA [14]. The greater efficacy of CPAP is currently interpreted to offset by inferior adherence relative to oral appliances, suggesting consequently similar effectiveness in comparison with CPAP in OSA treatment [16].

5 Oral Appliance and QOL

Oral appliances provide positive impact on quality of life measures in OSA patients [1, 3]. In comparison with no treatment or inactive control, oral appliances improve quality of life measures. Moreover, both oral appliances and CPAP are superior to inactive control or no treatment in improving quality of life measures. In one trial, overall Functional Outcomes of Sleep Questionnaire scores improved by 27.1% from baseline in those using a custom-made oral appliance while a −1.7% decline in those using a nontherapeutic appliance without mandibular advancement, although neither study group showed significant difference in the mean scores of the 36-Item Short Form Health Survey (SF-36) [17].

Some comparative studies have demonstrated that both oral appliances and CPAP are effective in improving quality of life and that oral appliances improve quality of life as much as CPAP compared to inactive control. According to a network meta-analysis of 23 randomized controlled trials, CPAP led to a 1.7-point increase in both the Mental Component Scores (MCS) and Physical Component Scores (PCS) of SF-36 when compared to inactive controls [18]. Meanwhile, oral appliances resulted in 2.4-point improvement in MCS and 1.5-point improvement in PCS compared to inactive controls. Notably, there were no significant differences in the treatment effects between CPAP and oral appliance with respect to the SF-36 scores. One direct comparative study between oral appliances and CPAP suggested that both were effective in improving QOL. Oral appliances performed better than CPAP for improving four of eight SF-36 general QOL domains and the overall mental component score [16]. Favorable outcome for quality of life measures may be partially accounted for a superior adherence of oral appliances to CPAP, particularly for mild to moderate OSA.

6 Oral Appliance and Cardiovascular Disease

OSA is associated with increased cardiovascular morbidity and mortality. However, both high quality and longitudinal studies are still required in relation to oral appliance therapy for OSA. In comparison with CPAP therapy, there are very few reports available on the effects of oral appliances on cardiovascular risk-related biomarkers, vascular endothelial function, and arteriosclerosis [1, 19]. On the other hand, oral appliances are found to lower the systolic, diastolic, and mean blood pressure of

OSA patients. The result of a meta-analysis showed that the mean reduction in systolic/diastolic blood pressure was 2.09/3.15 mmHg, respectively [3]. A network meta-analysis revealed that oral appliances were associated with a significant reduction in systolic blood pressure of 2.1 mmHg and diastolic blood pressure of 1.9 mmHg, respectively [20]. Further, oral appliances are reported to show equivalent effects to CPAP in decreasing systolic/diastolic blood pressure [3, 20, 21].

To date, there have been few long-term observational studies investigating the effects of oral appliances not only on the severity of OSA but also on cardiovascular mortality. In a study of mild to moderate OSA patients prescribed either oral appliance or CPAP, treatment was associated with a marked cardiovascular risk reduction of at least 38% after the median of 72 months follow-up [22]. An observational study focused on severe OSA patients for the median of 79 months follow-up, no difference in the cardiovascular mortality was found in those prescribed oral appliances and CPAP [23]. In a cohort where 154 consecutive Japanese OSA patients treated with auto-titrating CPAP, or with oral appliance, or untreated were followed-up for a median of 93 months, multivariate logistic regression demonstrated that reduction of body mass index and good adherence to treatment were predictors of improvement or unchanged AHI [24]. The findings of this Japanese study indicate that better control of OSA, regardless of whether it is through oral appliances or CPAP, may potentially have a positive impact on cardiovascular outcomes.

7 Side Effects of Oral Appliance

Oral appliances are generally well tolerated, however, they include both short-term and long-term side effects [25]. Discomfort and/or inconvenience of the device are the most common reasons for completely discontinuation of treatment, while limited perceived efficacy, such as inadequate reduction of snoring and apnea, is the primary reason for the discontinuation of treatment [26].

Typical short-term side effects involve excessive salivation, dry mouth, pain and discomfort and/or pain in the teeth and gums, abnormal occlusion in the morning, and jaw stiffness, most of which are usually mild and transient. Adjusting the appliance can reduce short-term side effects by decreasing pressure on the teeth and excessive forward movement of the mandible. In a randomized-controlled crossover study, short-term side effects of oral appliance were compared with those of CPAP by the use of visual analog scale [27]. Side-effects were similar in frequency and intensity, and self-reported compliance was higher with oral appliance with 70% of patients preferring oral appliance therapy. Contrary to short-term side effects, long-term side effects are irreversible, resulting significant negative effects on the occlusion. Sustained force on the teeth when using an oral appliance has the potential to cause retroclination of the upper incisors and proclination of the lower incisors, distal tipping of the maxillary molars and mesial tipping of the mandibular molars [28, 29] (Fig. 7.2). These dental changes also lead to downward rotation of the mandible. Some of these dental changes are observed not only in oral appliance users

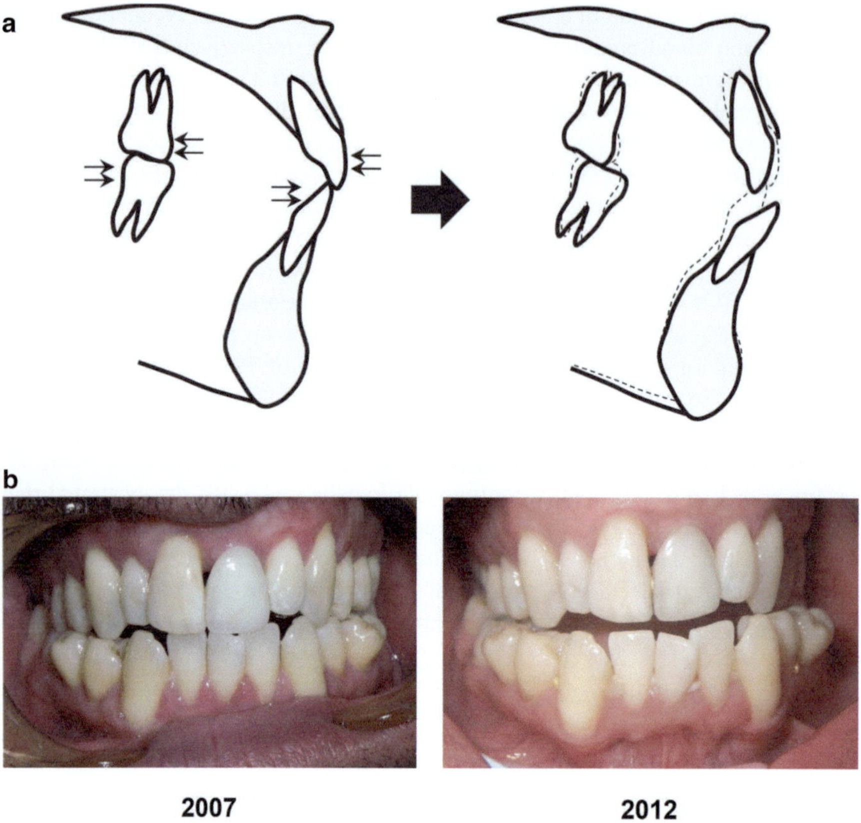

Fig. 7.2 A schematic illustration of possible and typical long-term dental side effects in oral appliance therapy (**a**) and an OSA case with unwanted teeth movements associated with long-term oral appliance use (**b**)(**a**) Sustained force on the teeth (small arrows) when using an oral appliance has the potential to cause retroclination of the upper incisors and proclination of the lower incisors, distal tipping of the maxillary molars and mesial tipping of the mandibular molars. (**b**) The patient (a teacher) got his first oral appliance in 1997 from a dentist. At that time, he was a severe Class II first molar relationship (i.e., lower first molar positioned dorsally relative to upper first molar). When another dentist saw him in 1999, he was status post uvulopalatopharyngoplasty and had a Gorge Gauge of +4 to −6 (i.e., maximal protrusive range of the mandible was 10 mm). *Note* the occlusal change by oral appliance use from 2007 to 2012. (Courtesy of Dr. B. Gail Demko)

but in CPAP patients [30]. It could be understandable that retroclination of upper incisors in CPAP patients can occur because of the considerable pressure on the upper lip and underlying maxillary incisors via a CPAP interface.

The described changes in dental occlusion may occur unnoticed and are generally not a significant cause of treatment discontinuation, as most individuals will obtain occlusal contacts as a result of developing a new occlusion [31]. However, every sleep dentist should make an effort not to overlook any short-term side effects that could turn into irreversible long-term adverse consequences. Innovation/renovation of devices to minimize or avoid reported side effects of both oral appliances and CPAP will be an adequate future direction of patient-centered OSA treatment. One key may be to newly develop devices that do not require either positive airway pressure or mandibular advancement for OSA by approaching the tongue position during sleep [32, 33].

8 Conclusion

Oral appliances are indicated for mild to moderate OSA patients who are not indicated for or cannot tolerate CPAP while many other different treatment modalities are currently available for OSA management. Oral appliance therapy is a lifelong treatment option for individuals with OSA. Success in the interdisciplinary management of OSA can be achieved through constant communication and follow-up with the sleep physician and sleep dentist [34].

Acknowledgments The authors would like to thank Dr. B. Gail Demko, DMD, who generously provided photographs in Fig. 7.2. Research partially discussed in this chapter was supported by grants from the Japanese Society for the Promotion of Science (Grant-in-Aid for Scientific Research KAKENHI;19K10236, 20K10085, 22K10069, 24K13038, 25K13118).

References

1. Akashiba T, Inoue Y, Uchimura N, Ohi M, Kasai T, Kawana F, Sakurai S, Takegami M, Tachikawa R, Tanigawa T, Chiba S, Chin K, Tsuiki S, Tonogi M, Nakamura H, Nakayama T, Narui K, Yagi T, Yamauchi M, Yamashiro Y, Yoshida M, Oga T, Tomita Y, Hamada S, Murase K, Mori H, Wada H, Uchiyama M, Ogawa H, Sato K, Nakata S, Mishima K, Momomura SI. Sleep apnea syndrome (SAS) clinical practice guidelines 2020. Respir Investig. 2022;60(1):3–32. https://doi.org/10.1016/j.resinv.2021.08.010.
2. Matsumoto T, Murase K, Tabara Y, Gozal D, Smith D, Minami T, Tachikawa R, Tanizawa K, Oga T, Nagashima S, Wakamura T, Komenami N, Setoh K, Kawaguchi T, Tsutsumi T, Takahashi Y, Nakayama T, Hirai T, Matsuda F, Chin K. Impact of sleep characteristics and obesity on diabetes and hypertension across genders and menopausal status: the Nagahama study. Sleep. 2018;41(7) https://doi.org/10.1093/sleep/zsy071.
3. Ramar K, Dort LC, Katz SG, Lettieri CJ, Harrod CG, Thomas SM, Chervin RD. Clinical practice guideline for the treatment of obstructive sleep apnea and snoring with oral appliance therapy: an update for 2015. J Clin Sleep Med. 2015;11(7):773–827. https://doi.org/10.5664/jcsm.4858.
4. Scherr SC, Dort LC, Almeida FR, Bennett KM, Blumenstock NT, Demko BG, Essick GK, Katz SG, McLornan PM, Phillips KS, Prehn RS, Rogers RR, Schell TG, Sheats RD, Sreshta FP. Definition of an effective oral appliance for the treatment of obstructive sleep apnea and snoring: a report of the American Academy of Dental Sleep Medicine. J Dent Sleep Med. 2014;1(1):39–50. https://www.aadsm.org/docs/jdsm7.10.10.sa1.pdf
5. Lowe AA. Oral appliances for sleep breathing disorders. In: Kryger MH, Roth T, Dement WC, editors. Principles and practice of sleep medicine. 3rd ed. Philadelphia: WB Saunders; 2000. p. 929–39.

6. Lowe AA. Dental appliances for the treatment of snoring and obstructive sleep apnea. In: Kryger MH, Roth T, Dement WC, editors. Principles and practice of sleep medicine. 2nd ed. Philadelphia: WB Saunders; 1994. p. 722–35.
7. Sharples L, Glover M, Clutterbuck-James A, et al. Clinical effectiveness and cost-effectiveness results from the randomised controlled trial of oral mandibular advancement devices for obstructive sleep apnoea-hypopnoea (TOMADO) and longterm economic analysis of oral devices and continuous positive airway pressure. Health Technol Assess. 2014;18(67):1–296. https://doi.org/10.3310/hta18670.
8. Pépin JL, Raymond N, Lacaze O, Aisenberg N, Forcioli J, Bonte E, Bourdin A, Launois S, Tamisier R, Molinari N. Heat-moulded versus custom-made mandibular advancement devices for obstructive sleep apnoea: a randomised non-inferiority trial. Thorax. 2019;74(7):667–74. https://doi.org/10.1136/thoraxjnl-2018-212726.
9. Tsuiki S, Fukuda T, Tanaka Y, Suzuki Y, Yanamoto S, Hasebe D, Kobayashi T, Iwanaga T, Inoko Y, Sato K. Current concept of titration of mandibular advancement oral appliances for obstructive sleep apnea. J Oral Sleep Med. 2018;5(1):1–11. (in Japanese). https://doi.org/10.24695/josm.5.1_1.
10. Tsuiki S, Kobayashi M, Namba K, Oka Y, Komada Y, Kagimura T, Inoue Y. Optimal positive airway pressure predicts oral appliance response to sleep apnoea. Eur Respir J. 2010;35(5):1098–105. https://doi.org/10.1183/09031936.00121608.
11. Ito E, Tsuiki S, Namba K, Takise Y, Inoue Y. Upper airway anatomical balance contributes to optimal continuous positive airway pressure for Japanese patients with obstructive sleep apnea syndrome. J Clin Sleep Med. 2014;10(2):137–42. https://doi.org/10.5664/jcsm.3438.
12. Tsuiki S, Lowe AA, Almeida FR, Kawahata N, Fleetham JA. Effects of mandibular advancement on airway curvature and obstructive sleep apnoea severity. Eur Respir J. 2004;23(2):263–8. https://doi.org/10.1183/09031936.04.00094304.
13. Narahara-Eno Y, Fukuda T, Taga H, Nakayama H, Inoue Y, Tsuiki S. Gradual reduction in the STOP score in patients with obstructive sleep apnea undergoing oral appliance therapy. J Prosthodont Res. 2021;65(3):360–4. https://doi.org/10.2186/jpr.JPR_D_20_00118.
14. Sharples LD, Clutterbuck-James AL, Glover MJ, Bennett MS, Chadwick R, Pittman MA, Quinnell TG. Meta-analysis of randomised controlled trials of oral mandibular advancement devices and continuous positive airway pressure for obstructive sleep apnoea-hypopnoea. Sleep Med Rev. 2016;27:108–24. https://doi.org/10.1016/j.smrv.2015.05.003.
15. Lettieri CJ, Almeida FR, Cistulli PA, et al. Oral appliances for the treatment of obstructive sleep apnea-hypopnea syndrome and for concomitant sleep bruxism. In: Kryger MH, Roth T, Dement WC, editors. Principles and practice of sleep medicine. 6th ed. Philadelphia: Elsevier; 2017. p. 1445–57.
16. Phillips CL, Grunstein RR, Darendeliler MA, Mihailidou AS, Srinivasan VK, Yee BJ, Marks GB, Cistulli PA. Health outcomes of continuous positive airway pressure versus oral appliance treatment for obstructive sleep apnea: a randomized controlled trial. Am J Respir Crit Care Med. 2013;187(8):879–87. https://doi.org/10.1164/rccm.201212-2223OC.
17. Blanco J, Zamarrón C, Abeleira Pazos MT, Lamela C, Suarez Quintanilla D. Prospective evaluation of an oral appliance in the treatment of obstructive sleep apnea syndrome. Sleep Breath. 2005;9(1):20–5. https://doi.org/10.1007/s11325-005-0003-4.
18. Kuhn E, Schwarz EI, Bratton DJ, Rossi VA, Kohler M. Effects of CPAP and mandibular advancement devices on health-related quality of life in OSA: a systematic review and meta-analysis. Chest. 2017;151(4):786–94. https://doi.org/10.1016/j.chest.2017.01.020.
19. de Vries GE, Wijkstra PJ, Houwerzijl EJ, Kerstjens HAM, Hoekema A. Cardiovascular effects of oral appliance therapy in obstructive sleep apnea: a systematic review and meta-analysis. Sleep Med Rev. 2018;40:55–68. https://doi.org/10.1016/j.smrv.2017.10.004.
20. Bratton DJ, Gaisl T, Schlatzer C, Kohler M. Comparison of the effects of continuous positive airway pressure and mandibular advancement devices on sleepiness in patients with obstructive sleep apnoea: a network meta-analysis. Lancet Respir Med. 2015;3(11):869–78. https://doi.org/10.1016/S2213-2600(15)00416-6.

21. Liu T, Li W, Zhou H, Wang Z. Verifying the relative efficacy between continuous positive airway pressure therapy and its alternatives for obstructive sleep apnea: a network meta-analysis. Front Neurol. 2017;8:289. https://doi.org/10.3389/fneur.2017.00289.
22. Buchner NJ, Sanner BM, Borgel J, Rump LC. Continuous positive airway pressure treatment of mild to moderate obstructive sleep apnea reduces cardiovascular risk. Am J Respir Crit Care Med. 2007;176(12):1274–80. https://doi.org/10.1164/rccm.200611-1588OC.
23. Anandam A, Patil M, Akinnusi M, Jaoude P, El-Solh AA. Cardiovascular mortality in obstructive sleep apnoea treated with continuous positive airway pressure or oral appliance: an observational study. Respirology. 2013;18(8):1184–90. https://doi.org/10.1111/resp.12140.
24. Sugiyama A, Shiota S, Yanagihara M, Nakayama H, Tsuiki S, Hayashida K, Inoue Y, Takahashi K. The role of long-term continuous positive airway pressure in the progression of obstructive sleep apnoea: a longitudinal cohort study. J Sleep Res. 2021;30(6):e13374. https://doi.org/10.1111/jsr.13374.
25. Sheats RD, Schell TG, Blanton AO, Braga PM, Demko BG, Dort LC, Farquhar D, Katz SG, Masse JF, Rogers RR, Scherr SC, Schwartz DB, Spencer J. Management of side effects of oral appliance therapy for sleep-disordered breathing. J Dent Sleep Med. 2017;4(4):111–25. https://doi.org/10.15331/jdsm.6746.
26. de Almeida FR, Lowe AA, Tsuiki S, Otsuka R, Wong M, Fastlicht S, Ryan F. Long-term compliance and side effects of oral appliances used for the treatment of snoring and obstructive sleep apnea syndrome. J Clin Sleep Med. 2005;1(2):143–52. https://doi.org/10.5664/jcsm.8978.
27. Gagnadoux F, Fleury B, Vielle B, Pételle B, Meslier N, N'Guyen XL, Trzepizur W, Racineux JL. Titrated mandibular advancement versus positive airway pressure for sleep apnoea. Eur Respir J. 34(4):914–20. https://doi.org/10.1183/09031936.00148208.
28. Almeida FR, Lowe AA, Sung JO, Tsuiki S, Otsuka R. Long-term sequellae of oral appliance therapy in obstructive sleep apnea patients: part 1. Cephalometric analysis. Am J Orthod Dentofacial Orthop. 2006;129(2):195–204. https://doi.org/10.1016/j.ajodo.2005.10.001.
29. Almeida FR, Lowe AA, Otsuka R, Fastlicht S, Farbood M, Tsuiki S. Long-term sequellae of oral appliance therapy in obstructive sleep apnea patients: part 2. Study-model analysis. Am J Orthod Dentofacial Orthop. 2006;129(2):205–13. https://doi.org/10.1016/j.ajodo.2005.04.034.
30. Doff MH, Finnema KJ, Hoekema A, Wijkstra PJ, de Bont LG, Stegenga B. Long-term oral appliance therapy in obstructive sleep apnea syndrome: a controlled study on dental side effects. Clin Oral Investig. 2013;17(2):475–82.
31. Martínez-Gomis J, Willaert J, Nogues L, Pascual M, Somoza M, Monasterio C. Five years of sleep apnea treatment with a mandibular advancement device. Side effects and technical complications. Angle Orthod. 2010;80(1):30–6. https://doi.org/10.2319/030309-122.1.
32. Fukuda T, Takei Y, Nakayama H, Inoue Y, Tsuiki S. Continuous tongue suction as a potential therapy for obstructive sleep apnea: a feasibility study. J Dent Sleep Med. 2020,7(3) https://doi.org/10.15331/jdsm.6746.
33. Fukuda T, Kohzuka Y, Almeida FR, Iijima T, Masuda R, Tsuiki S. Control of tongue position in patients with obstructive sleep apnea: concept and protocol for a randomized controlled crossover trial. Int J Environ Res Public Health. 2023;20(11):6026. https://doi.org/10.3390/ijerph20116026.
34. Taga H, Fukuda T, Katahira H, Taga M, Tsuiki S. Consequences and complications of side effects of oral appliance therapy for obstructive sleep apnea: Be true to the tooth. J Dent Sleep Med. 2025;12(1).

Chapter 8
Implantable Therapy: What is the Position of Implantable Equipment in the Treatments for OSA?

Motoo Yamauchi, Eriko Hamada, and Yukio Fujita

Abstract Continuous positive airway pressure (CPAP) is a standard therapy for moderate-to-severe obstructive sleep apnea (OSA). However, CPAP acceptance and adherence have been reported to be unsatisfactory. Although various strategies to improve CPAP adherence have been studied, a certain number of patients are intolerant or refuse CPAP treatment. Thus, currently, developments of alternative therapies for CPAP have been a hot topic including pharmacological and implantable therapies. In this chapter, the latter is focused on and introduces hypoglossal nerve stimulation (HNS) which is a current clinically available therapy.

Keywords Hypoglossal nerve stimulation · Obstructive sleep apnea · Continuous positive airway pressure · Upper airway muscular compensation

---

M. Yamauchi (✉)
Department of Clinical Pathophysiology of Nursing, Nara Medical University, Nara, Japan

Department of Respiratory Medicine, Nara Medical University Hospital, Nara, Japan
e-mail: motoo@naramed-u.ac.jp

E. Hamada
Department of Respiratory Medicine, Nara Medical University Hospital, Nara, Japan

Division of Pulmonary, Critical Care and Sleep Medicine, Case Western Reserve University, Cleveland, OH, USA
e-mail: hamadaso38@naramed-u.ac.jp

Y. Fujita
Department of Respiratory Medicine, Nara Medical University Hospital, Nara, Japan

K. Chin (ed.), *The Current State of Sleep Disordered Breathing in Japan and Around the World*, Respiratory Disease Series: Diagnostic Tools and Disease Managements, https://doi.org/10.1007/978-981-96-6030-8_8

1 Introduction

Continuous positive airway pressure (CPAP) has been established as a standard therapy for patients with moderate-to-severe obstructive sleep apnea (OSA). In Japan, the national health insurance system allows physicians to prescribe CPAP in case of apnea-hypopnea index (AHI) ≥ 20/hour. However, issues to be solved in the clinical practice for CPAP therapy include suboptimal CPAP adherence. Up to approximately 50% of patients with OSA have been reported to adhere to CPAP treatment [1]. Although various factors affect CPAP adherence, one topic would be an existing phenotype among OSA. Pathophysiology of OSA comprises four endotypes including arousal threshold, instability of ventilatory control system (loop gain), pharyngeal anatomy/collapsibility, and upper airway muscular compensation [2, 3]. The contribution of those four endotypes to the pathophysiology differs between individuals, thus there exists an OSA phenotype. CPAP is theoretically reasonable therapy since a pneumatic splint, which is a positive airway pressure, keeps the airway open, however, it is not always effective. In such a case, one may try another treatment option of which targets are abovementioned four endotypes. Recently, this situation has been inspiring researchers to develop personalized or recently called precision medicine of OSA using pharmacological and device-based approaches as well. For the latter approach, hypoglossal nerve stimulation (HNS) has been available across the world including Japan, also it is a hot topic right now among clinical practitioners as well as physician-scientists. In this chapter, HNS, which is an implantable therapy, will be addressed with the aspect of indication criteria, efficacy, clinical outcomes, and future direction of HNS.

2 Mechanisms of HNS to Improve OSA

As of April 2025, the clinically available HNS device is the only Inspire® system (Inspire Medical Systems Inc., Golden Valley, Minnesota, USA) in Japan and the United States. In 2014, the Food and Drug Administration (FDA) in the United States approved the Inspire® system as an FDA first-in-class therapy. As for Japan, the Inspire® system was approved in 2018 by the Pharmaceuticals and Medical Devices Agency (PMDA). PMDA is like the FDA in the United States and works together with the Ministry of Health, Labour, and Welfare. After this approval, the Ministry of Health, Labour, and Welfare made a careful review of this therapy and then eventually decided to start insurance reimbursement in June of 2021. At that point, among Asian countries, Japan was the first country to become able to use the Inspire® system for the treatment of OSA. Inspire® system has three components, which are a cuff electrode placed around the hypoglossal nerve, an implanted pulse generator (IPG), and a pressure sensor placed between the internal and external intercostal muscles to detect the respiratory phase (inhalation and exhalation).

(i) A Cuff Electrode Placed Around the Hypoglossal Nerve

The genioglossus (GG) and geniohyoid (GH) muscles are the main airway dilators, while the hyoglossus (HG) and styloglossus (SG) muscles cause tongue retrusion (Fig. 8.1) [4, 5]. Initially, a cuff electrode was placed around the proper distal branches of the hypoglossal nerve where tongue protrusion can be seen during intraoperative testing. Currently, cuff electrode placement is performed using a selective nerve integrity monitoring (NIM) system so that a selective stimulation site is identified to activate only the branch to obtain appropriate tongue protrusion [6].

(ii) Implanted Pulse Generator (IPG)

IPG is implanted into a subcutaneous pocket 3–4 cm below the clavicle. The placement of the IPG is usually within the soft tissues of the right upper chest. The lead from the cuff electrode around the hypoglossal nerve is tunneled subcutaneously, and then connected to the IPG. The IPG has a long-lasting battery (~11 years), and its settings are changed via a telemetry head placed on the skin above the IPG using the Inspire programmer (tablet).

(iii) Pressure Sensor That Detects Inhalation and Exhalation

A pressure sensor was used to be inserted between the fourth and fifth intercostal space with a separate incision from the one for IPG implantation. Right now, it has been inserted between the second and third intercostal space since 2021, so a pressure sensor insertion is done with the same incision as that for IPG implantation. Thus, an operation with three incisions has been taken over with the one with two incisions [7]. A pressure sensor lead is connected to the IPG. The function of the pressure sensor and the triggering of stimulation can be monitored wirelessly, and a respiratory trace displayed on the programmer.

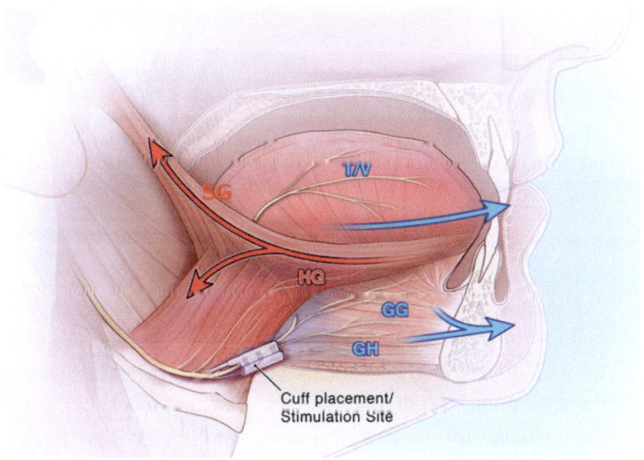

Fig. 8.1 The hypoglossal nerve branches into the styloglossus, hyoglossus, genioglossus, and geniohyoid muscles. A cuff electrode should be placed where it is able to stimulate the muscles (blue color) that cause tongue protrusion. The illustration is courtesy of Inspire Medical Systems Inc. *SG* styloglossus, *HG* hyoglossus, *GG* genioglossus, *GH* geniohyoid, *T/V* transverse and vertical intrinsic muscles

With these three components, the mechanisms of HNS can be described as follows. The pressure sensor identifies inspiration, and then IPG sends the electrical stimulation during each inspiration to the cuff electrode around the hypoglossal nerve. Stimulated hypoglossal nerve assists the upper airway compensation with tongue protrusion to keep the airway open.

3 Indication Criteria for the HNS in Japan and the United States

A fundamental principle of the indication for the HNS is that a patient must be confirmed to fail or cannot tolerate CPAP. Thus, HNS therapy is an alternative therapy for CPAP.

Others are shown in Table 8.1. The Japanese Ministry of Health, Labour and Welfare has defined the indication criteria as shown in the left column of Table 8.1, including that body mass index (BMI) is less than 30 kg/m^2, AHI is more than or equal to 20/hour, and age is older than or equal to 18 years old. Additionally, patients who do not have a complete concentric collapse at the level of the soft palate with drug-induced sleep endoscopy (DISE) are eligible, a pattern of anterior-posterior collapse is preferable. Also, central apneas must be less than or equal to 25% of the total number of apnea-hypopnea events.

Inclusion criteria in the United States are a bit different from the ones in Japan. The lower limit of AHI is 20/hour in Japan, while 15/hour in the United States, this lower limit of 20 comes from the cut-off value for the indication of CPAP therapy regulated in the national health insurance system in Japan. Also, in the United States, the FDA has been updating the criteria according to the results of the

Table 8.1 Inclusion criteria for hypoglossal nerve stimulation

	Ministry of health, labour, and welfare in Japan	U.S. Food and Drug Administration (FDA)
BMI, kg/m^2	< 30	≤ 40
AHI, /hour	≥ 20	≥ 15, ≤ 100
Age, years old	≥ 18	≥ 18
DISE	Do not have a complete concentric collapse at the soft palate level	Do not have a complete concentric collapse at the soft palate level
Apnea type predominance	Central apneas $\leq 25\%$ of the total number of apnea-hypopnea events	Central and mixed apneas $\leq 25\%$ of the total number of apnea-hypopnea events
Others	Do not have any anatomical finding that would compromise the performance of upper airway stimulation	Do not have any anatomical finding that would compromise the performance of upper airway stimulation Pediatric patients with Down syndrome between 13 and 18 years of age and AHI greater than 10 and less than 50

BMI body mass index, *AHI* apnea-hypopnea index, *DISE* drug-induced sleep endoscopy

ADHERE Registry (Adherence and Outcome of Upper Airway Stimulation for OSA International Registry) which is a post-market, multicenter, observational international registry that was designed to collect data related to the use and effectiveness of the HNS therapy. Recently, in June of 2023, the FDA has expanded the indications with an upper limit AHI to 100 (an increase from ≤65 to ≤100) and increased the upper limit BMI to 40 (an increase from ≤ 32 to ≤ 40). Furthermore, pediatric patients with Down syndrome have become eligible for HNS therapy.

4 Clinical Outcomes

The Stimulation Therapy for Apnea Reduction (STAR) trial was the pivotal Phase III study using a multicenter, prospective, single group, cohort design which led to FDA-approval of the Inspire® system [8]. The inclusion criteria for this trial included BMI ≤ 32 kg/m^2, AHI 20–50 events per hour, central and mixed apneic events ≤25% of all apnea-hypopnea events, and no observation of a complete concentric collapse at the retropalatal airway on DISE. Furthermore, patients with neuromuscular disease, hypoglossal-nerve palsy, severe restrictive or obstructive pulmonary disease, moderate-to-severe pulmonary arterial hypertension, severe valvular heart disease, New York Heart Association class III or IV heart failure, recent myocardial infarction or severe cardiac arrhythmias, persistent uncontrolled hypertension despite medication use, active psychiatric disease, and coexisting non-respiratory sleep disorders were excluded from the enrollment to this study. Eventually, participants were 126 OSA patients who had difficulty either accepting or adhering to CPAP therapy with a mean age of 54.5 years and a mean BMI of 28.4 kg/m^2. At the 12-month follow-up, the median AHI and oxygen desaturation index (ODI) decreased from the baseline value of 29.3 to 9.0, and 25.4 to 7.4, respectively. In addition, the median Functional Outcome of Sleep Questionnaire (FOSQ) score increased from 14.6 to 18.2, and the median Epworth Sleepiness Scale (ESS) score decreased from 11.0 to 6.0. In the STAR trial, the randomized, controlled therapy-withdrawal study was also performed with a subset of 46 consecutive treatment responders. In 23 patients of the withdrawal group, their AHI and ODI values at the point of 1 week of therapy off were significantly higher than those in the control (therapy-maintenance) group. Thus, the efficacy of the Inspire® system was proved with this STAR trial. After this trial, observational reports were published at the point of 3-year and 5-year follow-ups regarding the objective and subjective outcomes with the participants of the STAR trial. For the 12-month, 3-year, and 5-year outcomes, improvements in the median AHI, FOSQ, and ESS were maintained (AHI; 9.0, 6.0, 6.2, FOSQ; 18.2, 18.8, 18.7, ESS; 6.0, 6.0, 6.0, respectively) [8–10].

Adherence and Outcome of Upper Airway Stimulation for OSA International Registry (ADHERE Registry) is a post-market, multicenter, observational registry. The ADHERE Registry was established in 2016 and was designed to collect data on Inspire® system therapy across the United States and European countries. At the point of writing, enrollment has been already closed since the number of participants reached the target of 5000 samples. Now, the ADHERE Registry has kept observing follow-up outcomes. The most recent study has been reported in 2022 [11]. In this study, 1963 participants were analyzed. The average age and BMI were 60.2 years and 29.2 kg/m^2, and 72.8% were male. A total of 1921 participants had completed a post-titration (~6-month post-implant) visit and 1170 participants had completed a final (~12-month post-implant) visit. The median AHI, ODI, and ESS were reported to be significantly improved as compared with baseline values (AHI; 33.0, 7.8, 10.2, ODI; 22.9, 8.4, 9.4, ESS; 11.0, 7.0, 6.0, baseline, 6-month, 12-month, respectively). As for therapy usage, mean values at the 6-month and the 12-month were 6.4 and 5.7 hours/night, which exceeded the commonly used criteria for CPAP adherence of 4 hours/night. Self-reported patient satisfaction, which was collected by questionnaires regarding patients' experience, was quite high (more than 90% of all patients). Assessed items for patient satisfaction include "Subject rated Inspire® as better than CPAP," "Subject would choose Inspire® again," and "Subject would recommend Inspire® to friends or family," implying that Inspire therapy is a promising and convinced therapy option for the patients who are intolerant CPAP from the viewpoint of patient-oriented subjective effectiveness. More interestingly, this study includes an evaluation of outcomes based on OSA severity at baseline, that is, patients were divided into 5 subgroups comprised AHI $<$ 15 (Subgroup 1), 15 $\geq$ AHI $<$ 30 (Subgroup 2), 30 $\geq$ AHI $\leq$ 50 (Subgroup 3), 50 $>$ AHI $\leq$ 65 (Subgroup 4), and AHI $>$ 65 (Subgroup 5). The analyses using those five categories demonstrated that there were no significant differences between the subgroups in terms of treatment success, ESS score, and patient satisfaction. These updated data have contributed to the change in FDA indication criteria, as mentioned in the above section.

5 Current Position of HNS Treatment

As described in the above section of "Indication criteria for the HNS in Japan and the United States," HNS has not been the first-line therapy for patients with OSA, since it is one of the alternative therapies of CPAP. In case of CPAP failure and/or non-adherence, historically, other conventional treatments such as pharmacological therapy, oral appliance, weight loss, and positional therapy used to be considered depending on the OSA phenotype. As shown in Fig. 8.2, the OSA phenotype comprises four endotypes including low arousal threshold, oversensitive ventilatory control system (elevated loop gain), small and collapsible upper airway, and poor upper airway muscular compensation. In case the treatment target is an endotype of a low arousal threshold, hypnotics improve OSA by increasing the arousal threshold [12]. Also, Acetazolamide and supplemental oxygen have been reported to be effective for the OSA phenotype of which the endotype is elevated loop gain [13, 14]. Furthermore, in the case of having both endotypes of a low arousal threshold and elevated loop gain, a combination of hypnotics and supplemental oxygen improves OSA [15]. For the endotype of a small and collapsible upper airway, oral appliance,

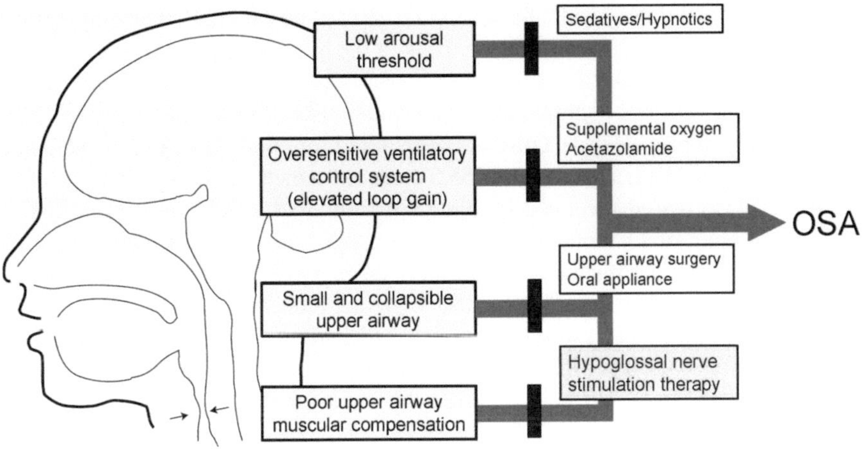

Fig. 8.2 Personalized therapy of which target is physiological endotype. Possible treatment options for each endotype are indicated. Among them, hypoglossal nerve stimulation therapy helps effectively against an endotype of poor upper airway muscular compensation. *OSA* obstructive sleep apnea

sleep surgery, and weight loss have been considered. Recently, weight loss using medication for type 2 diabetes such as glucagon-like peptide-1 (GLP-1) receptor agonists and sodium-glucose co-transporters 2 (SGLT2) inhibitors has been a topic being discussed for the treatment of OSA [16–18].

No promising treatment option for the endotype of poor upper airway muscular compensation had existed for a long time. Now, we've got NHS for this endotype. However, we have to keep in mind that HNS is not a one-size-fits-all approach for OSA patients, implying that HNS would not help against the other three endotypes. Even though a patient is satisfied with all the indication criteria for HNS, HNS is not necessarily effective for that patient. It has been reported that unfavorable response to HNS therapy was associated with endotypes of low arousal threshold and elevated loop gain [19]. Thus, evaluation of the pathophysiological trait (endotype) for each HNS therapy candidate is important for the expectation of treatment success. But the endotyping method should be established with further studies. Until then, the important thing would be careful looking at the raw respiratory signal in the PSG before implantation and preparing the additional therapy against residual apneic events after HNS intervention.

6 Other HNS Devices in Trials

Phase III clinical trials using other HNS devices have been ongoing to get approval from the FDA. Some of them were summarized in our previous review in 2020 [20]. After this review was published, one of the Phase III clinical trials with the aura6000™ (ImThera Medical, San Diego, CA, and LivaNova PLC, London, UK) was finished, and those results have been recently published [21]. The aura6000™ device places a 6-electrode cuff on the trunk of the hypoglossal nerve [22, 23]. This does not have a synchronizing trigger but rather the device cycles stimulation across the different electrodes continuously to activate muscles of the tongue to open the upper airway during sleep. A DISE is not required for eligibility. Participants were 138 OSA patients with a mean age of 55.5 years and a mean BMI of 29.8 kg/m^2. The aura6000™ decreased median AHI and ODI from 36.8 to 19.7 and from 35.8 to 19.5 at the point of 11 months of therapy. And the median FOSQ score increased from 14.7 to 18.0, and the median ESS score decreased from 11.7 to 6.7. When the AHI response rate was defined by a 50% or greater reduction in AHI to 20 or fewer events per hour, the AHI response rate was 42.5%, which fell short of the investigators' target of 50% in this trial. On the other hand, it was 66% in the STAR trial with Inspire® system. It should be noted that the inclusion criteria for this trial were broader than the one in the STAR trial. Nonetheless, the aura6000™ should be an HNS device that is close to getting the FDA approval next to the Inspire® system.

The Genio® system (Nyxoah SA, Mont-Saint-Guibert, Belgium) is another HNS device in the Phase III clinical trial (ClinicalTrials.gov Identifier: NCT02312479) that deploys bilateral implantation of very small electrodes at the insertion of the hypoglossal nerve into the base of the tongue and is externally charged and controlled by a disposable patch, worn on the patient's chin [24, 25]. It is approved for use in Europe.

7 Conclusions

The HNS is representative of implantable therapy for OSA and is one of the alternative therapies for OSA patients who are intolerant and/or nonadherent to CPAP. Currently, the Inspire® system is the only device that is clinically available in Japan and the United States. For easy access to the HNS therapy, it will be expected that other competitive devices become clinically available. Patient selection for the Inspire® system is very important, even if the patient satisfies the inclusion criteria. However, a method that can predict treatment success remains a further issue to be solved.

Conflicts of Interest Motoo Yamauchi has received a consultant fee from Inspire Medical Systems Inc. (Golden Valley, Minnesota, USA.)

References

1. Weaver TE, Grunstein RR. Adherence to continuous positive airway pressure therapy: the challenge to effective treatment. Proc Am Thorac Soc. 2008;5(2):173–8. https://doi.org/10.1513/pats.200708-119MG.

2. Wellman A, Eckert DJ, Jordan AS, Edwards BA, Passaglia CL, Jackson AC, et al. A method for measuring and modeling the physiological traits causing obstructive sleep apnea. J Appl Physiol (1985). 2011;110(6):1627–37. https://doi.org/10.1152/japplphysiol.00972.2010.
3. Wellman A, Edwards BA, Sands SA, Owens RL, Nemati S, Butler J, et al. A simplified method for determining phenotypic traits in patients with obstructive sleep apnea. J Appl Physiol (1985). 2013;114(7):911–22. https://doi.org/10.1152/japplphysiol.00747.2012.
4. Suurna MV, Jacobowitz O, Chang J, Koutsourelakis I, Smith D, Alkan U, et al. Improving outcomes of hypoglossal nerve stimulation therapy: current practice, future directions, and research gaps. Proceedings of the 2019 international sleep surgery society research forum. J Clinical Sleep Medicine: JCSM: Official Publication American Academy of Sleep Medicine. 2021;17(12):2477–87. https://doi.org/10.5664/jcsm.9542.
5. Schwab RJ, Wang SH, Verbraecken J, Vanderveken OM, Van de Heyning P, Vos WG, et al. Anatomic predictors of response and mechanism of action of upper airway stimulation therapy in patients with obstructive sleep apnea. Sleep. 2018;41(4) https://doi.org/10.1093/sleep/zsy021.
6. Heiser C, Hofauer B, Lozier L, Woodson BT, Stark T. Nerve monitoring-guided selective hypoglossal nerve stimulation in obstructive sleep apnea patients. Laryngoscope. 2016;126(12):2852–8. https://doi.org/10.1002/lary.26026.
7. Kent DT, Chio EG, Weiner JS, Heiser C, Suurna MV, Weidenbecher M. A noninferiority analysis of 3- vs 2-incision techniques for hypoglossal nerve stimulator implantation. Otolaryngology–head and neck surgery: Official J American Academy of Otolaryngology-Head and Neck Surgery. 2022;167(1):197–202. https://doi.org/10.1177/01945998211062150.
8. Strollo PJ Jr, Soose RJ, Maurer JT, de Vries N, Cornelius J, Froymovich O, et al. Upper-airway stimulation for obstructive sleep apnea. N Engl J Med. 2014;370(2):139–49. https://doi.org/10.1056/NEJMoa1308659.
9. Woodson BT, Soose RJ, Gillespie MB, Strohl KP, Maurer JT, de Vries N, et al. Three-Year Outcomes of Cranial Nerve Stimulation for Obstructive Sleep Apnea: The STAR Trial. Otolaryngology–Head Neck Surgery: Official J American Academy of Otolaryngology-Head and Neck Surgery. 2016;154(1):181–8. https://doi.org/10.1177/0194599815616618.
10. Woodson BT, Strohl KP, Soose RJ, Gillespie MB, Maurer JT, de Vries N, et al. Upper Airway Stimulation for Obstructive Sleep Apnea: 5-Year Outcomes. Otolaryngology–Head and Neck Surgery: Official J American Academy of Otolaryngology-Head and Neck Surgery. 2018;159(1):194–202. https://doi.org/10.1177/0194599818762383.
11. Bosschieter PFN, de Vries N, Mehra R, Manchanda S, Padhya TA, Vanderveken OM, et al. Similar effect of hypoglossal nerve stimulation for obstructive sleep apnea in 5 disease severity categories. J Clinical Sleep Med: JCSM: Official Publication of the American Academy Sleep Medicine. 2022;18(6):1657–65. https://doi.org/10.5664/jcsm.9956.
12. Eckert DJ, Owens RL, Kehlmann GB, Wellman A, Rahangdale S, Yim-Yeh S, et al. Eszopiclone increases the respiratory arousal threshold and lowers the apnoea/hypopnoea index in obstructive sleep apnoea patients with a low arousal threshold. Clin Sci (Lond). 2011;120(12):505–14. https://doi.org/10.1042/cs20100588.
13. Edwards BA, Sands SA, Eckert DJ, White DP, Butler JP, Owens RL, et al. Acetazolamide improves loop gain but not the other physiological traits causing obstructive sleep apnoea. J Physiol. 2012;590(5):1199–211. https://doi.org/10.1113/jphysiol.2011.223925.
14. Sands SA, Edwards BA, Terrill PI, Butler JP, Owens RL, Taranto-Montemurro L, et al. Identifying obstructive sleep apnoea patients responsive to supplemental oxygen therapy. Eur Respir J. 2018;52(3) https://doi.org/10.1183/13993003.00674-2018.
15. Edwards BA, Sands SA, Owens RL, Eckert DJ, Landry S, White DP, et al. The combination of supplemental oxygen and a hypnotic markedly improves obstructive sleep apnea in patients with a mild to moderate upper airway collapsibility. Sleep. 2016;39(11):1973–83. https://doi.org/10.5665/sleep.6226.
16. Grunstein RR, Wadden TA, Chapman JL, Malhotra A, Phillips CL. Giving weight to incretin-based pharmacotherapy for obesity-related sleep apnea: a revolution or a pipe dream? Sleep. 2023;46(10) https://doi.org/10.1093/sleep/zsad224.

17. Papaetis GS. GLP-1 receptor agonists, SGLT-2 inhibitors, and obstructive sleep apnoea: can new allies face an old enemy? Arch Med Sci Atheroscler Dis. 2023;8:e19–34. https://doi.org/10.5114/amsad/161170.
18. Blackman A, Foster GD, Zammit G, Rosenberg R, Aronne L, Wadden T, et al. Effect of liraglutide 3.0 mg in individuals with obesity and moderate or severe obstructive sleep apnea: the SCALE sleep apnea randomized clinical trial. Int J Obes. 2016;40(8):1310–9. https://doi.org/10.1038/ijo.2016.52.
19. Op de Beeck S, Wellman A, Dieltjens M, Strohl KP, Willemen M, Van de Heyning PH, et al. Endotypic mechanisms of successful hypoglossal nerve stimulation for obstructive sleep apnea. Am J Respir Crit Care Med. 2021;203(6):746–55. https://doi.org/10.1164/rccm.202006-2176OC.
20. Yamauchi M, Satoh M, Kitahara T, Ota I, Strohl K. Nerve stimulation for the treatment of obstructive sleep apnea. Sleep Biol Rhythms. 2020;18:77–87.
21. Schwartz AR, Jacobowitz O, Eisele DW, Mickelson SA, Miller MB, Oliven A, et al. Targeted hypoglossal nerve stimulation for patients with obstructive sleep apnea: a randomized clinical trial. JAMA Otolaryngol–Head Neck Sur. 2023;149(6):512–20. https://doi.org/10.1001/jamaoto.2023.0161.
22. Mwenge GB, Rombaux P, Dury M, Lengelé B, Rodenstein D. Targeted hypoglossal neurostimulation for obstructive sleep apnoea: a 1-year pilot study. Eur Respir J. 2013;41(2):360–7. https://doi.org/10.1183/09031936.00042412.
23. Friedman M, Jacobowitz O, Hwang MS, Bergler W, Fietze I, Rombaux P, et al. Targeted hypoglossal nerve stimulation for the treatment of obstructive sleep apnea: six-month results. Laryngoscope. 2016;126(11):2618–23. https://doi.org/10.1002/lary.25909.
24. Eastwood PR, Barnes M, MacKay SG, Wheatley JR, Hillman DR, Nguyên XL, et al. Bilateral hypoglossal nerve stimulation for treatment of adult obstructive sleep apnoea. Eur Respir J. 2020;55(1) https://doi.org/10.1183/13993003.01320-2019.
25. Lewis R, Pételle B, Campbell MC, MacKay S, Palme C, Raux G, et al. Implantation of the nyxoah bilateral hypoglossal nerve stimulator for obstructive sleep apnea. Laryngoscope Investig Otolaryngol. 2019;4(6):703–7. https://doi.org/10.1002/lio2.312.

Chapter 9
Telemedicine in Clinical Practice of Obstructive Sleep Apnea Patients: Is the Telemedicine Effective in the Treatment of OSA Patients?

Kimihiko Murase

Abstract Continuous positive airway pressure (CPAP) therapy is the primary treatment for obstructive sleep apnea (OSA), significantly improving symptoms like daytime sleepiness and fatigue. However, CPAP's benefits depend on the treatment adherence, and many patients discontinue CPAP use due to its discomfort and complexity. CPAP telemonitoring systems, which enable remote adherence tracking and feedback, have shown effectiveness in optimizing CPAP adherence in some clinical trials. In addition, combining CPAP adherence telemonitoring with remote feedback on lifestyle-related factors, such as body weight and blood pressure, shows promise in managing OSA patients' overall health. Future research should focus on optimizing telemedicine practices to enhance CPAP adherence and manage OSA complications effectively.

Keywords Obstructive sleep apnea · CPAP treatment adherence · CPAP telemonitoring system

1 CPAP Adherence in Clinical Practice of OSA

Obstructive sleep apnea (OSA) causes intermittent hypoxia and frequent arousals during sleep, leading to systemic inflammation and increased sympathetic nervous system activity. These events caused by OSA lead to hypertension and cardiovascular events [1]. Continuous positive airway pressure (CPAP) therapy is the main treatment for OSA and its introduction can dramatically improve main symptoms and severity of OSA, such as daytime sleepiness and fatigue [2]. However, CPAP

K. Murase (✉)
Department of Advanced Medicine for Respiratory Failure, Graduate School of Medicine, Kyoto University, Kyoto, Japan
e-mail: kmurase@kuhp.kyoto-u.ac.jp

K. Chin (ed.), *The Current State of Sleep Disordered Breathing in Japan and Around the World*, Respiratory Disease Series: Diagnostic Tools and Disease Managements, https://doi.org/10.1007/978-981-96-6030-8_9

therapy is not curative, and its clinical benefit requires continuous use of the device. Furthermore, maintaining optimal treatment adherence is an important clinical issue. In practice, many patients discontinue CPAP use due to the complexity of its use and discomfort. Only half of the patients maintain good treatment adherence at 3 months after initiation of CPAP therapy [3]. On the other hand, several large randomized controlled trials (RCTs) have examined whether CPAP therapy prevents cardiovascular events in patients with OSA, revealing no significant effects of CPAP compared to the control group [4, 5]. However, in sub-analyses of these studies, the occurrence of cardiovascular events was significantly lower in patients who used CPAP for more than or equal to 4 h per day, emphasizing the importance of optimizing CPAP adherence.

2 Clinical Practice Using CPAP Adherence Data

Although adherence to medication use is often self-reported by patients, CPAP is a medical device and its usage data is stored in the device, making it possible to obtain accurate and objective treatment adherence data. Furthermore, although there are some differences between CPAP devices according to the manufacturers, it is possible to ascertain various parameters such as "CPAP device settings" and "amount air leakage while wearing the CPAP mask" (Fig. 9.1). In addition, many devices can calculate the apnea-hypopnea index (AHI), which indicates the severity of OSA under CPAP use, providing a predictive tool for the effectiveness of CPAP treatment. Previous studies have compared the AHI calculated by CPAP equipment and polysomnography, which is the standard test for assessing the OSA severity, and demonstrated the accuracy of CPAP devices [6]. Although the algorithm for detecting respiratory events during sleep varies among devices, the parameters calculated by CPAP devices are useful for the physicians to provide guidance to the patients. In particular, when a patient complains of discomfort or other problems during CPAP use, the physicians can check air leakage and frequency of respiratory events. Based on these data, the physicians can re-instruct the patients about the mask fitting and consider changing the pressure settings. Furthermore, polysomnography can be performed while using the CPAP device to determine how the patient uses the CPAP device and to adjust the device settings.

CPAP adherence data is stored both in the device and on a memory card provided in the device. The patient carries the card when visiting the clinic, where the card data are extracted using a special software. Alternatively, the card can be sent to the equipment provider who transfer the data to the medical staff and patients. However, recent advancements in information technology have made it possible for medical staff and patients to monitor the data regarding CPAP adherence remotely via communication devices using telephone or Internet access.

Providing feedback on CPAP adherence data to patients may be effective in maintaining and improving subsequent adherence. The American Thoracic Society published a statement in 2013 stating that adherence data are calculated differently

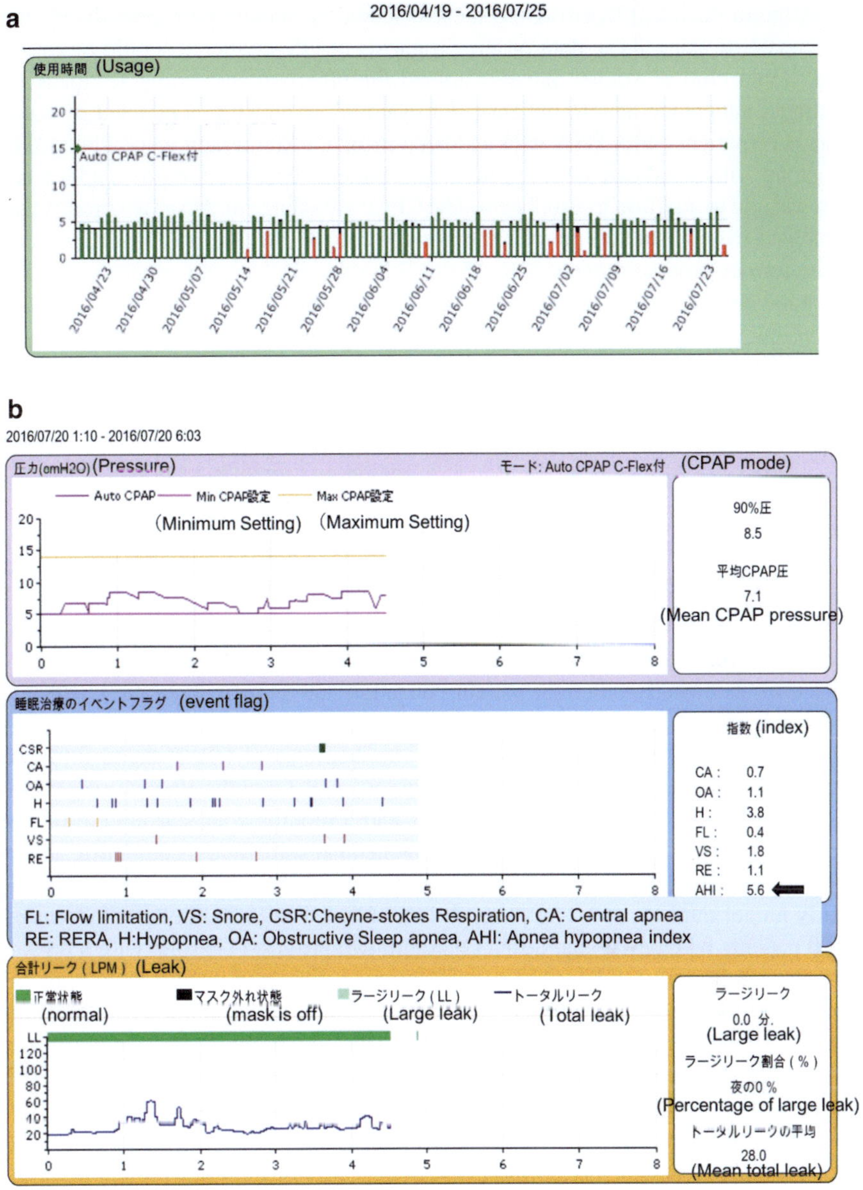

Fig. 9.1 Example of adherence data recorded on the memory card in the CPAP device. (**a**) Hours of CPAP use. Each bar indicates the number of hours of CPAP use every day. (**b**) CPAP data on an individual day. Top: CPAP pressure trend. The patient is using the auto-CPAP mode, and the CPAP pressure changes automatically as the patient's respiratory events occur during sleep. Middle row: Respiratory events while using CPAP. Each event is categorized as central apnea (CA), obstructive apnea (OA), and hypopnea (H). Each short vertical line represents the timing and type of respiratory events. Lower row: Air leakage from the mask during CPAP use

for different devices [7]. However, these calculations should be standardized, and the impact of using these data on the prognosis of OSA patients should be examined. Some clinical studies have examined the effects of providing feedback on treatment adherence data to patients. For example, in an RCT conducted by Kuna et al., 118 patients with OSA who had been using CPAP therapy were allocated to (1) group with usual care or (2) group where patients checked their own adherence on a website in addition to usual care. The CPAP adherence of these two groups was compared over a 3-month period. The average daily CPAP use was 3.8 ± 3.3 h/day in the former group, whereas it was 5.0 ± 3.2 h/day in the latter group, indicating that good adherence was maintained in the latter group [8]. In many clinical studies examining the clinical efficacy of CPAP, including the aforementioned RCT examining whether CPAP therapy prevents cardiovascular events, treatment adherence was considered as a key determinant of outcome. Moreover, improving and maintaining adherence is a key factor in the success of CPAP therapy [4, 5].

3 Maintaining and Improving CPAP Treatment Adherence with Support from Healthcare Professionals

Various approaches to maintain and improve treatment adherence of CPAP therapy have been evaluated, including patient education and support from the healthcare providers, CPAP pressure settings, masks and other interfaces. Sedakaoui et al. randomly assigned 379 patients with OSA who had started CPAP therapy to two groups: (1) patients who visit their physicians at 1 and 3 months after starting CPAP and (2) those who visit the physicians at 1 and 3 months after starting CPAP and were given regular telephone counselling by medical staff. When comparing adherence at 4 months after the start of CPAP therapy, the latter group reported a significantly longer duration of CPAP use [9]. In addition, Bouloukaki et al. randomized 3100 patients with newly diagnosed OSA into two groups: (1) group with a regular outpatient follow-up (standard care) and (2) group who received intensive support, including video lectures on OSA, telephone counselling and home visits by well-trained nurses, and active family involvement, in addition to standard care. Adherence was better in the latter group at 2 years after the start of CPAP [10]. Furthermore, the latter group also had a lower rate of cardiovascular events. In contrast, an RCT examining the effect of providing patients with an educational video on OSA at the time of CPAP initiation showed no significant improvement in adherence [11]. The impact of patient education and support from the healthcare providers on treatment adherence may vary significantly depending on patient background and the content and frequency of interventions. However, a meta-analysis examining the effects of behavioral therapy and healthcare provider support on CPAP adherence concluded that these interventions were generally effective in improving adherence [12].

4 Management of CPAP Therapy with Telemonitoring Systems

Currently, there is a growing interest in CPAP telemonitoring systems, in which healthcare professionals monitor CPAP adherence of patients remotely and provide education and support regarding CPAP use by telephone and email. These methods have been facilitated by advancements in communication technology, and their effectiveness has been examined in Europe and the USA since around 2010. Fox et al. randomly allocated 75 patients with OSA who had started CPAP therapy to two groups: (1) group with conventional outpatient care and (2) group with additional telephone coaching using the telemonitoring system. They evaluated the CPAP adherence for 3 months. In the group with telephone coaching, an investigator evaluated CPAP adherence via the telemonitoring system every weekday. When excessive air leaks or poor CPAP adherence was observed, patients were instructed on how to use the CPAP appropriately by telephone. As a result, adherence was significantly improved in the telemonitoring group than in the control group (191 vs. 105 min/day, $p < 0.01$) [13]. In addition, Hwang et al. conducted an RCT to examine the effectiveness of an automatic feedback system that uses a telemonitoring system for CPAP adherence and analyzed problems such as poor adherence or high air leakage. The information was sent to patients via text messages. This RCT verified the effectiveness of a remote education program in which a video explaining the pathophysiology of OSA, risks of leaving OSA untreated, and the importance of treatment was emailed to patients. The patients were encouraged to watch the video before CPAP initiation. In this trial, the patients were randomized into four groups: (1) usual care group, (2) remote patient education group, (3) group with automatic remote feedback, and (4) group with both remote education and automatic remote feedback. The CPAP adherence was evaluated for 3 months. In total, more than 550 patients were enrolled, and the mean daily CPAP use was significantly longer in the group with the automatic remote feedback (3.8 ± 2.5 h/day in the usual care group, 4.0 ± 2.4 h/day in the remote education group, 4.4 ± 2.2 h/day in the group with automatic remote feedback, and 4.8 ± 2.3 h/day in the group with both remote education and automatic remote feedback; $p < 0.01$). On the other hand, remote education did not show a significant impact on CPAP adherence. Interestingly, although automatic remote feedback system was scheduled to be discontinued at 3 months after randomization in this protocol, some patients unexpectedly continued to use the automatic feedback system even after the end of the RCT. This group showed better CPAP adherence than the group in which the automatic feedback system was discontinued as scheduled [14]. While CPAP adherence is likely to be improved by extensive education and support from medical staff, its cost-effectiveness should be examined. In the RCT performed by Turino et al., 100 patients with OSA who started CPAP were allocated to one of two groups: (1) group with CPAP telemonitoring and (2) group with usual care. The investigator compared not only CPAP adherence for 3 months period but also cost-effectiveness, revealing no difference in adherence between the two groups. However, healthcare costs were significantly lower in the telemonitoring group [15].

The positive effects of combined telemonitoring and feedback on CPAP adherence has been reported, but the impact of such systems has been studied intensively in groups of patients immediately after starting CPAP therapy, partly because long-term CPAP adherence is largely determined in the first few months after CPAP introduction.

5 CPAP Telemonitoring System in Japan

In Japan, CPAP treatment provided by public health insurance differs significantly from that in European and North American countries. In Japan, CPAP treatment for patients with OSA has been provided under public health insurance since 1998. In the Japanese governmental health insurance system, patients on CPAP therapy must visit physicians regularly even after long-term CPAP adherence has been established. Since the insurance system mandated the OSA patients to visit clinics every month to continue CPAP therapy, most sleep physicians continue to follow-up with patients every month even after the government modified the requirements regarding CPAP therapy in 2014. Because intensive supportive interventions for OSA patients can potentially increase CPAP adherence, reducing the frequency of visits may lead to worsening of adherence. Given that previous RCTs showed that the differences in the occurrence of cardiovascular events and the prognosis between good and poor CPAP adherence groups became significant several years after the start of CPAP treatment, it is important to provide patients with guidance and interventions to improve CPAP adherence over the long term. However, frequent follow-up visits may impose excessive burden on both patients and sleep units as well as increase the cost of managing patients with OSA.

In this situation, extending the intervals between face-to-face consultations and using a telemonitoring system as a substitute for these consultations to monitor adherence and provide remote guidance as appropriate regarding CPAP use may be a promising clinical pathway for maintaining and improving patient adherence without increasing the burden on the medical staff. Our group performed a clinical trial to evaluate the effects of this clinical pathway on CPAP adherence. In this trial, the patients who had been on CPAP therapy for at least 3 months and were visiting the clinic or hospital every month or every 2 months were randomized to one of the following three groups: (1) group with extension of the consultation interval from every 1 to 3 months, with telemonitoring used to monitor adherence once a month during the months without a visit and remote guidance provided by telephone when the CPAP adherence was poor (telemonitoring group); (2) group with extension of the consultation interval from every 1 to 3 months and no telemonitoring (3-month group); and (3) group with monthly consultations (1-month group). We observed changes in CPAP adherence for 6 months after the randomization. As a result, approximately 160 participants were allocated to each group, and the proportion of participants whose adherence worsened was 25.5% in the telemonitoring group, 33.1% in the 3-month group and 22.4% in 1-month group, showing the non-inferiority of the telemonitoring group to the 1-month group. In contrast, 3-month group did not demonstrate non-inferiority to the 1-month group. In this RCT, good adherence was defined as the use of CPAP device for more than 4 h per night on more than 70% of the days, but approximately 70% of patients demonstrated good adherence before the intervention, and only 30% of patients in the telemonitoring group were actually provided telephone guidance. In a sub-analysis of participants with poor adherence before the intervention, the CPAP adherence significantly improved in the telemonitoring and 1-month groups, suggesting that adherence improves with frequent support from healthcare professionals [16].

6 Telemonitoring System for Lifestyle-Related Diseases in OSA Patients

As discussed previously, telemonitoring of CPAP adherence and remote feedback by health professionals to patients regarding their adherence help the patients in optimizing treatment adherence. On the other hand, obesity is a major risk factor for OSA. Furthermore, weight tends to increase rather than decrease after CPAP induction [17, 18]. In addition, considering the high prevalence of lifestyle-related diseases such as hypertension and diabetes in patients with OSA, clinical pathways focusing on not only OSA but also lifestyle-related diseases are required after CPAP introduction [19]. With the availability of CPAP telemonitoring, expanding the scope of telemonitoring and remote feedback to body weight, blood pressure and physical activity is possible to improve lifestyle-related disease in OSA patients.

The effect of remote coaching on weight loss has been examined in some previous studies. For example, Spring et al. allocated 69 participants with a body mass index (BMI) of 25–40 kg/m^2 to two groups: (1) usual care group in which the participants received face-to-face guidance on weight loss at fortnightly visits and (2) remote coaching group in which the participants entered daily diet and activity data into the mobile application on a daily basis, and physicians and dietitians provided telephone coaching based on these data on a fortnightly basis. Weight was assessed every 3 months after the start of the intervention, and the researchers reported that the remote coaching group showed significantly greater weight loss than the usual care group in 1 year [20]. Steinberg et al. provided a scale to 91 participants with BMI 25–40 kg/m^2. The scale was used to send the data wirelessly and the investigators assigned the participants to a control group in which they were asked to measure their weight or to a telemonitoring group in which they received instructions on weight loss via email based on the weight measured at home. The study reported greater weight loss in the telemonitoring group than in the control group over a 6-month period [21].

On the other hand, few studies have examined the effect of telemonitoring of variables related to obesity and hypertension in addition to CPAP adherence. Pepin et al. randomized 306 patients with OSA who had a high risk of cardiovascular disease to the usual care group or group with telemonitoring of blood pressure and activity in addition to CPAP adherence. The outcomes were evaluated for 6 months. They reported that there were no differences between the two groups in terms of indices such as blood pressure and daily number of steps, but CPAP adherence was significantly better in the latter group [22]. We performed an RCT evaluating the clinical effects of telemonitoring weight, blood pressure, and physical activity in addition to CPAP adherence and providing remote feedback on these data from health professionals in OSA patients [23]. In this trial, we enrolled 168 OSA patients with obesity who were receiving CPAP therapy and provided them mobile health devices, namely an electronic scale, sphygmomanometer, and a wearable pedometer. The research staff instructed the participants to measure their body weight, blood pressure, and number of steps daily. In addition, the participants were asked to transmit the recorded data to a dedicated telemonitoring system via their smartphones using a dedicated mobile application. The participants were able to monitor the measured data on their smartphone (Fig. 9.2). Subsequently, the participants were randomized to (1) the usual CPAP telemonitoring group or (2) multimodal telemonitoring group. In both groups, the attending physicians checked the CPAP adherence remotely via the telemonitoring system and encouraged the participants to optimize their CPAP adherence every month. In addition, in the multimodal telemonitoring group, the physician encouraged the participants to lose weight by sharing the latest data from the mobile health devices. The participants were followed up for 6 months from randomization. The primary outcome was successful body weight reduction defined as achieving a body weight reduction of more than 3% from baseline to the end of the study. The percentage of participants who achieved the primary outcome was significantly higher in the multimodal telemonitoring group than in the usual CPAP telemonitoring group (39.3% vs. 25.0%, $p = 0.047$). Furthermore, both groups showed significant improvements in the percentages of days with ≥4 h/night of CPAP use from baseline to the study end (usual CPAP telemonitoring group, 72.7 ± 27.9% to 75.6 ± 26.1%, $p = 0.03$; multimodal telemonitoringgroup, 74.6 ± 27.7% to 77.0 ± 25.7%; $p = 0.046$) [23]. These data confirmed the beneficial impacts of CPAP telemonitoring and remote feedback on CPAP adherence and demonstrated that telemonitoring mobile health data related to body weight and physical activity can increase the success rate of body weight reduction.

7 Conclusion

Previous clinical trials have demonstrated that telemonitoring CPAP adherence data and providing remote feedback about the adherence data from healthcare professionals facilitates patients to optimize their CPAP adherence. Advancements in information technology offer great potential for telemedicine. Furthermore, the

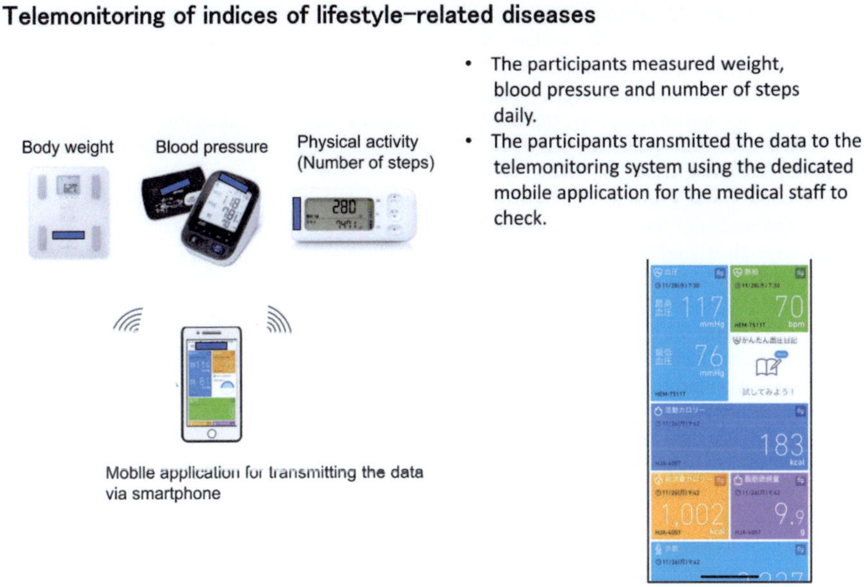

Fig. 9.2 The telemonitoring system used in our randomized clinical trial. The participants were instructed to measure their weight, blood pressure, and number of steps daily. In addition, they were asked to transmit the data to the telemonitoring system via the dedicated mobile application

corona virus pandemic is likely to enhance the importance of telemedicine, which allows physicians to evaluate patients remotely. However, in addition to the construction of stable communication systems and development of personal information protection systems and legal arrangements, there are a number of issues that need to be resolved, such as how and by whom the obtained medical data should be handled and which medical treatments should be administered based on these data. Further clinical investigations are needed to evaluate the impact of telemedicine on CPAP adherence and complications of OSA.

References

1. Tasali E, Ip MS. Obstructive sleep apnea and metabolic syndrome: alterations in glucose metabolism and inflammation. Proc Am Thorac Soc. 2008;5:207–17.
2. Jenkinson C, Davies RJ, Mullins R, Stradling JR. Comparison of therapeutic and subtherapeutic nasal continuous positive airway pressure for obstructive sleep apnoea: a randomised prospective parallel trial. Lancet. 1999;353:2100–5.
3. Rosen CL, Auckley D, Benca R, Foldvary-Schaefer N, Iber C, Kapur V, Rueschman M, Zee P, Redline S. A multisite randomized trial of portable sleep studies and positive airway pressure autotitration versus laboratory-based polysomnography for the diagnosis and treatment of obstructive sleep apnea: the HomePAP study. Sleep. 2012;35:757–67.
4. Barbé F, Durán-Cantolla J, Sánchez-de-la-Torre M, Martínez Alonso M, Carmona C, Barceló A, Chiner E, Masa JF, Gonzalez M, Marín JM, Garcia-Rio F, Diaz de Atauri J, Terán J, Mayos

M, de la Peña M, Monasterio C, del Campo F, Montserrat JM. Effect of continuous positive airway pressure on the incidence of hypertension and cardiovascular events in nonsleepy patients with obstructive sleep apnea: a randomized controlled trial. JAMA. 2012;307:2161–8.
5. Peker Y, Glantz H, Eulenburg C, Wegscheider K, Herlitz J, Thunström E. Effect of positive airway pressure on cardiovascular outcomes in coronary artery disease patients with nonsleepy obstructive sleep apnea. The RICCADSA randomized controlled trial. Am J Respir Crit Care Med. 2016;194:613–20.
6. Ueno K, Kasai T, Brewer G, Takaya H, Maeno K, Kasagi S, Kawana F, Ishiwata S, Narui K. Evaluation of the apnea-hypopnea index determined by the S8 auto-CPAP, a continuous positive airway pressure device, in patients with obstructive sleep apnea-hypopnea syndrome. J Clin Sleep Med. 2010;6:146–51.
7. Schwab RJ, Badr SM, Epstein LJ, Gay PC, Gozal D, Kohler M, Lévy P, Malhotra A, Phillips BA, Rosen IM, Strohl KP, Strollo PJ, Weaver EM, Weaver TE. An official American Thoracic Society statement: continuous positive airway pressure adherence tracking systems. The optimal monitoring strategies and outcome measures in adults. Am J Respir Crit Care Med. 2013;188:613–20.
8. Kuna ST, Shuttleworth D, Chi L, Schutte-Rodin S, Friedman E, Guo H, Dhand S, Yang L, Zhu J, Bellamy SL, Volpp KG, Asch DA. Web-based access to positive airway pressure usage with or without an initial financial incentive improves treatment use in patients with obstructive sleep apnea. Sleep. 2015;38:1229–36.
9. Sedkaoui K, Leseux L, Pontier S, Rossin N, Leophonte P, Fraysse JL, Didier A. Efficiency of a phone coaching program on adherence to continuous positive airway pressure in sleep apnea hypopnea syndrome: a randomized trial. BMC Pulm Med. 2015;15:102.
10. Bouloukaki I, Giannadaki K, Mermigkis C, Tzanakis N, Mauroudi E, Moniaki V, Michelakis S, Siafakas NM, Schiza SE. Intensive versus standard follow-up to improve continuous positive airway pressure compliance. Eur Respir J. 2014;44:1262–74.
11. Guralnick AS, Balachandran JS, Szutenbach S, Adley K, Emami L, Mohammadi M, Farnan JM, Arora VM, Mokhlesi B. Educational video to improve CPAP use in patients with obstructive sleep apnoea at risk for poor adherence: a randomised controlled trial. Thorax. 2017;72:1132–9.
12. Askland K, Wright L, Wozniak DR, Emmanuel T, Caston J, Smith I. Educational, supportive and behavioural interventions to improve usage of continuous positive airway pressure machines in adults with obstructive sleep apnoea. Cochrane Database Syst Rev. 2020;4:Cd007736.
13. Fox N, Hirsch-Allen AJ, Goodfellow E, Wenner J, Fleetham J, Ryan CF, Kwiatkowska M, Ayas NT. The impact of a telemedicine monitoring system on positive airway pressure adherence in patients with obstructive sleep apnea: a randomized controlled trial. Sleep. 2012;35:477–81.
14. Hwang D, Chang JW, Benjafield AV, Crocker ME, Kelly C, Becker KA, Kim JB, Woodrum RR, Liang J, Derose SF. Effect of telemedicine education and telemonitoring on continuous positive airway pressure adherence. The tele-OSA randomized trial. Am J Respir Crit Care Med. 2018;197:117–26.
15. Turino C, de Batlle J, Woehrle H, Mayoral A, Castro-Grattoni AL, Gómez S, Dalmases M, Sánchez-de-la-Torre M, Barbé F. Management of continuous positive airway pressure treatment compliance using telemonitoring in obstructive sleep apnoea. Eur Respir J. 2017;49:1601128.
16. Murase K, Tanizawa K, Minami T, Matsumoto T, Tachikawa R, Takahashi N, Tsuda T, Toyama Y, Ohi M, Akahoshi T, Tomita Y, Narui K, Nakamura H, Ohdaira T, Yoshimine H, Tsuboi T, Yamashiro Y, Ando S, Kasai T, Kita H, Tatsumi K, Burioka N, Tomii K, Kondoh Y, Takeyama H, Handa T, Hamada S, Oga T, Nakayama T, Sakamaki T, Morita S, Kuroda T, Hirai T, Chin K. A randomized controlled trial of telemedicine for long-term sleep apnea continuous positive airway pressure management. Ann Am Thorac Soc. 2020;17:329–37.
17. Drager LF, Brunoni AR, Jenner R, Lorenzi-Filho G, Benseñor IM, Lotufo PA. Effects of CPAP on body weight in patients with obstructive sleep apnoea: a meta-analysis of randomised trials. Thorax. 2015;70:258–64.

18. Tachikawa R, Ikeda K, Minami T, Matsumoto T, Hamada S, Murase K, Tanizawa K, Inouchi M, Oga T, Akamizu T, Mishima M, Chin K. Changes in energy metabolism after continuous positive airway pressure for obstructive sleep apnea. Am J Respir Crit Care Med. 2016;194:729–38.
19. Matsumoto T, Murase K, Tabara Y, Gozal D, Smith D, Minami T, Tachikawa R, Tanizawa K, Oga T, Nagashima S, Wakamura T, Komenami N, Setoh K, Kawaguchi T, Tsutsumi T, Takahashi Y, Nakayama T, Hirai T, Matsuda F, Chin K. Impact of sleep characteristics and obesity on diabetes and hypertension across genders and menopausal status: the Nagahama study. Sleep. 2018;41 https://doi.org/10.1093/sleep/zsy071.
20. Spring B, Duncan JM, Janke EA, Kozak AT, McFadden HG, DeMott A, Pictor A, Epstein LH, Siddique J, Pellegrini CA, Buscemi J, Hedeker D. Integrating technology into standard weight loss treatment: a randomized controlled trial. JAMA Intern Med. 2013;173:105–11.
21. Steinberg DM, Tate DF, Bennett GG, Ennett S, Samuel-Hodge C, Ward DS. The efficacy of a daily self-weighing weight loss intervention using smart scales and e-mail. Obesity (Silver Spring). 2013;21:1789–97.
22. Pépin JL, Jullian-Desayes I, Sapène M, Treptow E, Joyeux-Faure M, Benmerad M, Bailly S, Grillet Y, Stach B, Richard P, Lévy P, Muir JF, Tamisier R. Multimodal remote monitoring of high cardiovascular risk patients with OSA initiating CPAP: a randomized trial. Chest. 2019;155:730–9.
23. Murase K, Minami T, Hamada S, Gozal D, Takahashi N, Nakatsuka Y, Takeyama H, Tanizawa K, Endo D, Akahoshi T, Moritsuchi Y, Tsuda T, Toyama Y, Ohi M, Tomita Y, Narui K, Matsuyama N, Ohdaira T, Kasai T, Tsuboi T, Gon Y, Yamashiro Y, Ando S, Yoshimine H, Takata Y, Yoshihisa A, Tatsumi K, Momomura SI, Kuroda T, Morita S, Nakayama T, Hirai T, Chin K. Multimodal telemonitoring for weight reduction in patients with sleep apnea: a randomized controlled trial. Chest. 2022;162:1373–83.

Part III
SAS in Patients with CVD

Chapter 10
Sleep Apnea in Patients with Atrial Fibrillation and Heart Failure: What Should We Know About the Correlation Between Sleep Apnea Syndrome and AF or Heart Failure?

Takatoshi Kasai and Shoichiro Yatsu

Abstract This chapter explores the intricate relationship between sleep apnea, either obstructive or central, and two prevalent cardiovascular diseases: atrial fibrillation and heart failure. We investigated the pathophysiology, clinical implications, and management strategies associated with the coexistence of these conditions to shed light on the interconnected nature of cardiovascular and sleep disorders.

Keywords Adaptive servo ventilation · Central sleep apnea · Cheyne-Stokes breathing · Continuous positive airway pressure · Obstructive sleep apnea

---

T. Kasai (✉)
Department of Cardiovascular Biology and Medicine, Juntendo University Graduate School of Medicine, Tokyo, Japan

Cardiovascular Respiratory Sleep Medicine, Juntendo University Graduate School of Medicine, Tokyo, Japan

Sleep and Sleep-Disordered Breathing Center, Juntendo University Hospital, Tokyo, Japan

Department of Cardiovascular Management and Remote Monitoring, Juntendo University Graduate School of Medicine, Tokyo, Japan
e-mail: kasai-t@mx6.nisiq.net

S. Yatsu
Department of Cardiovascular Biology and Medicine, Juntendo University Graduate School of Medicine, Tokyo, Japan

K. Chin (ed.), *The Current State of Sleep Disordered Breathing in Japan and Around the World*, Respiratory Disease Series: Diagnostic Tools and Disease Managements, https://doi.org/10.1007/978-981-96-6030-8_10

1 Introduction

Cardiovascular diseases and sleep disorders have emerged as significant health challenges in contemporary society [1]. Particularly, sleep apnea (SA), including both obstructive and central SA (OSA and CSA, respectively) in patients with cardiovascular diseases, such as atrial fibrillation (AF) and heart failure (HF), are known to profoundly impact morbidity and mortality [2–4]. Thus, understanding SA in the context of AF and HF is crucial for improving the prognosis of these patients. However, the beneficial effects of SA treatment on cardiovascular outcomes remain unclear. Recently, the clinical importance of SA treatment in patients with AF and HF has garnered attention, shedding new light on their intricate relationships and their implications for underlying cardiovascular diseases. In this section, the relationships between these factors and the treatment of SA under these conditions are reviewed.

2 SA in Patients with AF

2.1 Prevalence, Risk Factors of SA in AF and Their Bidirectional Relationships

The prevalence of SA in patients with AF is notably high up to 50–70% and it mainly consists of OSA [4–6]. However, as the AF burden increases (i.e., an increase in the frequency of paroxysmal, persistent, or permanent AF), OSA severity will also increase. CSA is also prevalent in patients with AF (up to 30%) [4, 7]. As the AF burden further increases, CSA will also develop and worsen in such patients [4].

High prevalence of SAs in patients with AF may be due to the common risk factors associated with AF and OSA. These factors include obesity, advanced age, male sex, habitual drinking, and heart failure. OSA has been identified as a potential trigger and exacerbating factor for AF. Intermittent hypoxia and increased sympathetic activity associated with OSA can induce oxidative stress, inflammation, and changes in autonomic tone, all of which may promote the initiation and perpetuation of AF [3, 4]. Additionally, repetitive episodes of apneas and hypopneas during sleep may lead to significant hemodynamic changes, impacting cardiac structure and function [8, 9]. As the AF burden increases, systemic congestion occurs along the upper airway mucosal edema and/or overnight rostral fluid shifts from the legs, which contributes to the development and/or worsening of OSA [4, 10–13].

Risk factors of CSA in patients with AF include advanced age and male sex, and presence of HF especially ischemic cardiomyopathy, all of which are the predisposing factors of both AF and CSA [4]. In addition, as mentioned above, persistent and longstanding AF may be associated with a higher likelihood of developing CSA [4]. In addition to the pulmonary congestion, an irregular heart rhythm and hemodynamic changes in AF contribute to the instability of respiratory control through the sympathetic nerve overactivation [4]. Cheyne-Stokes breathing (CSB), characterized by a periodic waxing and waning of breathing with central apneas and by a long cycle length, is often observed in AF patients with CSA especially in HF state [4]. Such oscillations in respiratory effort cause hemodynamic change, leading to the development and worsening of HF. HF itself and its worsening also increases the AF burden. Thus, the relationships between AF and SA are dynamic and bidirectional, where each condition can influence the other and potentially exacerbate the severity of both conditions [4]. Understanding such bidirectional relationships is crucial for comprehensive patient care and targeted treatment strategies.

2.2 *Impact of SA on Cardiovascular Outcomes in Patients with AF*

As mentioned earlier, the presence of SA in patients with AF may increase the AF burden, leading to the deterioration of cardiac function and development, and worsening of HF. Till date, no longitudinal data suggests that the presence of SA in patients with AF is associated with an increased risk of incident HF. In terms of other major clinical outcomes of AF and stroke, since SA may enhance platelet activity and increase coagulability, and because SA is an independent risk factor for stroke, the presence of SA may also increase the risk of stroke in patients with AF [4, 14, 15]. However, no data has clearly shown a relationship between SA and incident stroke in patients with AF. Furthermore, the effect of SA on the long-term mortality of patients with AF remains unclear. However, the presence of SA is associated with adverse clinical outcomes, particularly AF recurrence following AF treatment such as cardioversion and catheter ablation [4–6]. Thus, addressing SA becomes crucial in managing and potentially preventing further cardiovascular complications in patients with AF.

2.3 *Treatment of SA in Patients with AF*

For OSA, lifestyle modifications and weight management should be considered, even in patients with AF [16]. They are particularly important because they may be effective not only for OSA, but also for AF outcomes. Therefore, multidisciplinary approaches involving both cardiology and sleep medicine are essential for comprehensive patient care. However, the problem is that such an approach is usually difficult to continue and it takes long term to obtain satisfactory results. Similarly, in the general population, continuous positive airway pressure (CPAP) is usually considered the first-line therapy for OSA, even in patients with AF. Although, whether CPAP for OSA in patients with AF improves long-term clinical outcomes such as incident HF, incident stroke, and cardiovascular mortality remains to be elucidated, several observational studies strongly suggest that CPAP therapy for OSA is effective in reducing AF recurrence following cardioversion and catheter ablation [4]. However, this should be confirmed by further randomized controlled trials (RCT). In terms of the AF burden in patients with paroxysmal AF, in one RCT, CPAP failed to show a clinical benefit in reducing the AF burden and the number and duration of AF episodes [17]. Notably, adherence to CPAP did not influence the results in this study. However, the actual AF burden was lower than anticipated and thus may be underpowered in this case. Furthermore, since OSA was diagnosed using respiratory polygraphy, central respiratory events may not have been correctly evaluated. The CPAP machine suggested that their SA was sufficiently suppressed (i.e., apnea-hypopnea index [AHI] <5) on average; the AHI on CPAP might have varied or was insufficiently suppressed in some cases or on some occasions because of the development/worsening of CSA. An RCT assessing whether sufficient suppression of the SA in patients with AF by adaptive servo ventilation (ASV), which is an advanced form of positive airway pressure and the most effective therapy that adapts to the patient's respiratory patterns to suppress both OSA and CSA, can reduce cardiac sympathetic nerve activity as assessed by ^{123}I-MIBG myocardial scintigraphy which is now underway [18].

3 Sleep Apnea in Patients with Heart Failure

3.1 *Prevalence, Risk Factors of SA in HF and Their Bidirectional Relationships*

The prevalence of SA is notably high in patients with HF [2–4]. Studies indicate that a substantial proportion of patients with HF, either with a reduced or preserved ejection fraction (HFrEF and HFpEF, respectively), experience various forms of SA, including OSA, CSA, and CSB. Estimates suggest that up to 50–70% of patients with HF, either HFrEF or HFpEF, may have coexisting SA [2–4, 19]. Both OSA and CSA are prevalent in HF populations, although the predominant type may vary according to HF status. In patients with advanced or acute HF, CSA is generally more prevalent than OSA [20].

Risk factors for OSA in patients with HF include obesity, advanced age, male sex, and high left ventricular filling pressure [2–4]. OSA may result in the development and worsening of HF, possibly through intermittent hypoxia, oxidative stress, inflammation, augmented sympathetic activity, and exaggerated negative intrathoracic pressure [2, 3, 21]. Additionally, incident hypertension, AF, and ischemic cardiomyopathy in association with OSA lead to the development/worsening of HF [3]. Once HF is developed, OSA remains or worsens due to upper airway mucosal edema association with systemic congestion and/or overnight rostral fluid shift from the legs [10–13].

Risk factors for CSA in patients with HF include obesity, advanced age, male sex, presence of AF, low arterial carbon dioxide level, high left ventricular filling pressure, and use of diuretics [20, 22]. As HF worsens, CSA with CSB becomes apparent due to pulmonary congestion, instability of respiratory control in association with sympathetic nerve overactivation, and circulatory delay due to impaired cardiac output [4].

Similar to AF, the relationship between HF and SA is dynamic and bidirectional, where each condition can influence the other, potentially altering the type of SA and exacerbating the severity of both conditions. Such bidirectional relationships are important when considering treatment strategies.

3.2 Impact of SA on Cardiovascular Outcomes in Patients with HF

The presence of OSA in patients with HF may deteriorate cardiac function, leading to worsening of HF. Our study suggests that in patients with HF, OSA leads to an overnight reduction in cardiac output proportional to OSA severity [23]. This may be explained by repetitive intermittent hypoxia, alteration of hemodynamics in association with exaggerated negative intrathoracic pressure, and elevated blood pressure and arterial stiffness in association with augmented sympathetic nerve activity. Longitudinal observational studies have suggested that the presence of OSA in patients with HFrEF is associated with worse cardiovascular outcome [24]. However, limited data clearly showing the relationship between OSA and poor clinical outcomes are available for patients with HFpEF [25].

The presence of CSA in patients with HF may also be associated with deterioration of cardiac function and worsening of HF [2, 4]. Many studies have shown relationships between CSA and poor clinical outcome [2]. Similar to OSA, CSA causes repetitive intermittent hypoxia, alteration of hemodynamics in association with enhanced intrathoracic pressure swings during the hyperventilation phase of CSB, and sympathetic overactivity [2]. Many studies have shown relationships between the presence of CSA or CSB and increased mortality risk in patients with HFrEF. However, data showing the relationship between the presence of CSA or CSB and poor clinical outcomes are scarce in patients with HFpEF.

3.3 Treatment of SA in Patients with HF

Studies have suggested that treatment with SA can improve SA-related symptoms such as excessive daytime sleepiness, non-restorative sleep, chocking/gasping during sleep, and quality of life, even in HF patients with either OSA or CSA. [2–4, 26] SA in patients with HF should be treated properly. In addition, studies, including

RCT, have suggested that treatment with SA, either OSA or CSA, can improve cardiac function in patients with HF [2]. SA in patients with HF should also be treated keeping this aim in mind. Treatments for SA in patients with HF are divided into two targets, one for SA and the other for underlying HF, on account of the bidirectional relationship [4]. In this perspective, SA necessitates a comprehensive and tailored approach to the management of patients with HF. Addressing SA in the context of HF involves a range of therapeutic strategies aimed at improving both sleep quality and cardiac function, leading to an improved quality of life. However, till date no treatment option for SA has clearly shown to improve the prognosis for such patients.

3.3.1 Treatment Targeted for HF

Medication for HF

Specific medications for HF such as diuretics, beta-blockers, angiotensin converting enzyme (ACE) inhibitors, mineral corticoid receptor (MR) blockers, angiotensin receptor neprilysin inhibitors (ARNI) can also be effective for alleviating the AHI in patients with HF [2–4, 27–30]. In HF patients with OSA and fluid retention, a combination of the mineral corticoid receptor blocker, spironolactone, and loop diuretics has shown to alleviate AHI through the decongestion around the upper airway mucosa or the reduction of overnight rostral fluid shift from the legs [31]. Since CSA in patients with HF is caused by the HF itself, optimization of HF treatment based on guidelines for HF is essential for the CSA in patients with HF, either HFrEF or HFpEF. In OSA patients with HF, diuretics may alleviate CSA in HF patients by improving pulmonary congestion. A small observational study suggested that the ACE inhibitor captopril reduced the AHI in patients with HF by improving cardiac function. In patients with HFrEF and CSA, the beta-blocker carvedilol significantly alleviated AHI through the improvement of cardiac function and possibly through the reduction of enhanced ventilatory response, which is an important pathogenetic factor for CSA/CSB [2, 4]. Recent studies have investigated the effect of ARNI on SA in patients with HFrEF. Although an RCT comparing the AHI before and after 8 weeks of treatment in HFrEF patients with mostly OSA showed no significant reduction in AHI, there were two observational studies in which HFrEF patients with mostly CSA showed a significant reduction in AHI [28–30].

Other HF Treatments

Cardiac resynchronization therapy (CRT) has been reported to alleviate SA, mainly CSA in patients with HF [4]. Improvements in CSA have been reported after percutaneous or surgical coronary intervention in patients with ischemic cardiomyopathy, and after mitral valvuloplasty in patients with mitral regurgitation [4, 32]. Following transcatheter aortic valve implantation for aortic stenosis, the AHI reduced especially in patients with CSA [4, 33]. Furthermore, following left ventricular assist device implantation or heart transplantation in patients with severe HF, CSA generally alleviated [4]. Once all these interventions improve pulmonary congestion, cardiac function and hemodynamics, CSA will disappear. It should be noted that when HF improves with optimized therapy, the CSA may decrease or disappear, and OSA sometimes becomes apparent. Exercise is an important non-pharmacological treatment for HF and SA as OSA or CSA can be alleviated by exercise training in patients with HF [4]. Reduction of overnight rostral fluid shift from the legs may be a mechanism to alleviate OSA and CSA [4, 10, 12]. The pathogenesis of CSA is associated with hyperventilation, and exercise training has been reported to improve hyperventilation during exertion and CO_2 chemoreceptor hyperactivity. This may be another mechanism underlying the alleviation of the CSA after exercise training.

3.3.2 Treatment Targeted for SA

CPAP

Even in patients with HF, CPAP is a standard and effective treatment for OSA that reduces the AHI and improves nocturnal oxygenation. In patients with HFrEF, short-term RCTs have reported that CPAP improved cardiac function in patients with predominant OSA, and meta-analyses have confirmed such effects [2–4]. Our group reported more improvement of left ventricular function in the younger and the more obese patients [34]. Observational studies have shown that CPAP for HF patients with predominant OSA might improve the long-term prognosis [35]. No RCTs have investigated the prognostic efficacy of CPAP in patients with HF and predominant OSA. Japanese guidelines for SA in patients with cardiovascular disease suggest that patients with OSA-related symptoms, such as daytime sleepiness, should be treated even in patients with HF, and CPAP therapy should be considered for HFrEF patients with OSA to improve left ventricular function [36].

CPAP has been shown to have a short-term effect not only in suppressing CSA in patients with HFrEF but also in reducing sympathetic nerve activity, improving left ventricular function, and exercise tolerance [2, 4]. However, in the Canadian Continuous Positive Airway Pressure for Patients with Central Sleep Apnea and Heart Failure Trial (CANPAP), an RCT investigating the effect of CPAP on the prognosis of HFrEF patients with CSA, CPAP failed to show prognostic benefit (Table 10.1) [37]. A post-hoc analysis of the CANPAP indicated one reason to this effect that the group of patients whose AHI alleviated as <15 with CPAP at 3 months after starting CPAP (CPAP responder) had a better prognosis than those in the control group and that the group of patients whose AHI still ≥15 with CPAP at 3 months after starting CPAP (CPAP non responder) had rather worse prognosis than those in the control group [42]. Similar observation was reported by our group, suggesting that in patients with HFrEF, a presence of unsuppressed SA (i.e., AHI ≥15) even on

Table 10.1 Randomized controlled trials investigating effects of positive airway pressure on clinical outcomes in patients with HF

	Year	N	LVEF SA type	Duration (month)	Primary endpoint	Other endpoints
CANPAP [37]	2005	258	<40% AHI ≥ 15 Predominant CSA	24	Death + heart transplantation >No difference	LVEF↑ Post-hoc analysis: AHI < 15 on CPAP was better outcome vs. controls
SERVE-HF [38]	2015	1325	≤45% AHI ≥ 15 Predominant CSA	31	Death + CV intervention + HF hospitalization >No difference	All-cause mortality↑ CV mortality↑
SAVIOR-C [39]	2015	213	<40% No criteria for SA	6	LVEF >No difference	Clinical events (death + hospitalization) tended to be better in ASV ($P = 0.283$). Composite clinical response (changes in NYHA class+clinical events) ASV was better in ASV ($P = 0.002$).
CAT-HF [40]	2017	126	ADHF (HFrEF & HFpEF) AHI ≥ 15 by portable monitor	6	Global rank endpoint (death + HF hospitalization +6MWD) >No difference	HFrEF: no difference HFpEF: better in ASV ($P = 0.036$)
ADVENT-HF [41]	2023	731	≤45% AHI ≥ 15 (OSA&CSA)	43	Death + CV hospitalization + AF/AFL requiring anticoagulation + ICD shock >No difference overall and in OSA-/CSA-predominant subgroups	All-cause mortality: no difference overall and in OSA-/CSA-predominant subgroups CV mortality: no difference overall and in OSA-/CSA-predominant subgroups MLHFQ score improved in ASV overall and in OSA-/CSA-predominant subgroups

(continued)

Table 10.1 (continued)

AF atrial fibrillation, *AFL* atrial flutter, *AHI* apnea-hypopnea index, *ASV* adaptive servo ventilation, *CPAP* continuous positive airway pressure, *CSA* central sleep apnea, *CV* cardiovascular, *HF* heart failure, *HFpEF* heart failure with preserved ejection fraction, *HFrEF* heart failure with reduced ejection fraction, *ICD* implantable cardioverter defibrillator, *MLHFQ* Minnesota living with heart failure questionnaire, *NYHA* New York Heart Association, *OSA* obstructive sleep apnea, *SA* sleep apnea, *6 MWD* 6-min walk distance

CPAP was associated with worse prognosis as compared to those with suppressed SA by CPAP (i.e., AHI <15) [43].

With respect to SA management in patients with HFpEF, CPAP should be considered, particularly if the patient presents with OSA. Several reports have suggested reductions in left ventricular myocardial mass and right and left atrial volumes with CPAP in patients with OSA, which can improve cardiac function, hemodynamics, and congestive status [4]. However, such data focused on HFpEF are scarce. Although CPAP is likely to be useful for OSA associated with HFpEF, no clear evidence has been established to indicate the improvement in cardiac function and prognosis of HFpEF with OSA. As a CSA treatment, CPAP can also be used if the CSA is effectively suppressed by CPAP in patients with HFpEF.

ASV

ASV is particularly useful in treating CSA/CSB since it provides ventilatory support during periods of reduced respiratory effort and it also provides automated end-expiratory positive pressure to keep the upper airway open to alleviate OSA [2].

In terms of ASV as an OSA treatment in patients with HF, several short-term RCTs showed that ASV provided more improvements of cardiovascular functions and quality of life along with better adherence to devices as compared with CPAP in HF patients with coexisting OSA and CSA/CSB [2, 4]. In a multicenter RCT of ASV in HF patients with moderate or severe OSA or CSA and left ventricular ejection fraction (LVEF) <45% (ADVENT-HF), the overall analysis did not confirm a significant effect of SA treatment with ASV on cardiovascular events, and the same was true in the subgroup analysis of OSA-predominant patients (Table 10.1) [41]. However, in secondary endpoints, quality of life was significantly improved by ASV in patients with OSA-predominant patients [41].

RCTs and meta-analyses have indicated that ASV improves LVEF and exercise tolerance and lowers B-type natriuretic peptide (BNP) level in HFrEF patients with CSA [2, 4]. In addition, the use of ASV in patients with residual CSA on CPAP showed improvement in both CSA and LVEF, in addition to the better adherence to ASV than CPAP [44]. Observational studies have demonstrated reductions in cardiac mortality and heart failure rehospitalization rates [2, 4]. However, the SERVE-HF study, a large RCT examining the prognostic value of ASV in HF patients with LVEF ≤45% and predominant CSA with AHI ≥15, found that the primary endpoints of total deaths, life-saving cardiovascular interventions were similar, and the secondary endpoints of all-cause death and cardiovascular death were rather increased in the ASV group (Table 10.1) [38]. Based on this, European and US societies indicated that ASV should not use in HFrEF patients with predominant CSA. The CAT-HF trial (Table 10.1), in which SA (either OSA or CSA, and AHI ≥15) was detected in patients hospitalized with acute decompensated HF and randomly assigned them to the ASV or control group, was stopped early due to the results of SERVE-HF [40]. However, the SERVE-HF study has also raised a number of issues, including the large number of crossover patients between the two groups, and problems with the intention-to-treat analysis. Although the ADVENT-HF trial failed to show mortality benefit in HFrEF patients with SA, and in subgroups with predominant OSA or CSA, in that trial, ASV was not associated with worse prognosis even in the subgroup of predominant CSA, and rather there was a non-significant but modest trend for less cardiovascular events in the ASV intervention group in the CSA subgroup [41]. It is noteworthy that the trend was different to the results of the SERVE-HF trial.

In HFpEF patients with SA including CSA, 6-month treatment with ASV improved left ventricular diastolic function, arterial stiffness, and endothelial function, and reduced cardiac death and heart failure rehospitalization rates [45]. Similarly, in CSA-predominant HFpEF patients, ASV reduced estimated pulmonary artery pressure and BNP level, and improved right heart function. In a subgroup analysis of the CAT-HF study, ASV improved the outcomes in patients with HFpEF [40].

In Japan, the SAVIOR-C trial (Table 10.1), a multicenter RCT conducted in patients with HFrEF, showed a significant improvement in the ASV group in the clinical composite response, a composite of symptoms, and HF exacerbation at 6 months. However, this was a secondary endpoint [39]. This is one explanation that even after the SERVE-HF trial, the use of ASV is not contraindicated in HFrEF patients with predominant CSA in Japan. In particular, the clinical composite response in the SAVIOR-C trial was evaluated at 6 months, and the impact of ASV therapy over a longer period is still unknown. Therefore, switching to CPAP should be considered as soon as possible after the introduction of ASV. Considering the results of the ADVENT-HF trial, this statement should be revised. Considering the secondary endpoint of the SAVIOR-C study (i.e., improvement in clinical composite response) and considering that ASV has been used in real clinical practice to improve not only symptoms but also to stabilize cardiac function in patients with severe HF whose congestive symptoms have not improved despite standard treatment and in many Japanese studies, ASV has shown beneficial effects on cardiovascular function, hemodynamics and outcomes, it is possible to use ASV to relieve congestion and continue it after discharge from the hospital under insurance reimbursement.

Oxygen Therapy

Nocturnal supplemental oxygen can be prescribed for patients with HF or CSA. Oxygen therapy helps maintain adequate blood oxygen levels during sleep, probably reducing strain on the cardiovascular system. Short-term studies on nocturnal oxygen therapy have reported the disappearance of CSA, suppression of sympathetic nerve activity, improvement in exercise tolerance, and reduction in plasma BNP concentration in patients with HF [2, 4]. A Japanese multicenter study (chronic heart failure nocturnal home oxygen therapy study) was conducted to evaluate the effect of nocturnal oxygen therapy in HFrEF patients with CSA and it was found that the oxygen group did not show a reduction in the composite cardiovascular events of HF hospitalization and cardiovascular death. In contrast, in a recent RCT conducted in Japan, 3 months of nocturnal oxygen therapy resulted in a mild decrease in AHI and a non-significant improvement in LVEF compared to ASV. A large RCT of oxygen therapy in HFrEF patients with CSA is underway [46], and further studies on its efficacy, including cardiovascular death and adverse events, in patients with HFpEF are warranted in the future.

Phrenic Nerve Stimulation

This emerging therapy involves the implantation of a device that stimulates the phrenic nerve during sleep, thereby improving the CSA/CSB in patients with HF. The Remedē System Pivotal Trial, an RCT conducted in HFrEF patients with CSA, showed >50% reduction in the AHI at 6 months and a 36-month safety and tolerability profile [47, 48]. A post-hoc analysis of the Remedē System Pivotal Trial reported a significant improvement in LVEF in HF patients at 12 months post-PNS compared with baseline [49], and a significant improvement in LVEF at 12 months post-PNS compared with baseline [50]. PNS may improve outcomes such as death and HF hospitalizations in HF patients through improvement of CSA without affecting patient adherence [48]. Future studies should examine cardiac function and prognosis in large RCTs of CSA associated with HF or CVD.

4 Conclusion

There was an obvious bidirectional relationship between SA and AF and HF, suggesting that each can contribute to the development or exacerbation of the other. For instance, individuals with untreated SA are at an increased risk of developing AF, and SA can aggravate existing AF and it may contribute to its progression. Treating SA, often with CPAP, may help manage AF and possibly improve outcomes. SA is highly prevalent and is similar to AF in patients with HF, and untreated SA can contribute to the progression. Congestion in association with HF can lead to the development and worsening of SA, either OSA or CSA. Treatment with SA, mainly positive airway pressure, has positive effects on HF itself and probably on clinical outcomes. Thus, screening for SA in patients with AF or HF is crucial for managing underlying AF and HF. Since SA is a disease that occurs across multiple fields of medicine, a multidisciplinary approach involving cardiologists, respiratory physicians, otorhinolaryngologists, and sleep specialists, including nurses and technicians, is often beneficial for comprehensive care and patient-centered approaches. Adherence to treatments, such as CPAP, is essential for improving both sleep-related symptoms and cardiovascular outcomes. Thus, recognizing and addressing SA in patients with AF or HF is important for comprehensive cardiovascular care, and it can have positive effects on overall health outcomes.

Funding Source This study was partly supported by JSPS KAKENHI (Grant number: JP21K08116, JP21K16034); a Grant-in-Aid for Scientific Research (Grant number: 20FC1027, 23FC1031) from the Ministry of Health, Labour and Welfare of Japan; and a research grant from the Japanese Center for Research on Women in Sport, Juntendo University. None of the funding sources played any other role in this chapter.

Disclosures Dr. Kasai is affiliated with a department endowed by Philips, ResMed, and Fukuda Denshi and with a department funded by Paramount Bed based on collaborative research agreement.

References

1. Lloyd-Jones DM, Allen NB, Anderson CAM, Black T, Brewer LC, Foraker RE, et al. Life's essential 8: updating and enhancing the American Heart Association's construct of cardiovascular health: a presidential advisory from the American Heart Association. Circulation. 2022;146:e18–43.
2. Kasai T. Sleep apnea and heart failure. J Cardiol. 2012;60:78–85.
3. Kasai T, Bradley TD. Obstructive sleep apnea and heart failure: pathophysiologic and therapeutic implications. J Am Coll Cardiol. 2011;57:119–27.
4. Kasai T, Floras JS, Bradley TD. Sleep apnea and cardiovascular disease: a bidirectional relationship. Circulation. 2012;126:1495–510.
5. Sato A, Naito R, Kasai T. Screening for sleep apnea in atrial fibrillation prior to catheter ablation. Circ J. 2021;85:261–3.
6. Sato A, Matsumoto H, Kasai T. Home sleep apnea test for patients undergoing atrial fibrillation ablation: an alternative for polysomnography? J Arrhythm. 2023;39:799–800.
7. Bitter T, Langer C, Vogt J, Lange M, Horstkotte D, Oldenburg O. Sleep-disordered breathing in patients with atrial fibrillation and normal systolic left ventricular function. Dtsch Arztebl Int. 2009;106:164–70.
8. Maeno K, Kasai T, Kasagi S, Kawana F, Ishiwata S, Ohno M, et al. Relationship between atrial conduction delay and obstructive sleep apnea. Heart Vessel. 2013;28:639–45.
9. Maeno K, Kasagi S, Ueda A, Kawana F, Ishiwata S, Ohno M, et al. Effects of obstructive sleep apnea and its treatment on signal-averaged P-wave duration in men. Circ Arrhythm Electrophysiol. 2013;6:287–93.
10. Kasai T, Motwani SS, Yumino D, Gabriel JM, Montemurro LT, Amirthalingam V, et al. Contrasting effects of lower body positive pressure on upper airways resistance and partial pressure of carbon dioxide in men with heart failure and obstructive or central sleep apnea. J Am Coll Cardiol. 2013;61:1157–66.

11. Kasai T, Motwani SS, Elias RM, Gabriel JM, Taranto Montemurro L, Yanagisawa N, et al. Influence of rostral fluid shift on upper airway size and mucosal water content. J Clin Sleep Med. 2014;10:1069–74.
12. Kasai T. Fluid retention and rostral fluid shift in sleep-disordered breathing. Curr Hypertens Rev. 2016;12:32–42.
13. da Silva BC, Kasai T, Coelho FM, Zatz R, Elias RM. Fluid redistribution in sleep apnea: therapeutic implications in edematous states. Front Med (Lausanne). 2017;4:256.
14. Chin K, Ohi M, Kita H, Noguchi T, Otsuka N, Tsuboi T, et al. Effects of NCPAP therapy on fibrinogen levels in obstructive sleep apnea syndrome. Am J Respir Crit Care Med. 1996;153:1972–6.
15. Barcelo A, Pierola J, de la Pena M, Frontera G, Yanez A, Alonso-Fernandez A, et al. Impaired circadian variation of platelet activity in patients with sleep apnea. Sleep Breath. 2012;16:355–60.
16. Akashiba T, Inoue Y, Uchimura N, Ohi M, Kasai T, Kawana F, et al. Sleep apnea syndrome (SAS) clinical practice guidelines 2020. Respir Investig. 2022;60:3–32.
17. Traaen GM, Aakeroy L, Hunt TE, Overland B, Bendz C, Sande LO, et al. Effect of continuous positive airway pressure on arrhythmia in atrial fibrillation and sleep apnea: a randomized controlled trial. Am J Respir Crit Care Med. 2021;204:573–82.
18. Kasai T. Short-term effect of positive airway pressure therapy in patients with atrial fibrillation (AF) and sleep-disordered breathing (SDB) (SYNERGY-AF). 2019 [updated 2019; cited]. Available from: https://jrct.niph.go.jp/en-latest-detail/jRCTs032180344.
19. Bitter T, Faber L, Hering D, Langer C, Horstkotte D, Oldenburg O. Sleep-disordered breathing in heart failure with normal left ventricular ejection fraction. Eur J Heart Fail. 2009;11:602–8.
20. Suda S, Kasai T, Matsumoto H, Shiroshita N, Kato M, Kawana F, et al. Prevalence and clinical correlates of sleep-disordered breathing in patients hospitalized with acute decompensated heart failure. Can J Cardiol. 2018;34:784–90.
21. Sato A, Kato T, Kasai T, Ishiwata S, Yatsu S, Matsumoto H, et al. Relationship between inflammatory biomarkers and sleep-disordered breathing in patients with heart failure. Sleep Biol Rhythms. 2021;19:55–61.
22. Yumino D, Wang H, Floras JS, Newton GE, Mak S, Ruttanaumpawan P, et al. Prevalence and physiological predictors of sleep apnea in patients with heart failure and systolic dysfunction. J Card Fail. 2009;15:279–85.
23. Kasai T, Yumino D, Redolfi S, Su MC, Ruttanaumpawan P, Mak S, et al. Overnight effects of obstructive sleep apnea and its treatment on stroke volume in patients with heart failure. Can J Cardiol. 2015;31:832–8.
24. Wang H, Parker JD, Newton GE, Floras JS, Mak S, Chiu KL, et al. Influence of obstructive sleep apnea on mortality in patients with heart failure. J Am Coll Cardiol. 2007;49:1625–31.
25. Arikawa T, Toyoda S, Haruyama A, Amano H, Inami S, Otani N, et al. Impact of obstructive sleep apnoea on heart failure with preserved ejection fraction. Heart Lung Circ. 2016;25:435–41.
26. Tan JWC, Leow LC, Wong S, Khoo SM, Kasai T, Kojodjojo P, et al. Asian Pacific Society of Cardiology consensus statements on the diagnosis and management of obstructive sleep apnoea in patients with cardiovascular disease. Eur Cardiol. 2022;17:e16.
27. Fox H, Bitter T, Horstkotte D, Oldenburg O. Resolution of cheyne-stokes respiration after treatment of heart failure with sacubitril/valsartan: a first case report. Cardiology. 2017;137:96–9.
28. Passino C, Sciarrone P, Vergaro G, Borrelli C, Spiesshoefer J, Gentile F, et al. Sacubitril-valsartan treatment is associated with decrease in central apneas in patients with heart failure with reduced ejection fraction. Int J Cardiol. 2021;330:112–9.
29. Jaffuel D, Nogue E, Berdague P, Galinier M, Fournier P, Dupuis M, et al. Sacubitril-valsartan initiation in chronic heart failure patients impacts sleep apnea: the ENTRESTO-SAS study. ESC Heart Fail. 2021;8:2513–26.

30. Owens RL, Birkeland K, Heywood JT, Steinhubl SR, Dorn J, Grant D, et al. Sleep outcomes from AWAKE-HF: a randomized clinical trial of sacubitril/valsartan vs enalapril in patients with heart failure and reduced ejection fraction. J Card Fail. 2021;27:1466–71.
31. Bucca CB, Brussino L, Battisti A, Mutani R, Rolla G, Mangiardi L, et al. Diuretics in obstructive sleep apnea with diastolic heart failure. Chest. 2007;132:440–6.
32. Takahashi M, Kasai T, Dohi T, Maeno K, Kasagi S, Kawana F, et al. Conversion from predominant central sleep apnea to obstructive sleep apnea following valvuloplasty in a patient with mitral regurgitation. J Clin Sleep Med. 2011;7:523–5.
33. Doi S, Kasai T, Yatsu S, Miyazaki S, Fujimoto S, Okazaki S, et al. Changes in polysomnographic findings following transcatheter aortic valve implantation in a patient with aortic stenosis. J Cardiol Cases. 2020;21:75-8.
34. Naito R, Kasai T, Dohi T, Takaya H, Narui K, Momomura SI. Factors associated with the improvement of left ventricular systolic function by continuous positive airway pressure therapy in patients with heart failure with reduced ejection fraction and obstructive sleep apnea. Front Neurol. 2022;13:781054.
35. Kasai T, Narui K, Dohi T, Yanagisawa N, Ishiwata S, Ohno M, et al. Prognosis of patients with heart failure and obstructive sleep apnea treated with continuous positive airway pressure. Chest. 2008;133:690–6.
36. Tsutsui H, Isobe M, Ito H, Ito H, Okumura K, Ono M, et al. JCS 2017/JHFS 2017 guideline on diagnosis and treatment of acute and chronic heart failure – digest version. Circ J. 2019;83:2084–184.
37. Bradley TD, Logan AG, Kimoff RJ, Series F, Morrison D, Ferguson K, et al. Continuous positive airway pressure for central sleep apnea and heart failure. N Engl J Med. 2005;353:2025–33.
38. Cowie MR, Woehrle H, Wegscheider K, Angermann C, d'Ortho MP, Erdmann E, et al. Adaptive servo-ventilation for central sleep apnea in systolic heart failure. N Engl J Med. 2015;373:1095–105.
39. Momomura S, Seino Y, Kihara Y, Adachi H, Yasumura Y, Yokoyama H, et al. Adaptive servo-ventilation therapy for patients with chronic heart failure in a confirmatory, multicenter, randomized, controlled study. Circ J. 2015;79:981–90.
40. O'Connor CM, Whellan DJ, Fiuzat M, Punjabi NM, Tasissa G, Anstrom KJ, et al. Cardiovascular outcomes with minute ventilation-targeted adaptive servo-ventilation therapy in heart failure: the CAT-HF trial. J Am Coll Cardiol. 2017;69:1577–87.
41. Bradley TD, Logan AG, Lorenzi Filho G, Kimoff RJ, Duran Cantolla J, Arzt M, et al. Adaptive servo-ventilation for sleep-disordered breathing in patients with heart failure with reduced ejection fraction (ADVENT-HF): a multicentre, multinational, parallel-group, open-label, phase 3 randomised controlled trial. Lancet Respir Med. 2024;12:153–66.
42. Arzt M, Floras JS, Logan AG, Kimoff RJ, Series F, Morrison D, et al. Suppression of central sleep apnea by continuous positive airway pressure and transplant-free survival in heart failure: a post hoc analysis of the Canadian Continuous Positive Airway Pressure for Patients with Central Sleep Apnea and Heart Failure Trial (CANPAP). Circulation. 2007;115:3173–80.
43. Naito R, Kasai T, Tomita Y, Kasagi S, Narui K, Momomura SI. Clinical outcomes of chronic heart failure patients with unsuppressed sleep apnea by positive airway pressure therapy. Front Cardiovasc Med. 2023;10:1156353.
44. Kasai T, Kasagi S, Maeno K, Dohi T, Kawana F, Kato M, et al. Adaptive servo-ventilation in cardiac function and neurohormonal status in patients with heart failure and central sleep apnea nonresponsive to continuous positive airway pressure. JACC Heart Fail. 2013;1:58–63.
45. Yoshihisa A, Suzuki S, Yamaki T, Sugimoto K, Kunii H, Nakazato K, et al. Impact of adaptive servo-ventilation on cardiovascular function and prognosis in heart failure patients with preserved left ventricular ejection fraction and sleep-disordered breathing. Eur J Heart Fail. 2013;15:543–50.
46. The impact of low flow nocturnal oxygen therapy on hospital admissions and mortality in patients with heart failure and central sleep apnea (LOFT-HF). [cited]. Available from: https://clinicaltrials.gov/ct2/show/NCT03745898.

47. Costanzo MR, Ponikowski P, Javaheri S, Augostini R, Goldberg L, Holcomb R, et al. Transvenous neurostimulation for central sleep apnoea: a randomised controlled trial. Lancet. 2016;388:974–82.
48. Fox H, Oldenburg O, Javaheri S, Ponikowski P, Augostini R, Goldberg LR, et al. Long-term efficacy and safety of phrenic nerve stimulation for the treatment of central sleep apnea. Sleep. 2019;42:zsz158.
49. Costanzo MR, Ponikowski P, Coats A, Javaheri S, Augostini R, Goldberg LR, et al. Phrenic nerve stimulation to treat patients with central sleep apnoea and heart failure. Eur J Heart Fail. 2018;20:1746–54.
50. Ponikowski P, Javaheri S, Michalkiewicz D, Bart BA, Czarnecka D, Jastrzebski M, et al. Transvenous phrenic nerve stimulation for the treatment of central sleep apnoea in heart failure. Eur Heart J. 2012;33:889–94.

Chapter 11
SAS in Stroke and Coronary Artery Disease: What is Known About a Possible Association Between Coronary Artery Disease or Stroke and SAS

Yasuhiro Tomita

Abstract Coronary artery disease (CAD) and cerebrovascular disease (CVD) are serious conditions that have the potential to result in mortality. These disorders develop in the presence of hypertension and arteriosclerosis.

Studies have demonstrated that obstructive sleep apnea (OSA) can actively contribute to the advancement of arteriosclerosis and elevate blood pressure. There is speculation that OSA may contribute to the development of coronary artery disease and cerebrovascular disease. Also, studies have shown that sleep-disordered breathing (SDB), not only OSA but also central sleep apnea (CSA), becomes more common right after acute coronary syndrome (ACS) and in the early stages after a stroke. Hence, it is crucial to take into account the timing of SDB assessments while addressing the simultaneous presence of these conditions.

This chapter will first examine epidemiological research investigating the likelihood of individuals with OSA acquiring CAD and CVD. Additionally, it will analyze the progression of SDB following the occurrence of an acute phase of ACS or stroke. This study aims to look into the possible benefits of continuous positive airway pressure (CPAP) therapy in lowering the risk of developing CAD or CVD in people who have been diagnosed with OSA. Furthermore, it will underscore the significance of treating OSA following the occurrence of these illnesses. Lastly, it will investigate the potential mechanisms that explain the connection between OSA and these diseases.

Keywords Acute coronary syndrome (ACS) · Atherosclerosis · Cerebrovascular disease (CVD) · Coronary artery disease (CAD) · Stroke · Primary prevention · Secondary prevention

Y. Tomita (✉)
Sleep Center, Toranomon Hospital, Tokyo, Japan

K. Chin (ed.), *The Current State of Sleep Disordered Breathing in Japan and Around the World*, Respiratory Disease Series: Diagnostic Tools and Disease Managements, https://doi.org/10.1007/978-981-96-6030-8_11

1 Coronary Artery Disease

Coronary artery disease (CAD) impacts the coronary arteries, which are responsible for delivering oxygen and nutrients to the heart muscle. In the event that the arteries undergo constriction or blockage, the heart may encounter inadequate blood circulation, leading to a variety of complications. CAD can be categorized into two main types: effort angina and vasospastic angina. Effort angina is a medical disorder characterized by the gradual narrowing of the coronary arteries due to the accumulation of cholesterol and lipids on the arterial walls. This constriction restricts the flow of blood to the heart, resulting in symptoms such as angina or chest discomfort. Vasospastic angina is characterized by a brief constriction of the coronary arteries, which causes a sharp decrease in blood flow to the heart. This phenomenon may occur throughout the nighttime hours and could lead to attacks of angina. Although the symptoms of vasospastic angina may appear similar to those of stable angina, the fundamental cause of these two diseases differs.

Vasospastic angina typically begins during sleep, specifically during REM sleep, which occurs in the early morning. Increased activity and variations in the sympathetic nervous system, parasympathetic nervous system, and serotonin levels are characteristics of REM sleep. During this period, it is hypothesized that the coronary arteries are more prone to experiencing spasms. Nevertheless, there is a scarcity of studies on the correlation between vasospastic angina and OSA, and many aspects of the mechanism remain undisclosed. This chapter will mostly focus on effort angina.

Two further primary kinds of effort angina include stable angina and acute coronary syndrome (ACS). Stable angina is a condition that arises when the coronary arteries constrict as a result of atherosclerosis, leading to insufficient blood flow to the cardiac muscle. Exercise, or exerting oneself, is a common way to start it. Typically, chest pain or discomfort that worsens with exercise and goes away with rest characterizes stable angina. ACS is a medical disorder that occurs when there is a rapid blockage or decrease in blood flow in the coronary arteries. Plaque rupture is typically the cause of this blockage. The symptoms of ACS, such as chest pain or discomfort, resemble those of stable angina but persist even during periods of rest. ACS is more prevalent during the nocturnal and predawn periods.

1.1 CAD with a Background of OSA

The following are risk factors for CAD: smoking, male gender, dyslipidemia, diabetes, and hypertension. Patients with CAD often exhibit several risk factors, and it is possible for some to also have OSA in conjunction with these. Cohort research has shown that people with OSA have a greater likelihood of developing CAD in the future.

The Wisconsin Cohort Study [39] found that individuals with severe OSA (AHI > 30) had a hazard ratio of 3.8 (1.6–9.0) for overall mortality and 5.2 (1.4–19.2) for mortality related to cardiovascular events, compared to individuals without OSA (AHI < 5/h) during a period of 18 years. In addition, a subsequent study conducted over a period of 24 years [14] found that those with severe OSA had a hazard ratio of 2.6 for developing coronary artery disease or heart failure compared to those without OSA.

The Sleep Heart Health Study (SHHS) [34] likewise demonstrated a progressive rise in cardiovascular incidents based on the severity of SAS. The risk ratio for CAD was 1.27 when comparing the group with the highest severity (AHI > 11.0/h) to the group with the lowest severity (AHI < 1.3/h). The chances ratio for this was lower in comparison to heart failure (2.38) and stroke (1.58). The SHHS cohort was surveyed again in 2010 [9], and it was shown that the group with AHI ≥ 30 had a 1.68 times greater incidence of CAD compared to the control group. Nevertheless, OSA was determined to be a distinct hazard for cardiovascular events solely in males below the age of 70, with no correlation detected in older males or females.

The correlation between CAD and OSA is somewhat weaker than that observed with other cardiovascular conditions, such as hypertension. More precisely, there is a limited connection between CAD and mild OSA, and it is anticipated that severe OSA in males who are not elderly may be linked to the occurrence of CAD.

A study investigating the timing of the occurrence of ACS in individuals revealed a significant prevalence of OSA in patients whose ACS onset was during nocturnal sleep. Similarly, patients with OSA who had an implanted cardioverter-defibrillator (ICD) had a much higher risk of fatal arrhythmias while they slept at night. The occurrence of sudden death during the nighttime is more frequent when there is the presence of OSA, suggesting a cause-and-effect relationship [8]. If an ACS occurs, particularly during nocturnal sleep, there is a high likelihood of a correlation with OSA.

1.2 *Progress of SDB After ACS Onset*

The prevalence of SDB is elevated in patients with a prior diagnosis of CAD, particularly in ACS cases. Based on a study carried out on Japanese patients with ACS [40], it was shown that 57% of these patients had SDB, which is defined as having an AHI greater than 10 per hour. This study conducted a longitudinal observation of patients over a period of approximately 7 months. The findings revealed that patients with SDB experienced a significantly higher number of events, including cardiac death, recurrent myocardial infarction, and target vessel revascularization. The hazard ratio for these events was 11.6 times higher, with a confidence interval ranging from 2.2 to 62.2. Extensive studies have been conducted on stable-effort angina. Several studies indicate that SDB increases the likelihood of cardiovascular events and stent restenosis following percutaneous coronary intervention (PCI) treatment. However, contrasting findings have been reported in other studies where a distinct disparity is not observed. Presently, there is a lack of agreement over this issue. The importance of SDB treatment in secondary prevention following ACS will be addressed in a later section.

The incidence of SDB in ACS is documented to be greater than that in stable angina. Moruzzi et al. found that the occurrence rate of AHI ≥10 was around 22% in cases of acute myocardial infarction, which is roughly double the rate observed in chronic CAD. Additionally, they observed an occurrence rate of nearly 36% in cases with ACS [25]. This may suggest that SDB is associated with more unstable conditions of the coronary arteries or that unstable conditions like ACS can worsen SDB. In a study by Tsukamoto et al., polysomnography done on days 3–5 after ACS showed that both OSA and CSA got worse temporarily compared to polysomnography done during the chronic phase [37]. SDB is thought to be caused by a number of things, such as CSA from unstable blood flow and increased sympathetic nerve activity in conditions like ACS, changes in sleep architecture from having to rest a lot in cardiac care units, and OSA getting worse when lying on your back. Hayashi et al. [13] noted a significant decrease in the average AHI from 22.0 to 18.5 when comparing the 14th day from the onset of ACS to 2 months after the commencement. The observed enhancement might be attributable to a notable improvement in CSA and a tendency for OSA to remain. This suggests that CSA arises as a consequence of ACS onset and gradually ameliorates with time.

1.3 Primary Prevention of CAD Using CPAP

I have been examining the potential correlation between severe OSA and the likelihood of developing CAD, including ACS. Observational studies can offer insights into the potential of continuous positive airway pressure (CPAP) therapy to mitigate the risk of developing CAD.

Based on a Spanish observational study, it was found that patients with OSA who received CPAP treatment had a similar occurrence of cardiovascular events compared to a control group without OSA [20]. This study presents compelling evidence that the treatment of severe OSA is crucial in order to enhance the prognosis. Nevertheless, a randomized controlled trial carried out by Barbe et al. yielded inconclusive results regarding the preventative impact of CPAP on cardiovascular events [3]. Post-hoc subgroup analysis demonstrated a notable reduction in cardiovascular events, specifically among patients who utilized CPAP for a duration exceeding 4 h. Extended utilization of CPAP is recommended to potentially enhance the prognosis of CAD, with a strong emphasis on adhering to CPAP therapy to anticipate improvements in cardiovascular outcomes.

1.4 Secondary Prevention for CAD Patients Using CPAP

Multiple observational studies have provided evidence about the significance of CPAP therapy in the secondary prevention of CAD following its onset. These studies have investigated the potential of positive pressure treatments, such as CPAP, to enhance the prognosis of CAD associated with OSA. According to a study by Milleron et al. [22], CAD patients who received OSA treatment had a noticeably lower rate of events over a 7.2-year follow-up period than the group who did not. Cassar et al. [6] looked into the effects of CPAP therapy on patients with post-PCI OSA in a separate investigation. The study revealed that the group of patients who received CPAP treatment experienced a considerably lower rate of cardiovascular mortality in comparison to the group that did not receive any treatment. Nevertheless, this specific investigation did not reveal any notable disparity in cardiovascular events between the two groups.

The SAVE trial [21], a randomized controlled trial published in 2016, included 2717 individuals between the ages of 45 and 75 who had a previous diagnosis of CAD or CVD complicated by OSA. These individuals did not exhibit an abnormal level of sleepiness during the day, as indicated by an Epworth Sleepiness Scale (ESS) score of less than 15. The participants were randomized to either the CPAP group or the non-CPAP group. The occurrence of cardiovascular death, myocardial infarction, stroke, unstable angina, heart failure, or transient ischemic attack was assessed as the endpoint. The investigation revealed that the utilization of CPAP did not enhance the prognosis of cardiovascular events. A drawback of the SAVE trial was the relatively low average CPAP usage time of approximately 3.3 h, indicating that inadequate adherence to CPAP treatment may have compromised its efficacy. Furthermore, the results may have been influenced by the exclusion criteria for severe daytime sleepiness (ESS $\geq$15) and severe hypoxemia ($SpO2 \leq 80\%$ recorded for more than 10% of the time).

The RICCADSA study [29] examined 244 individuals who had recently undergone treatment for CAD and were diagnosed with moderate to severe OSA with an AHI greater than 15 per hour. These individuals did not experience excessive daytime sleepiness, as indicated by an ESS score of less than 10. The participants were allocated at random to either the CPAP group or the non-CPAP group, and their progress was monitored for a median duration of 57 months. There was no significant difference in the occurrence of major composite cardiovascular outcomes between the two groups. Nevertheless, after conducting an analysis that accounts for treatment adjustments, it was seen that patients who utilized CPAP for over 4 h experienced a notable decrease in cardiovascular risk, in contrast to patients who used the devices for less than 4 h or did not receive any treatment. Like the SAVE study, there were concerns regarding the relatively brief average usage duration of CPAP, suggesting that low adherence may have impacted the findings. The removal of people who experience extreme daytime sleepiness and the small number of severe cases may have an impact on the findings. This is significant because severe

OSA is known to have a stronger correlation with negative cardiovascular outcomes when compared to mild or moderate OSA.

The ISSACC study [32] was a multicenter study carried out at 15 institutions in Spain, with a specific focus on patients with ACS. Within the timeframe of 24–72 h after being admitted to the hospital, a total of 2834 patients underwent respiratory polygraphy. Out of these patients, 1264 were diagnosed with OSA and were randomly divided into two groups: the CPAP group and the usual care group. The patients were monitored for a median duration of 3.35 years, and there was no disparity in the occurrence of cardiovascular events between the two groups. The average duration of CPAP therapy utilization was 2.78 h. The relatively shorter mean CPAP usage duration observed in this study could perhaps account for the absence of a statistically significant disparity in incident frequency. Additional investigation is required to assess the impact of CPAP in individuals with severe hypoxemia linked to ischemic heart disease or those who utilize CPAP for a duration exceeding 4 h.

1.5 Possible Mechanism Between OSA and CAD

Atherosclerotic plaque buildup in the coronary arteries is the main cause of CAD. VH-IVUS is able to quantify the number of these plaques. Tan et al. [36] conducted a study on 118 patients with CAD who underwent angiography and VH-IVUS. The study found that 34.4% of these patients had moderate to severe OSA with an AHI of more than 15. Within this group of patients, those with OSA or mild OSA had smaller atheroma volumes in comparison to patients without OSA. The observed correlation remained statistically significant even after controlling for age, BMI, hypertension, diabetes, smoking, and hyperlipidemia. In patients with coronary artery disease, moderate to severe OSA was independently associated with a larger atheroma volume within the coronary arteries. Intravascular ultrasonography and coronary artery CT scans have both shown a correlation between OSA and the development of coronary artery atherosclerosis in additional studies. There is a high association between the severity of OSA and the severity of coronary artery atherosclerosis. A meta-analysis study found a significant correlation between the severity of OSA and the extent of coronary artery calcification [11].

The plaques found in the coronary arteries are indicative of one of the arterial modifications linked to systemic atherosclerosis. Arterial stiffening has been verified to advance not just in the coronary arteries but also in other arteries among people with OSA. Episodic periods of low oxygen levels and subsequent reoxygenation produced by OSA trigger inflammation and oxidative stress in the body, leading to impaired functioning of the endothelium (Drager et al., J Am Coll Cardiol. 2013 Aug 13;62(7):569–76). Endothelial dysfunction is the initial stage of arterial calcification, and the presence of arterial calcification in the coronary arteries can be referred to as coronary artery disease. Elevated levels of inflammatory markers, including high-sensitivity C-reactive protein, interleukin-6, and tumor necrosis factor-alpha, have been observed in individuals with OSA [38]. Vascular endothelial function tests, such as flow-mediated vasodilation (FMD) and reactive hyperemia peripheral arterial tonometry (RH-PAT), indicate that endothelial function improves in individuals with OSA after CPAP treatment. This suggests the existence of reversible variables [5, 11]. ACS arises in the presence of coronary artery atherosclerosis, and it is hypothesized that the instability of plaque and anomalies in blood clotting caused by OSA play a role. Moreover, the presence of SDB is likely to contribute to the occurrence of ACS as a result of the high probability of concomitant polycythemia. Polycythemia elevates the likelihood of thrombosis development, which can contribute to the occurrence of thrombosis in ACS. Nighttime low oxygen levels cause more erythropoietin to be made, which is thought to play a part in the development of polycythemia [28, 41]. There is a belief that increased platelet aggregation and activation of the coagulation system during nocturnal breathing events affect thrombus formation [23].

Although the explanation for the increased susceptibility of coronary arteries to arterial stiffening in people with OSA can be provided, it should be noted that not all patients experience positive outcomes from OSA treatment in randomized controlled trials. Previous discussions have indicated that the effectiveness of treatment is restricted when the duration of CPAP usage is short, and individuals with lower levels of daytime sleepiness may encounter challenges in feeling the advantages. There is a hypothesis suggesting that the AHI may not accurately predict cardiovascular events in OSA. This is because the AHI measures the number of recurrent respiratory episodes rather than the severity of intermittent hypoxia. A study proposed that a hypoxic burden index, which measures the severity of intermittent hypoxia, would be a more suitable measure [1]. Prognostic predictions based on indicators such as ΔHR, which measures the pulse-rate response linked to respiratory events [2], and pulse wave amplitude drops (PWADs), which indicate sympathetic activations and vasoreactivity, have recently gained significant interest [35].

2 Stroke

Stroke is categorized as cerebral infarction or cerebral hemorrhage, with hypertension being a significant contributing factor to both. Cerebral infarction, commonly known as ischemic stroke, happens when the blood vessels in the brain get obstructed. Hypertension causes endothelial damage, leading to the formation of thrombi within the blood vessels. The formation of this blood clot obstructs the blood flow in the brain's blood vessels, leading to cerebral infarction. Cerebral hemorrhage is the result of the rupture of blood vessels in the brain. Hypertension compromises the integrity of blood vessel walls, rendering them more vulnerable to rupture.

Cerebral infarction is often categorized into two main types: atherosclerotic and embolic. Atherosclerotic cerebral infarction refers to the pathological process in which the walls of blood vessels thicken and narrow. During this condition, there is a blockage in the flow of blood, which can lead to the formation of blood clots or plaques within the blood vessels. The primary factors are thought to be lifestyle-related, including hypertension, elevated cholesterol levels, smoking, and diabetes. Embolic cerebral infarction refers to the obstruction of blood vessels by emboli. Atrial fibrillation, a heart arrhythmia, is the primary reason. Atrial fibrillation raises the risk of thrombus formation in the heart, which then lets them move through the circulatory system and block blood vessels in the brain, leading to a cerebral infarction.

OSA is considered to be a cause of both atherosclerosis and atrial fibrillation, and it is speculated that intervention for OSA, which often coexists, is important for the prevention of cerebral infarction.

2.1 Stroke with a Background of OSA

OSA can heighten the likelihood of developing vascular conditions, such as stroke. There is much documentation indicating that snoring, which is a prominent symptom of OSA, is a separate and significant factor that increases the risk of stroke [27].

The SHHS cohort study examined the occurrence of new ischemic strokes in 5442 individuals without a prior history of stroke. The study had a median observation period of 8.7 years [30]. The group of individuals with the highest OAHI (>19) had a hazard ratio of 2.86 (95% confidence interval, 1.1–7.3) compared to the group without OSA (OAHI<4). The correlation was notably robust among males, with an estimated 6% increase in the risk of stroke for every 1/h rise in OAHI. The risk in females was considerably heightened when considering just severe cases (defined as OAHI >25).

Similar to ACS, the timing of stroke onset has also been investigated [24]. Out of the individuals who experienced stroke symptoms upon waking up, 72.5% (29 out of 40 persons) had OSA, which was a higher occurrence compared to the group that had a stroke during the daytime (45%, or 30 out of 67 individuals). This implies a potential correlation between OSA and stroke events that happen while sleeping.

2.2 Progress of SDB After Stroke Onset

The prevalence of SDB with an AHI greater than 5 was found to be 72% in a meta-analysis of 2343 patients with ischemic or hemorrhagic stroke and transient ischemic attack [16]. The incidence of SDB with an AHI greater than 20 was 38%, indicating a higher occurrence relative to the general population. The study indicates that the prevalence of SDB did not alter significantly depending on the timing of testing after stroke. However, the majority of the research included in the study was performed within 1 month of the stroke's beginning.

The occurrence of SDB diminishes as the stroke advances. A comparative study conducted on the occurrence of SDB during different phases of stroke recovery revealed that the prevalence of SDB with an AHI of 15 or higher per hour was 50.3% in the acute phase (within 1 month), 44.3% in the subacute phase (within 3 months), and 33.1% in the chronic phase (3 months or later) [12]. Another study [26] found that severe SDB decreased after 3 months, while mild SDB increased. Moreover, both OSA and CSA are frequently reported in stroke patients. Specifically, in the immediate phase up to 3 months following a stroke, the occurrence of OSA reduces, whereas the occurrence of CSA tends to stay the same.

2.3 *Primary Prevention of Stroke Using CPAP*

A meta-analysis has been conducted to assess whether CPAP therapy can mitigate the likelihood of future stroke in individuals diagnosed with OSA [18]. The analysis included nine randomized controlled trials and four cohort studies. The cohort trials demonstrated a substantial decrease in the likelihood of experiencing a stroke when undergoing CPAP therapy. Nevertheless, the randomized controlled trials did not see a statistically significant disparity, resulting in contradictory findings when compared to the cohort studies. Analysis of subgroups, categorized by adherence to CPAP treatment and the degree of OSA at the time of diagnosis, showed a noteworthy decrease in the risk of stroke in the subgroup with high CPAP adherence and in the subgroup with moderate to severe OSA. The significance of adhering to CPAP treatment was also noted in the main prevention of CAD. The results of this study are consistent with the SHHS cohort study, which showed a correlation between more severe OSA and a higher likelihood of experiencing a stroke.

2.4 *Secondary Prevention for Stroke Patients Using CPAP*

The neurological prognosis is of paramount importance in cases of stroke. OSA has been found to be linked with deteriorating neurological outcomes following a stroke, as demonstrated by prospective cohort research [19, 26]. The 2020 European statement [4] emphasizes that untreated OSA can result in deteriorated clinical out comes and heightened overall mortality. OSA exacerbates neurological outcomes following a stroke through many processes, such as hypoxia, harm to the penumbra region of cerebral infarction, and necrosis in places that can be restored. Hence, it is crucial to promptly detect and treat OSA at its first stage. Nevertheless, establishing a link between diagnosis and treatment in practice can prove to be difficult during the acute period.

CPAP therapy is beneficial for the secondary prevention of stroke. Nevertheless, according to statistics, a mere 22% of people with OSA undergo therapy following a stroke [7]. Stroke patients, particularly the elderly or those with hand paralysis, typically rely on caregivers for help with tasks such as fitting a mask and other aspects of using CPAP. The study examined 191 patients with cerebral infarction and OSA who needed CPAP treatment. The rates of CPAP usage at 3 months, 6 months, 12 months, 24 months, and 60 months after the stroke occurred were 58%, 53%, 48%, 45%, and 39%, respectively. These findings indicate a gradual decline in CPAP usage over time [17]. Significantly, the most substantial dropouts happened within the initial 3 months. Given the potential for variations in the severity of OSA between the subacute and chronic phases, it would be advantageous to reassess and potentially revise the treatment approach throughout the chronic phase.

CPAP has been utilized in clinical trials to address the difficulties of OSA following a stroke and evaluate the neurological outlook. However, these investigations are often conducted on a limited scale and have yielded few notable findings. Research conducted on individuals who used CPAP for a duration of 1–2 months and for a short period of time each night did not demonstrate any notable enhancement in neurological function [15, 33]. Nonetheless, a randomized controlled trial that compared a group of 22 participants using CPAP with a control group showed that the CPAP group experienced enhanced neurological function after 1 month. The CPAP group had an average CPAP usage time of around 5 h [31]. A subsequent randomized controlled trial, conducted over a period of 1 year and with participants who demonstrated good adherence to CPAP therapy (with an average usage time of 4.2 h and a mean usage rate of 76% of days), found no significant disparity in the occurrence of vascular events between the CPAP group (34 participants) and the control group (36 participants) [10].

2.5 The Possible Mechanism Between OSA and Stroke

It is crucial to acknowledge the significant correlation between stroke and OSA. The connection is thought to be attributable to shared risk factors as well as the specific characteristics and coexisting medical conditions of OSA. Indeed, certain risk factors associated with stroke, such as male gender, obesity, hypertension, and diabetes, also contribute to the likelihood of OSA. These findings indicate that the frequent occurrence of comorbidity between stroke and OSA is probably due to the fact that they share similar underlying mechanisms.

In cases of obstructive sleep apnea (OSA) accompanied by high blood pressure and nocturnal dyspnea, the blood pressure can rapidly rise to levels exceeding 200 mmHg. These nocturnal blood pressure elevations are expected to be associated with nocturnal strokes. Atrial fibrillation, frequently coexisting with OSA, is a major factor in the occurrence of ischemic stroke.

Atherosclerosis, which is also discussed in the CAD section, is an additional factor that contributes to the link between stroke and OSA, in addition to the shared risk factors. OSA is known to be associated with atherosclerosis, a condition characterized by the buildup of plaque in the arteries. Cerebral artery atherosclerosis can lead to a stroke.

Additionally, it is noteworthy that individuals who have experienced a stroke frequently spend an increased amount of time in a supine posture, which entails reclining on their backs. The combination of this posture and the reduced movement of the paralyzed chest can result in a reduction in lung capacity. The reduction in lung capacity can be detrimental for those with OSA since it can exacerbate the underlying mechanisms of the disorder. Hence, it is unsurprising that OSA is more commonly detected during the acute phase of stroke. Stroke can directly impact respiratory control and potentially lead to breathing instability during sleep, depending on the specific area of disability. The respiratory instability mentioned can contribute to the development of both OSA and CSA.

To summarize, the relationship between stroke and OSA is intricate and influenced by multiple factors. The phenomenon encompasses shared risk factors, the influence of atherosclerosis, and the respiratory consequences of post-stroke impairments. Gaining insight into these associations is essential for delivering holistic treatment to individuals with stroke and OSA.

References

1. Azarbarzin A, Sands SA, Stone KL, et al. The hypoxic burden of sleep apnoea predicts cardiovascular disease-related mortality: the osteoporotic fractures in men study and the sleep heart health study. Eur Heart J. 2018;40:1149–57. https://doi.org/10.1093/eurheartj/ehy624.
2. Azarbarzin A, Sands SA, Younes M, et al. The sleep apnea–specific pulse-rate response predicts cardiovascular morbidity and mortality. Am J Respir Crit Care Med. 2021;203:1546–55. https://doi.org/10.1164/rccm.202010-3900oc.
3. Barbé F, Durán-Cantolla J, Sánchez-de-la-Torre M, et al. Effect of continuous positive airway pressure on the incidence of hypertension and cardiovascular events in nonsleepy patients with obstructive sleep apnea. JAMA. 2012;307:2161. https://doi.org/10.1001/jama.2012.4366.
4. Bassetti CLA, Randerath W, Vignatelli L, et al. EAN/ERS/ESO/ESRS statement on the impact of sleep disorders on risk and outcome of stroke. Eur J Neurol. 2020;27:1117–36. https://doi.org/10.1111/ene.14201.
5. Bayram NA, Ciftci B, Keles T, et al. Endothelial function in normotensive men with obstructive sleep apnea before and 6 months after CPAP treatment. Sleep. 2009;32:1257–63. https://doi.org/10.1093/sleep/32.10.1257.
6. Cassar A, Morgenthaler TI, Lennon RJ, et al. Treatment of obstructive sleep apnea is associated with decreased cardiac death after percutaneous coronary intervention. J Am Coll Cardiol. 2007;50:1310–4. https://doi.org/10.1016/j.jacc.2007.06.028.
7. Festic N, Alejos D, Bansal V, et al. Sleep apnea in patients hospitalized with acute ischemic stroke: underrecognition and associated clinical outcomes. J Clin Sleep Med. 2018;14:75–80. https://doi.org/10.5664/jcsm.6884.
8. Gami AS, Howard DE, Olson EJ, Somers VK. Day–night pattern of sudden death in obstructive sleep apnea. N Engl J Med. 2005;352:1206–14. https://doi.org/10.1056/nejmoa041832.
9. Gottlieb DJ, Yenokyan G, Newman AB, et al. Prospective study of obstructive sleep apnea and incident coronary heart disease and heart failure. Circulation. 2010;122:352–60. https://doi.org/10.1161/circulationaha.109.901801.
10. Gupta A, Shukla G, Afsar M, et al. Role of positive airway pressure therapy for obstructive sleep apnea in patients with stroke: a randomized controlled trial. J Clin Sleep Med. 2018;14:511–21. https://doi.org/10.5664/jcsm.7034.

11. Hao W, Wang X, Fan J, et al. Association between apnea-hypopnea index and coronary artery calcification: a systematic review and meta-analysis. Ann Med. 2021;53:302–17. https://doi.org/10.1080/07853890.2021.1875137.
12. Hasan F, Gordon C, Wu D, et al. Dynamic prevalence of sleep disorders following stroke or transient ischemic attack. Stroke. 2021;52:655–63. https://doi.org/10.1161/strokeaha.120.029847.
13. Hayashi H, Fukuma N, Kato K, et al. Clinical backgrounds and the time course of sleep-disordered breathing in patients after myocardial infarction. J Nippon Med Sch. 2013;80:192–9. https://doi.org/10.1272/jnms.80.192.
14. Hla KM, Young T, Hagen EW, et al. Coronary heart disease incidence in sleep disordered breathing: the Wisconsin sleep cohort study. Sleep. 2015;38:677–84. https://doi.org/10.5665/sleep.4654.
15. Hsu C-Y. Sleep-disordered breathing after stroke: a randomised controlled trial of continuous positive airway pressure. J Neurol Neurosurg Psychiatry. 2006;77:1143–9. https://doi.org/10.1136/jnnp.2005.086686.
16. Johnson KG, Johnson DC. Frequency of sleep apnea in stroke and TIA patients: a meta-analysis. J Clin Sleep Med. 2010;06:131–7. https://doi.org/10.5664/jcsm.27760.
17. Kendzerska T, Wilton K, Bahar R, Ryan CM. Short- and long-term continuous positive airway pressure usage in the post-stroke population with obstructive sleep apnea. Sleep Breathing. 2019;23:1233–44. https://doi.org/10.1007/s11325-019-01811-9.
18. Lin H-J, Yeh J-H, Hsieh M-T, Hsu C-Y. Continuous positive airway pressure with good adherence can reduce risk of stroke in patients with moderate to severe obstructive sleep apnea: an updated systematic review and meta-analysis. Sleep Med Rev. 2020;54:101354. https://doi.org/10.1016/j.smrv.2020.101354.
19. Lisabeth LD, Sánchez BN, Lim D, et al. Sleep-disordered breathing and poststroke outcomes. Ann Neurol. 2019;86:241–50. https://doi.org/10.1002/ana.25515.
20. Marin J, Carrizo S, Vicente E, Agusti A. Long-term cardiovascular outcomes in men with obstructive sleep apnoea-hypopnoea with or without treatment with continuous positive airway pressure: an observational study. Lancet. 2005;365:1046–53. https://doi.org/10.1016/s0140-6736(05)74229-x.
21. McEvoy RD, Antic NA, Heeley E, et al. CPAP for prevention of cardiovascular events in obstructive sleep apnea. N Engl J Med. 2016;375:919–31. https://doi.org/10.1056/nejmoa1606599.
22. Milleron O. Benefits of obstructive sleep apnoea treatment in coronary artery disease: a long-term follow-up study. Eur Heart J. 2004;25:728–34. https://doi.org/10.1016/j.ehj.2004.02.008.
23. Minoguchi K, Yokoe T, Tazaki T, et al. Silent brain infarction and platelet activation in obstructive sleep apnea. Am J Respir Crit Care Med. 2007;175:612–7. https://doi.org/10.1164/rccm.200608-1141oc.
24. Mohammad Y, Almutlaq A, Al-Ruwaita A, et al. Stroke during sleep and obstructive sleep apnea: there is a link. Neurol Sci. 2019;40:1001–5. https://doi.org/10.1007/s10072-019-03753-2.
25. Moruzzi P, Sarzi-Braga S, Rossi M, Contini M. Sleep apnoea in ischaemic heart disease: differences between acute and chronic coronary syndromes. Heart. 1999;82:343–7. https://doi.org/10.1136/hrt.82.3.343.
26. Ott SR, Fanfulla F, Miano S, et al. SAS care 1: sleep-disordered breathing in acute stroke an transient ischaemic attack—prevalence, evolution and association with functional outcome at 3 months, a prospective observational polysomnography study. ERJ Open Res. 2020;6:00334–2019. https://doi.org/10.1183/23120541.00334-2019.
27. Partinen M, Palomaki H. Snoring and cerebral infarction. Lancet. 1985;326:1325–6. https://doi.org/10.1016/s0140-6736(85)92625-x.
28. Pathak R, Giri S, Karmacharya P, Aryal MR. Obstructive sleep apnea syndrome and secondary polycythemia: analysis of the nationwide inpatient sample. Sleep Med. 2015;16:205–6. https://doi.org/10.1016/j.sleep.2014.09.012.

29. Peker Y, Glantz H, Eulenburg C, et al. Effect of positive airway pressure on cardiovascular outcomes in coronary artery disease patients with nonsleepy obstructive sleep apnea. The RICCADSA randomized controlled trial. Am J Respir Crit Care Med. 2016;194:613–20. https://doi.org/10.1164/rccm.201601-0088oc.
30. Redline S. Obstructive sleep apnea–hypopnea and incident stroke: the sleep heart health study. Am J Respir Crit Care Med. 2010;182:1332–3. https://doi.org/10.1164/ajrccm.182.10.1332b.
31. Ryan CM, Bayley M, Green R, et al. Influence of continuous positive airway pressure on outcomes of rehabilitation in stroke patients with obstructive sleep apnea. Stroke. 2011;42:1062–7. https://doi.org/10.1161/strokeaha.110.597468.
32. Sánchez-de-la-Torre M, Sánchez-de-la-Torre A, Bertran S, et al. Effect of obstructive sleep apnoea and its treatment with continuous positive airway pressure on the prevalence of cardiovascular events in patients with acute coronary syndrome (ISAACC study): a randomised controlled trial. Lancet Respir Med. 2020;8:359–67. https://doi.org/10.1016/S2213-2600(19)30271-1.
33. Sandberg O, Franklin KA, Bucht G, et al. Nasal continuous positive airway pressure in stroke patients with sleep apnoea: a randomized treatment study. Eur Respir J. 2001;18:630–4. https://doi.org/10.1183/09031936.01.00070301.
34. Shahar E, Whitney CW, Redline S, et al. Sleep-disordered breathing and cardiovascular disease. Am J Respir Crit Care Med. 2001;163:19–25. https://doi.org/10.1164/ajrccm.163.1.2001008.
35. Solelhac G, Sánchez-de-la-Torre M, Blanchard M, et al. Pulse wave amplitude drops index: a biomarker of cardiovascular risk in obstructive sleep apnea. Am J Respir Crit Care Med. 2023;207:1620–32. https://doi.org/10.1164/rccm.202206-1223oc.
36. Tan A, Hau W, Ho H-H, et al. OSA and coronary plaque characteristics. Chest. 2014;145:322–30. https://doi.org/10.1378/chest.13-1163.
37. Tsukamoto K, Ohara A. Temporal worsening of sleep-disordered breathing in the acute phase of myocardial infarction. Circ J. 2006;70:1553–6. https://doi.org/10.1253/circj.70.1553.
38. Yokoe T, Minoguchi K, Matsuo H, et al. Elevated levels of C-reactive protein and Interleukin-6 in patients with obstructive sleep apnea syndrome are decreased by nasal continuous positive airway pressure. Circulation. 2003;107:1129–34. https://doi.org/10.1161/01.cir.0000052627.99976.18.
39. Young T. Sleep disordered breathing and mortality: eighteen-year follow-up of the Wisconsin sleep cohort. Sleep. 2008; https://doi.org/10.5665/sleep/31.8.1071.
40. Yumino D, Tsurumi Y, Takagi A, et al. Impact of obstructive sleep apnea on clinical and angiographic outcomes following percutaneous coronary intervention in patients with acute coronary syndrome. Am J Cardiol. 2007;99:26–30. https://doi.org/10.1016/j.amjcard.2006.07.055.
41. Zhang X-B, Zeng Y-M, Zeng H-Q, et al. Erythropoietin levels in patients with sleep apnea: a meta-analysis. Eur Arch Otorrinolaringol. 2017;274:2505–12. https://doi.org/10.1007/s00405-017-4483-1.

Part IV
The Social Issue

Chapter 12
Use of Hypnotics

Yuuki Matsumoto, Naohisa Uchimura, and Hiroyuki Mori

Abstract Sleeping pills should not initially be used in the treatment of OSA patients with insomnia. The treatment of OSA itself should be prioritized. If insomnia is present despite the proper use of CPAP, we suggest the use of sleeping pills. Problems with the use of sleeping pills may include the aggravation OSA, for example, decreased respiratory events due to decreased upper airway hypotonia and decreased ventilatory response, along with prolonged respiratory event time. It has been reported that orexin receptor antagonists can mildly suppress a decrease in average SpO2, but as they are new drugs, there are still not many reports on them.

Keywords OSA · CPAP · Sleeping pills

The following research question and the answer along with its explanation are based on references [1] and [2].

Clinical Question 1
Do you prescribe sleeping pills for insomnia in OSA patients?

- Sleeping pills should not initially be used in the treatment of OSA patients with insomnia. The treatment of OSA itself should be prioritized.

Clinical Question 2
What are the side effects of hypnotic treatment for insomnia in OSA patients?

This chapter is based on the guidelines published in *Sleep and Biological Rhythms* (https://doi.org/10.1007/s41105-021-00353-6) and *Respiratory Investigation* (https://doi.org/10.1016/j.resinv.2021.08.010).

Y. Matsumoto (✉)
Kurume University School of Nursing, Kurume, Japan
e-mail: yuuki_m@kurume-u.ac.jp

N. Uchimura · H. Mori
Department of Neuropsychiatry, Kurume University School of Medicine, Kurume, Japan

K. Chin (ed.), *The Current State of Sleep Disordered Breathing in Japan and Around the World*, Respiratory Disease Series: Diagnostic Tools and Disease Managements, https://doi.org/10.1007/978-981-96-6030-8_12

- The results differ depending on the drug; however, an increase in the number of events, along with extension of the event time, has been reported, particularly in severe cases.

Clinical Question 3
Are sleeping pills effective for improving adherence in patients using CPAP?

- If insomnia is present despite the proper use of CPAP, we suggest the use of sleeping pills.

Clinical Question 4
What are the side effects of hypnotic treatment for CSA?

- While reports on the number of events before and after use for CSA, sleep construction, sleepiness, etc. do exist, the number of reports is too small to require further investigation.

Explanation
(a) Insomnia Treatment and Sleeping Pills for OSA

Insomnia is an insurance-covered indication for sleeping pills, but if used for the treatment of OSA itself, it will not be covered by insurance.

It is said that the probability of insomnia observed in OSA is 39–55%, which is not small, and sleeping pills are often taken because insomnia adversely affects CPAP adherence. Problems with the use of sleeping pills may include the aggravation OSA, for example, decreased respiratory events due to decreased upper airway hypotonia and decreased ventilatory response, along with prolonged respiratory event time [3, 4].

A randomized controlled trial of triazolam 0.25 mg and a placebo, conducted in 12 patients with severe OSA, found a significant increase in hypopnea/apnea time and a decrease in the minimum SpO_2 observed during non-REM sleep, indicating that sleeping pills exhibited adverse effects for severe OSA [5].

It is said that ramelteon, a melatonin receptor agonist, along with zolpidem and eszopiclone, which are non-benzodiazepine hypnotics, has no muscle relaxant effect and can be taken relatively safely. On the other hand, there are many reports indicating that even benzodiazepine hypnotics do not aggravate the condition in moderate OSA.

Randomized controlled trials of ramelteon 16 mg (double the dose in Japan) and a placebo in 26 patients with mild to moderate OSA have indicated no adverse effects on AHI or SpO_2 [6], while randomized controlled trials using the benzodiazepine hypnotics flurazepam, temazepam, nitrazepam and zolpidem, and ramelteon have indicated improved sleep, with no significantly adverse effects on OSA [7].

A randomized controlled trial, with a placebo using the benzodiazepine hypnotic nitrazepam 10 mg, in 14 mild to moderate OSA patients, found that the nitrazepam administration group exhibited an increase in total sleep time, with no worsening AHI and minimum SpO_2 [8].

Although there is still little research on suvorexant, which is an orexin receptor antagonist, a study of 26 patients with mild to moderate OSA, who received 40 mg, which is twice the usual dose in the United States and Japan, also reported that the decrease in AHI and mean SpO_2 was clinically very mild [9].

However, while many studies target mild to moderate OSA, it is important for severe OSA patients to take sleeping pills for control along with treatment such as CPAP (refer to next section "(b) CPAP treatment and hypnotics").

Lemborexant, also an orexin receptor antagonist, is the newest sleep medication on the market. Although few studies have been reported on this drug, a randomized controlled trial of 33 patients with moderate to severe OSA reported no significant changes in AHI or peripheral oxygen saturation after single or multiple 10 mg doses of Lemborexant [10].

(b) CPAP Treatment and Hypnotics

Randomized controlled trials of a placebo and zolpidem 10 mg, in patients with severe OSA receiving CPAP therapy, have indicated that zolpidem does not diminish the therapeutic effect of CPAP [11], with reports also indicating that the use of sleeping pills improved sleep parameters and CPAP adherence during titration. A study in which eszopiclone 3 mg was administered to 226 OSA patients, in order to compare with a placebo, found that the eszopiclone group exhibited an increase in total sleep time and sleep efficiency, a decrease in sleep latency and interrupted sleep time, and residual AHI [12], while another randomized controlled trial of a placebo and eszopiclone 3 mg in 98 OSA patients found that the group receiving eszopiclone 3 mg during CPAP titration had significantly higher CPAP usage and overnight usage time 4–6 weeks after CPAP introduction [13]. A randomized controlled trial of eszopiclone 3 mg and placebo in 160 severe OSA patients indicated that the eszopiclone group had significantly higher CPAP usage and overnight use time [14]. Furthermore, a meta-analysis of the effect of non-benzodiazepine sedative hypnotics use on CPAP adherence in patients with OSA found the best adherence with eszopiclone [15].

As mentioned above, the combined use of CPAP and sleeping pills is considered to be effective for improving compliance.

(c) CSA/CSB Treatment and Sleeping Pills

The indication for sleeping pills is insomnia, so if sleeping pills are used as a treatment for CSA and CSB, they will not be covered by insurance.

Biberdorf et al. used 15 mg of temazepam (not yet released in Japan, one of the metabolites of diazepam) for CSB associated with moderate to severe congestive heart failure in seven patients in order to alleviate the rate of sleep stage 1, AHI in sleep stage 1, wakefulness time during sleep, and daytime sleepiness, reporting that no exacerbation of CSB was observed [16]. Bonnet also reported that triazolam 0.125 mg and 0.25 mg was administered to five male patients with central apnea in order to increase the total sleep time and decrease the central apnea index and the number of awakenings [17]. Quadri et al. administered zolpidem 10 mg to patients with idiopathic central sleep apnea in order to find improvements in arousal response, sleep stage, central apnea index, and ESS score without observing the aggravation of obstructive apnea index or arterial oxygen saturation [18]. Furthermore, although it is a case report, Grimaldi et al. reduced the number of central apnea events by administering zolpidem 10 mg to a 47-year-old male patient who could not continue CPAP or BiPAP due to idiopathic central apnea syndrome and reported that the effect was still sustained for the following 2 years [19]. While sleeping pills have the potential to reduce respiratory events for CSA and CSB, the number of reports is small and future studies are needed.

References

1. Akashiba T, Inoue Y, Uchimura N, et al. Sleep Apnea syndrome (SAS) clinical practice guidelines 2020. Respir Investig. 2022;60:3–32.
2. Akashiba T, Inoue Y, Uchimura N, et al. Sleep Apnea syndrome (SAS) clinical practice guidelines 2020. Sleep Biol Rhythms. 2022;20:5–37.
3. Luyster FS, Buysse DJ, Strollo PJ Jr. Comorbid insomnia and obstructive sleep apnea: challenges for clinical practice and research. J Clin Sleep Med. 2010;6:196–204.
4. Lavie P. Insomnia and sleep-disordered breathing. Sleep Med. 2007;8:S21–5.
5. Berry RB, Kouchi K, Bower J, et al. Triazolam in patients with obstructive sleep apnea. Am J Respir Crit Care Med. 1995;151:450–4.
6. Kryger M, Wang-Weigand S, Roth T. Safety of ramelteon in individuals with mild to moderate obstructive sleep apnea. Sleep Breath. 2007;11:159–64.
7. Sériès F. Workshop participants: can improving sleep influence sleep-disordered breathing? Drugs. 2009;69:77–91.
8. Höijer U, Hedner J, Ejnell H, et al. Nitrazepam in patients with sleep apnoea: a double-blind placebo-controlled study. Eur Respir J. 1994;7:2011–5.
9. Sun H, Palcza J, Card D, et al. Effects of suvorexant, an orexin receptor antagonist, on respiration during sleep in patients with obstructive sleep apnea. J Clin Sleep Med. 2016;12:9–17.
10. Cheng JY, Lorch D, Lowe AD, et al. A randomized, double-blind, placebo-controlled, crossover study of respiratory safety of lemborexant in moderate to severe obstructive sleep apnea. J Clin Sleep Med. 2024;20:57–65.
11. Berry RB, Patel PB. Effect of zolpidem on the efficacy of continuous positive airway pressure as treatment for obstructive sleep apnea. Sleep. 2006;29:1052–6.
12. Lettieri CJ, Quast TN, Eliasson AH, et al. Eszopiclone improves overnight polysomnography and continuous positive airway pressure titration: a prospective, randomized, placebo-controlled trial. Sleep. 2008;31:1310–6.
13. Lettieri CJ, Collen JF, Eliasson AH, et al. Sedative use during continuous positive airway pressure titration improves subsequent compliance: a randomized, double-blind, placebo-controlled trial. Chest. 2009;136:1263–8.
14. Lettieri CJ, Shah AA, Holley AB, et al. Effects of a short course of eszopiclone on continuous positive airway pressure adherence: a randomized trial. Ann Intern Med. 2009;151:696–702.
15. Wang D, Tang Y, Chen Y, et al. The effect of non-benzodiazepine sedative hypnotics on CPAP adherence in patients with OSA: a systematic review and meta-analysis. Sleep. 2021;44:zsab077.

16. Biberdorf DJ, Steens R, Millar TW, et al. Benzodiazepines in congestive heart failure: effects of temazepam on arousability and cheyne-stokes respiration. Sleep. 1993;16:529–38.
17. Bonnet MH, Dexter JR, Arand DL. The effect of triazolam on arousal and respiration in central sleep apnea patients. Sleep. 1990;13:31–41.
18. Quadri S, Drake C, Hudgel DW. Improvement of idiopathic central sleep apnea with zolpidem. J Clin Sleep Med. 2009;5:122–9.
19. Grimaldi D, Provini F, Vetrugno R, et al. Idiopathic central sleep apnoea syndrome treated with zolpidem. Neurol Sci. 2008;29:355–7.

Chapter 13
Obstructive Sleep Apnea and Driving Risk: What Should We Know About Patients with OSA and Driving?

Yuichi Inoue

Abstract Since around 1990, it has been reported that the risk of motor vehicle accidents (MVAs) among patients with obstructive sleep apnea (OSA) is higher compared to general drivers, with a quite high accident rate among professional drivers. The primary causes are considered to be excessive daytime sleepiness (EDS) brought about by frequent nighttime sleep disruptions and intermittent hypoxemia due to apneic events and its related declines in various driving-related functions. Additionally, factors such as fatigue, age, and some psychological disturbance may contribute to the occurrence of accidents. Real-world driving tests would be ideal for predicting the risk of accidents in individuals with OSA. However, since it is impossible to implement such tests widely, other evaluations, including the Epworth Sleepiness Scale, which assesses subjective sleepiness; the Maintenance of Wakefulness Test, which evaluates the ability to stay awake objectively; and driving simulator tests, are conducted either individually or in combination. For professional drivers, where accident prevention is of utmost importance, it is desirable to conduct home sleep apnea tests for those with OSA risk factors such as obesity. For OSA drivers who are at risk of MVAs, treatment with nasal continuous positive airway pressure (CPAP) is desirable, as the treatment suppresses EDS in most of the affected individuals. However, a certain number of cases show residual sleepiness even after the treatment. In such cases, the use of wake-promoting drugs should be considered. Additionally, to reduce the risk of driving accidents caused by drivers with OSA, it would be desirable to create effective guidelines and to establish a close network between companies that employ drivers, the agencies involved in issuing and renewing driver's licenses, and medical institutions in the future.

Keywords Obstructive sleep apnea · Motor vehicle accidents · Sleepiness · Epworth Sleepiness Scale · Maintenance of wakefulness test · Driving simulator · Nasal continuous positive airway pressure · Residual sleepiness

---

Y. Inoue (✉)
Department of Somnology, Tokyo Medical University, Tokyo, Japan
e-mail: inoue@somnology.com

K. Chin (ed.), *The Current State of Sleep Disordered Breathing in Japan and Around the World*, Respiratory Disease Series: Diagnostic Tools and Disease Managements, https://doi.org/10.1007/978-981-96-6030-8_13

1 Introduction

According to the statement by the World Health Organization (WHO), road traffic accident is the eighth leading cause of death for people of all ages and lead to 1.35 million injuries worldwide [1]. Vehicular driving is a skill that requires complex integrated higher cortical function, alertness, concentration, and coordination. Although some environmental factors or mechanical issues may contribute to motor vehicular accidents (MVAs), most accidents occur due to the driver's problems. 10–30% of fatal accidents have been attributed to sleepiness at the wheel, [2] and car crashes related to falling asleep often cause death and severe injury. Death of the drivers occurred in 11.4% of sleepiness-related accidents, in contrast with 5.6% of accidents unrelated to sleep [3]. Reportedly, sleepiness-related MVAs may result from falling asleep while driving and behavioral impairment attributable to sleepiness [4]. As for the cause of excessive daytime sleepiness (EDS), there has been an interest in sleep disorders having the potential to affect daytime alertness and executive functioning that may affect driving performance, with the driving risk of obstructive sleep apnea (OSA) being of particular importance. Untreated OSA has been reported to be associated with excessive daytime sleepiness, cognitive dysfunction, impaired productivity at the workplace, and an increased risk of MVA, possibly resulting in injury and fatality [5]. From these, OSA has been accepted as an economic burden on health systems in many counties, [6] and many driving license regulations taking into account the situation in each country have been developed to reduce MVAs among drivers affected by the disorder [7–9].

2 Sleepiness, OSA, and Driving Risk

The risk of driving accidents in OSA has been of interest in many countries since the 1980s [10]. Results of previous meta-analyses of driving accident risk for OSA drivers are presented (Table 13.1). Ellen and colleagues first revealed that the risk was consistently elevated in the included studies [11]. Subsequent studies with similar designs also showed similar results (Table 13.1) [12–17]. Of particular importance among these was the higher risk of accidents among OSA occupational drivers, with a higher percentage of on-the-job accidents than for other occupations [18, 19].

Some but not all studies have shown the association of OSA severity manifested as the apnea-hypopnea index or oxygen desaturation during sleep to subjective EDS [20]. On the other hand, sleepiness has been reported to be associated with prolonged sleep time and fragmented sleep, reflecting the increased sleep pressure coming from poor sleep quality. Interestingly, obesity and metabolic variables were often associated with sleepiness, and depression may exert an independent role in the pathogenesis of EDS. However, definitive indicators that could predict the risk of accidents have not been identified so far. This may be due to the fact that

Table 13.1 Summary of results of meta-analyses on risk of MVA in patients with OSA, and effects of CPAP (partially revised from the report by Bonsignore et al. [12]

Author, Year, Ref	Study Type	Studies	Results
Ellen et al. (2006) [11]	Systematic review of literature until 2006	30 studies, 27 in noncommercial drivers, 3 in commercial drivers	Increased risk of MVA in OSA. Studies did not consistently find that sleepiness and OSA severity were correlated with crash risk
Tregear et al. (2009) [13]	Systematic review and meta-analysis (until May 2009)	18 retrospective studies, 2 in commercial drivers	Crash rate associated with OSA between 1.21 and 4.89.Predictors of risk: body mass index, AHI, oxygen saturation. ESS not significant. No control for exposure in most studies, and significant heterogeneity
Tregear et al. (2010) [14]	Systematic review and meta-analysis (until May 2009)	9 observational studies on effects of CPAP	CPAP decrease the risk for accidents in patients with OSA (RR, 0.28; 95% CI, 0.22–0.35). ESS decreased after 1 night of CPAP and driving performance improved after 2–7 d of treatment
Antonopoulos et al. (2011) [15]	Meta-analysis (until July 2011)	10 studies on MVA, 5 studies on near miss accidents, 6 studies on performance at driving simulator	CPAP reduced the risk of real (OR, 0.21; 95% CI,0.12–0.35) and near-miss (OR, 0.09; 95% CI,0.04–0.21) accidents in patients with OSA, and improved performance at simulated driving (OR, 0.09; 95% CI, 0.04–0.21)
Garbarino et al. (2016) [16]	Systematic review and meta-analysis (until Sept 2015)	10 studies (7 in the meta-analysis) on occupational accidents including professional driving	Increased risk in patients with OSA (OR, 2.18; 95% CI, 1.53–3.10). Risk associated with driving higher compared with other occupational activities
Patil et al. (2019) [17]	Meta-analysis on effects of CPAP in several domains, including driving risk (until April 2015)	4 RCTs on driving simulator performance,10 studies on MVA in noncommercial drivers	No improvement in performance at driving simulators in RCTs. Significant reduction in car accident risk after CPAP (OR, 0.09; 95% CI, 0.04–0.21)

occupational drivers spent more time behind the wheel than the general drivers and thus were more exposed to the risk [20]. The risk of driving accidents in OSA drivers has been demonstrated in studies of diverse cohorts, i.e., healthcare workers, transportation operators, and occupational drivers [21]. Along with this research trend, attention to driving accidents has expanded to encompass overall work operations, and meta-analyses have shown that OSA workers have a higher incidence of work-related injuries compared to non-OSA workers [22]. From these, OSA patients who experience EDS are often noted to bear significant economic and social burdens [23]. In view of this situation, the American Academy of Sleep Medicine recommends that healthcare providers ask patients about motor vehicle crashes and near-miss crashes during the initial evaluation for OSA [24].

Interestingly, recent studies have shown that the differences in driving accident risk among OSA drivers compared to the healthy population become less compared with those in previous studies. Furthermore, it was recently estimated that OSA could be held responsible for only about 7% of total MVAs [25]. The cause of this phenomenon is unclear, but the possibility cannot be ruled out that the increased awareness of the accident risk may have contributed to the suppression of new accidents of this kind. A more rigorous examination of the case backgrounds and search for the cause of the accident may also contribute to this phenomenon [26] Nevertheless, since OSA drivers have still been reported to have significantly higher MVA rates in studies reported later than 2020, there is no doubt that the presence of the disorder is one of the risk factors in the occurrence of MVAs. Future studies should also clarify the vehicular accident risk in female drivers and elderly OSA drivers, who may show a high driving risk but both of whom are less likely to be engaged in occupational driving, which may be compensated by a low driving distance per year and/or preventive behaviors such as avoiding driving at night.

3 Factors Related to the Occurrence of MVAs in OSA Drivers (Fig. 13.1)

OSA is characterized by recurrent airway obstruction during sleep, leading to sleep fragmentation and subsequent excessive sleepiness during wake-time hours [27]. Intermittent hypoxia brought about by repeated episodes of apnea or hypopnea may also lead to neuroinflammation and oxidative stress, contributing to increased daytime sleepiness [28, 29]. Excessive daytime sleepiness may not only cause transient loss of consciousness at the wheel due to dozing off, including microsleep at the wheel, but also reduce concentration and slow both cognitive processing and reaction time [30].

Delays in processing and reaction times have been associated with an increased risk of accidents or injuries, including motor vehicle accidents (MVAs) [31]. OSA patients exhibited much longer reaction times, leading to increased stopping distances and doubled number of collisions on a road safety platform [32].

In general, accidents related to drowsiness tend to be single-vehicle crashes when they occur at night, while rear-end collisions are more common when they happen during the day [33]. On the other hand, accumulated fatigue, distractibility, emotional instability, or depression, which are not infrequently associated with OSA, may also deteriorate driving performance. In particular, symptoms of depression have been reported to be positively associated with poor driving performance [34]. Age is another important risk factor for car accidents, particularly in patients

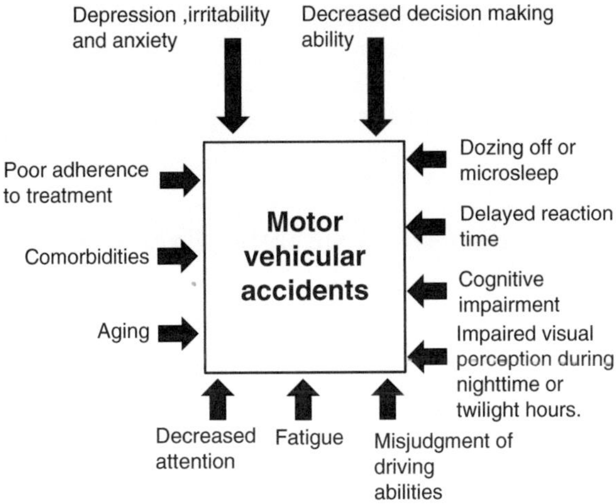

Fig. 13.1 The factors associated with motor vehicular accidents in drivers with obstructive

with OSA. Doherty et al. found that higher sleep apnea severity was associated with a higher incidence of adverse driving behavior, such as hard acceleration, braking, and speeding [35]. These findings were also observed in cognitively unimpaired old individuals.

The reduced performance in multi-tasking should also be considered as the cause of MVAs in OSA drivers. Previous reports suggested that OSA patients showed a reduced performance for divided attention during driving simulator trials compared to controls [36]. Another report evaluated the driving performance of OSA patients with tasks that consisted of avoiding an aquatic obstacle during simple conditions, distraction conditions, and anticipation conditions [37]. During these conditions, subject patients showed an increase in reaction time and a lengthening of the vehicle stopping distance in comparison with controls. Of note, after nasal continuous positive airway pressure (CPAP) therapy, the patients showed a significant reduction in reaction time, as well as a reduction in stopping distance in the distraction and anticipation driving conditions.

It is challenging to determine which OSA patients have impaired driving ability. Vakulin et al. [38] reported that brain mitochondrial bioenergetics in the frontal brain regions are impaired in OSA patients who are vulnerable to driving impairment following sleep loss by using H magnetic resonance spectra. In order to reduce accidents, these vulnerable patients should not only be encouraged to use CPAP therapy at night, as described below but should also be instructed to take a nap as needed. Although this result should be confirmed in larger future studies, such a research approach may provide a potential way to identify at-risk OSA phenotype when assessing fitness to drive.

MVAs in OSA drivers are assumed to be mainly caused by elevated daytime sleepiness (EDS), unexpected microsleep episodes, lack of attention, and fatigue. When comprehensively reviewing previous research, EDS could be the most significant risk factor for MVAs [12]. However, the involvement of other factors in close proximity to sleepiness should not be ignored. In particular, sleep deprivation is frequent in commercial drivers and clearly increases the risk of accidents [26]. To prevent accidents caused by sleep deprivation, it will be necessary to ensure that drivers take measures such as resting or taking a nap while driving long distances.

4 Measures for Evaluating Excessive Sleepiness and Driving Risk

Theoretically, an assessment of real-world driving performance using an on-road driving test would be most reliable for the evaluation of sleepiness-related decline in the driving performance of OSA drivers. This method undoubtedly offers the advantage of providing realistic assessments, as it closely mirrors actual driving conditions, allowing the collection of comprehensive data on various aspects of driving performance, such as lane deviations, speed variability, and reaction times, all of which may be altered by elevated sleepiness [39, 40]. However, the method is resource-intensive, requiring vehicles, supervisors, and standardized courses, thus raising costs. Among these, standardization is challenging due to varying driving conditions across different locations and times, which can affect the consistency of study results. Therefore, the method of combining subjective and objective sleepiness measures with a result of a driving simulator test is often the most effective approach for assessing driving ability in OSA patients (Table 13.2).

Validated subjective scales have been used to assess self-reported sleepiness in both clinical and research settings differently. Among these, the Epworth Sleepiness Scale (ESS) is well validated and most commonly used for assessing excessive daytime sleepiness in OSA drivers [41]. The ESS consists of only eight questions, making it quick and easy for drivers to complete, causing minimal burden. For this reason, we can collect a large amount of accumulated data, encouraging the comparison of the results with other studies and clinical data [42]. The ESS relies on self-reporting, heavily depending on the individual's subjective perception. If the self-awareness is inaccurate, the evaluation results can also be inaccurate [43].

While useful for evaluating long-term sleepiness, it is not suitable for capturing short-term changes. Sleepiness while driving can vary based on the time of day and specific daily conditions, so the ESS alone may not accurately assess the condition on the day of driving. In addition, many older adults are reported to be not able to answer all of the ESS items; thereby, their ESS score may underscore sleepiness severity in this population [44]. The prevalence of pathological ESS score (>10) in patients with OSA remains less than 50% [45, 46], and there are not a few cases where subjective sleepiness is underestimated [47]. Considering these points, the ESS should be used as part of a comprehensive assessment of driving sleepiness, alongside other objective evaluation methods and clinical assessments.

There are several objective measures for evaluating different aspects of sleepiness. The multiple sleep latency test (MSLT), maintenance of wakefulness test

Table 13.2 Evaluation measures of sleepiness-related driving risk in drivers with obstructive sleep apnea (OSA)

Measure	Strengths	Weakness
Epworth Sleepiness Scale (ESS)	Quick to administer with subjective assessment. Widely used with abundant comparative data. Cost-effective	Depends on subjective evaluation Risk of underestimation or overestimation Limited information on specific driving risk
Maintenance of Wakefulness Test (MWT)	Objective evaluation of sleepiness with standardized protocol. Can assess treatment effectiveness	Requires specialized facilities. Test environment may not fully reflect daily driving situations
Driving Simulator	Simulates real driving conditions Measures reaction times and errors Detailed evaluation of driving skills and judgement Provides consistent and repeatable results	High cost Differences from actual driving conditions Stress for patients unfamiliar with the simulator May not fully reflect psychological factors
On road testing	Actual driving habits and behaviors in real-world conditions Evaluates overall driving behavior (lane deviation, signal response, speed adjustment, following distance) Provides real-time feedback to improve driver awareness and skills	Higher costs and longer time commitments Influences from weather, traffic, and road conditions can affect results Difficulty in standardization

(MWT) [48], and Oxford Sleep Resistance (OSLER) test [49] are the candidates for the measures of driver's sleepiness, but all have obvious limitations. In particular, the MSLT assesses an individual's sleep propensity during the day, and intuitively, it is not appropriate to assess a patient's fitness to drive because the test cannot measure the ability to stay awake [50]. This characteristic is supported by the fact that there is no difference in mean sleep latency on MSLT between individuals involved in MVAs and those who were not [51].

Since the MWT is an objective measure of the ability of an individual to stay awake, it may theoretically reflect situational alertness when driving (i.e., trying to maintain alertness). The same is true for the OSLER test, a behavioral equivalent of the MWT. A relationship between driving ability and the mean sleep latency of MWT in patients with untreated OSA has been reported [52, 53]. A pathological sleep latency on the MWT may predict simulator driving impairment; sleepy patients showing mean sleep latencies lower than the cutoff value (19 min) had a larger number of inappropriate line crossings than controls [53]. In France, the Maintenance of Wakefulness Test (MWT) is used as a critical component in the assessment of professional drivers with obstructive sleep apnea (OSA) to determine their fitness to drive [54].

However, since the environment in which the MWT is conducted is different from the real driving environment, and the MWT result does not reflect motivation to drive, the suitability of the test to real-world performance and/or risks has been questioned [55–57]. In addition, microsleep episodes that frequently occur during MWT (Maintenance of Wakefulness Test) sessions may be considered to be related to brief dozing off at the wheel [58] However, there has been no consensus on the interpretation of microsleep in this test.

The Psychomotor Vigilance Test (PVT) is a test designed to assess an individual's attention and reaction time. Typically, the subject is required to respond as quickly as possible to visual stimuli that appear at specific intervals. PVT has the advantage of being easy to quantitatively measure sustained attention and fatigue/sleepiness because it can be conducted in about 10 min using a button-pushing task [59]. However, PVT may not be sufficient to assess other cognitive functions or driving skills, and the test has limitations in fully assessing the risk of fatigue/sleepiness accumulation in long-hours driving.

The driving simulator is an important test in assessing overall driving performance parameters, including lane position variability, number of crashes, and reaction times, possibly providing an objective assessment of drowsiness-related driving impairments [60]. Simulated driving performance significantly correlates with objective measures of sleepiness like MWT and MSLT. This demonstrates a certain predictive validity of simulators for detecting sleepy vs alert drivers. However, simulators may not fully replicate real-world driving environments' complex and dynamic nature, and their performance does not always correlate with actual driving performance. Schreier et al. reported that simulated driving did not reliably predict real-life motor vehicle accidents, especially not on an individual level, despite the moderate relationship between simulated and real-road test driving performance [61]. In addition, simulators may overestimate some driving abnormalities compared to real-world driving [1]. Considering these, it seems that we should not rely too much on the result of simulator tests to predict MVA risk due to sleepiness.

5 Effect of OSA Treatment on MVA Risk

CPAP is known to be the most reliable treatment for controlling EDS in patients with OSA, and a meta-analytic study by Bratton et al. showed a 2.5-point reduction in ESS scores after this treatment [62]. Previous studies have agreed on the positive effect of OSA treatment, especially CPAP, in reducing the risk of MVA, and several reports have indicated that the risk was reduced to a level quite similar to the general population [63, 64]. It has also been found that the risk of near-miss accidents in truck drivers decreased to a normal level after two consecutive years of treatment [65]. Moreover, a meta-analysis found a significant reduction in MVAs with the treatment brought obvious benefits in financial and human costs [66]. Reportedly, CPAP improves subjective sleepiness even after one night of treatment [67, 68]. Improvements in vigilance were confirmed after 1 year of CPAP treatment, and the treatment was reported to be associated with objectively improved reaction time and sustained attention in drivers with OSA [69]. Meta-analyses reported by

Antonopoulos and his colleagues demonstrated a sizeable protective effect of CPAP on road traffic accidents, both in real road conditions and virtual environments [15]. Taking these into consideration, there would be high potential benefits for OSA patients who adhere to CPAP therapy and also for public health and safety, as driving accidents pose a risk to others on the road. Although the cost of diagnosing OSA and CPAP treatment can be a financial burden for patients, benefits to individuals and public health clearly outweigh potential harm. Thus, CPAP therapy in OSA drivers is recommended to reduce motor vehicle accidents. Compliance with CPAP treatment would be a significant problem in preventing MVA in OSA drivers. In a truck drivers' cohort, participants with OSA who were nonadherent to CPAP had a fivefold greater crash rate compared with controls, but the rate was quite similar between adherent drivers and controls [71]. A statement from the European Respiratory Society indicated that documented use of CPAP for at least 4 h for at least 70% of nights is enough evidence to consider a treated CPAP patient fit to drive [70].

Nevertheless, despite the decrease in MVA rates with CPAP therapy in OSA, there is evidence that the driving performance in OSA patients remains poorer than that of matched controls even after CPAP therapy in a driving simulator experiment study [71]. In addition, high-quality data is currently not available to indicate what kind of OSA patients are most likely to experience reduction in MVA risk with CPAP therapy [72].

Of note, residual EDS is found in about 6% to 13% of effectively CPAP-treated patients [73] without potential behavioral factors, and the responsible mechanisms of this condition remain uncertain. Wake-promoting drugs such as modafinil [74] or pitolisant [75], both of which are used in neurological disorders such as narcolepsy or idiopathic hypersomnia, have been reported to be effective in CPAP-treated patients with residual EDS. However, the preventive effect of treatment with these drugs on MVA is currently lacking so far. Besides, we should consider the possibility that the treatment for EDS without concomitant OSA treatment might have a detrimental effect on other consequences of OSA, such as cardiovascular diseases.

Oral appliance therapy is known to be effective for mild to moderate OSA [76] and is often used in cases that are intolerant to CPAP therapy, resulting in quite successful outcomes. However, the effect of this treatment on MVA risk in OSA drivers has not been established, and its application to occupational OSA drivers possibly having excessive daytime sleepiness should be made with caution [77].

In any case, a high degree of obesity is certainly a predictive factor for OSA [78], so it is important to conduct proactive screening tests, especially for obese professional drivers. The OSA screening with an authorized questionnaire may be appropriate in achieving these objectives. However, the screening accuracy of currently available standard OSA questionnaires, such as the Berlin questionnaire and the STOP-BANG, remains relatively low in this special population, and the use of the home sleep apnea test would be recommended for the screening [79]. Furthermore, the possibility cannot be ruled out that fatigue due to long working hours and insufficient sleep resulting from a demanding work schedule exists behind the MVAs of OSA drivers [16, 26], so it will be necessary to search for these factors as well. In addition, in-car or driver-worn real-time monitoring for drowsiness, including the lane departure warning system, driver status monitoring system, attention assist system, etc. may offer some advantages in the real-time detection of subtle changes that might limit accident risk.

6 Conclusion

The problem of fitness to drive in individuals with OSA has been extensively investigated in the last 30 years, and the high likelihood of increased driving risk with the disorder has been affirmed. This led to the development of guidelines in many countries [80–83]. However, it is difficult to strictly limit the driving of OSA drivers because only less than half of patients with OSA report EDS, and there is currently no definitive biomarker that can define the risk of MVA. It will be necessary to determine whether or not the driver can drive based on a combination of factors such as past accident history, severity of sleepiness coming from the disorder, and sleep hygiene status. Education of all relevant stakeholders is an important component of effective regulation, including educating affected individuals on the benefit of diagnosis and treatment, employers, especially in the companies that hold a large number of vocational drivers, on the benefit of screening, and the police on the report of motor vehicle accidents where sleepiness is one of the important contributing factors [84]. Furthermore, the double agency involved in treating OSA drivers' sleepiness and notifying the authorities is a significant burden for physicians, so it will be essential to establish a safe and effective notification system [85]. Furthermore, improving the accuracy of drivers' drowsiness monitoring systems will also be an important issue in preventing accidents.

References

1. Dwarakanath A, Elliott MW, et al. Assessment of sleepiness in drivers: current methodology and future possibilities. Sleep Med Clin. 2019;14(4):441–51.
2. Ohayon MM. Determining the level of sleepiness in the American population and its correlates. J Psychiatr Res. 2012;46(4):422–7.
3. Garbarino S, Nobili L, Beelke M, et al. The contributing role of sleepiness in highway vehicle accidents. Sleep. 2001;24(2):203–6.
4. Dinges DF. An overview of sleepiness and accidents. J Sleep Res. 1995;4(S2):4–14.
5. Kales SN, Straubel MG. Obstructive sleep apnea in North American commercial drivers. Ind Health. 2014;52(1):13–24.
6. Alakörkkö I, Törmälehto S, Leppänen T, et al. The economic cost of obstructive sleep apnea: a systematic review. Sleep Med Rev. 2023;72:101854.
7. Garbarino S. Excessive daytime sleepiness in obstructive sleep apnea: implications for driving licenses. Sleep Breath. 2020;24(1):37–47.
8. Ayas N, Skomro R, Blackman A, et al. Obstructive sleep apnea and driving: a Canadian thoracic society and Canadian sleep society position paper. Can Respir J. 2014;21(2):114–23.

9. McNicholas WT. Sleepiness and driving: the role of official regulation. Sleep Med Clin. 2019;14(4):491–8.
10. Aldrich MS. Automobile accidents in patients with sleep disorders. Sleep. 1989;12(6):487–94.
11. Ellen RL, Marshall SC, Palayew M, et al. Systematic review of motor vehicle crash risk in persons with sleep apnea. J Clin Sleep Med. 2006;15:193–200.
12. Bonsignore MR, et al. Sleep, apnea, sleepiness, and driving risk. Sleep Med Clin. 2019;14(4):431–9.
13. Tregear S, Reston J, Schoelles K, et al. Obstructive sleep apnea and risk of motor vehicle crash: systematic review and meta-analysis. J Clin Sleep Med. 2009;5:573–81.
14. Tregear S, Reston J, Schoelles K, et al. Continuous positive airway pressure reduces risk of motor vehicle crash among drivers with obstructive sleep apnea. Sleep. 2010;33:1373–80.
15. Antonopoulos CN, Sergentanis TN, Daskalopoulou SS, et al. Nasal continuous positive airway pressure (nCPAP) treatment for obstructive sleep apnea, road traffic accidents and driving simulator performance: a meta-analysis. Sleep Med Rev. 2011;15:301–10.
16. Garbarino S, Durando P, Guglielmi O, et al. Sleep apnea, sleep debt and daytime sleepiness are independently associated with road accidents. A cross-sectional study on truck drivers. PLoS One. 2016;11:e0166262.
17. Patil SP, Ayappa IA, Caples SM, et al. Treatment of adult obstructive sleep apnea with positive airway pressure: an American academy of sleep medicine systematic review, meta-analysis, and GRADE assessment. J Clin Sleep Med. 2019;15:15301–34.
18. Garbarino S, Guglielmi O, Sanna A, et al. Risk of occupational accidents in workers with obstructive sleep apnea: systematic review and meta-analysis. Sleep. 2016;39(6):1211–8.
19. Komada Y, Nishida Y, Inoue Y, et al. Elevated risk of motor vehicle accident for male drivers with obstructive sleep apnea syndrome in the Tokyo metropolitan area. Tohoku J Exp Med. 2009;219(1):11–6.
20. Purtle MW, Renner CH, McCann DA, et al. Driving with undiagnosed obstructive sleep apnea (OSA): high prevalence of OSA risk in drivers who experienced a motor vehicle crash. Traffic Inj Prev. 2020;21(1):38–41.
21. Das AM, Chang JL, Berneking M, et al. Obstructive sleep apnea screening, diagnosis, and treatment in the transportation industry. J Clin Sleep Med. 2022;18(10):2471–9.
22. Chou KT, et al. Risk of work-related injury in workers with obstructive sleep apnea: a systematic review and meta-analysis. J Sleep Res. 2022;31(1):e13446.
23. Léger D, Stepnowsky C. The economic and societal burden of excessive daytime sleepiness in patients with obstructive sleep apnea. Sleep Med Rev. 2020;51:101275.
24. Kapur VK, Auckley DH, Chowdhuri S, et al. Clinical practice guideline for diagnostic testing for adult obstructive sleep apnea: an american academy of sleep medicine clinical practice guideline. J Clin Sleep Med. 2017;13(3):479–504.
25. Garbarino S, Pitidis A, Giustini M, et al. Motor vehicle accidents and obstructive sleep apnea syndrome: a methodology to calculate the related burden of injuries. Chron Respir Dis. 2015;12(4):320–8.
26. Matsui K, Sasai-Sakuma T, Inoue Y, et al. Insufficient sleep rather than the apnea-hypopnea index can be associated with sleepiness-related driving problems of Japanese obstructive sleep apnea syndrome patients residing in metropolitan areas. Sleep Med. 2017;33:19–22.
27. Peppard PE, Young T, Barnet JH, et al. Increased prevalence of sleep-disordered breathing in adults. Am J Epidemiol. 2013;177(9):1006–101.
28. Veasey SC, Davis CW, Fenik P, Zhan G, Hsu YJ, Pratico D, Gow A. Sleep. 2004;27(2):194–201.
29. Gozal D, Daniel JM, Dohanich GP. Behavioral and anatomical correlates of chronic episodic hypoxia during sleep in the rat. J Neurosci. 2001;21(7):2442–50.
30. George CF. Sleep apnea, alertness, and motor vehicle crashes. J Neurosci. 2001;21(7):2442–50. Am J Respir Crit Care Med, 176 (10) (2007), pp. 954–956
31. Hiestand D, Phillips B. Obstructive sleep apnea syndrome: assessing and managing risk in the motor vehicle operator. Curr Opin Pulm Med. 2011;17(6):412–8.

32. Mazza S, Pépin J-L, Naëgelé B, et al. Driving ability in sleep apnoea patients before and after CPAP treatment: evaluation on a road safety platform. Eur Respir J. 2006;28(5):1020–8.
33. Abe T, Komada Y, Inoue Y, et al. Short sleep duration and long spells of driving are associated with the occurrence of Japanese drivers' rear-end collisions and single-car accidents. J Sleep Res. 2010;19(2):310–6.
34. Tsoutsi V, Papadakaki M, Yannis G, et al. Driving behaviour in depression based on subjective evaluation and data from a driving simulator. Int J Environ Res Public Health. 2023;20(8):5609.
35. Doherty JM, Roe CM, Murphy SA, et al. Adverse driving behaviors are associated with sleepapnea severity and age in cognitively normal older adults at risk for Alzheimer's disease. Sleep. 2022;45(6):zsac070.
36. Huang Y, Hennig S, Fietze I, et al. The psychomotor vigilance test compared to a divided attention steering simulation in patients with moderate or severe obstructive sleep apnea. Nat Sci Sleep. 2020;12:509–24.
37. Mazza S, Pépin JL, Naëgelé B, et al. Driving ability in sleep apnoea patients before and after CPAP treatment: evaluation on a road safety platform. 2006;28(5):1020–8.
38. Vakulin A, Green MA, D'Rozario AL, et al. Brain mitochondrial dysfunction and driving simulator performance in untreated obstructive sleep apnea. J Sleep Res. 2022;31(2):e13482.
39. Filtness AJ, et al. Objective and subjective measures of sleepiness, and their associations with on-road driving events in patients with obstructive sleep apnea. J Clin Sleep Med. 2012;8(3):249–57.
40. Philip P, et al. Maintenance of wakefulness test, obstructive sleep apnea syndrome, and driving risk. Ann Int Med. 2010;151(8):528–36.
41. Johns MW. A new method for measuring daytime sleepiness: the Epworth sleepiness scale. Sleep. 1991;14(6):540–5.
42. Gonçalves MT, Malafaia S, Moutinho Dos Santos J, et al. Epworth sleepiness scale: a meta-analytic study on the internal consistency. Sleep Med. 2023;109:261–9.
43. Chin K, Fukuhara S, Takahashi K, et al. Response shift in perception of sleepiness in obstructive sleep apnea-hypopnea syndrome before and after treatment with nasal CPAP. Sleep. 2004;27(3):490–3.
44. Onen F, Moreau T, Gooneratne NS, et al. Limits of the Epworth sleepiness scale in older adults. Sleep Breath. 2013;17(1):343–50.
45. Mehrtash M, Bakker JP, Ayas N. Predictors of continuous positive airway pressure adherence in patients with obstructive sleep apnea. Lung. 2019;197(2):115–21.
46. Saaresranta T, Hedner J, Bonsignore MR, et al. Clinical phenotypes and comorbidity in european sleep apnoea patients. PLoS One. 2016;11(10):e0163439.
47. Chervin RD, Aldrich MS. The Epworth Sleepiness Scale may not reflect objective measures of sleepiness or sleep apnea. Neurology. 1999;52(1):125–31.
48. Littner MR, Kushida C, Wise M, et al. Practice parameters for clinical use of the multiple sleep latency test and the maintenance of wakefulness test. Sleep. 2005;28(1):113–21.
49. Huang Y, Aumüller P, Fietze I, et al. Comparison of the Oxford sleep resistance test and the multiple sleep latency test. Physiol Meas. 2020;41(10):104005.
50. Wise MS. Objective measures of sleepiness and wakefulness: application to the real world? J Clin Neurophysiol. 2006;23(1):39–49.
51. Young T, Blustein J, Finn L, et al. Sleep-disordered breathing and motor vehicle accidents in a population-based sample of employed adults. Sleep. 1997;20(8):608–13.
52. Philip P, Chaufton C, Taillard J, et al. Maintenance of WakefulnessTest scores and driving performance in sleep disorder patients and controls. Int J Psychophysiol. 2013;89(2):195–202.
53. Philip P, Sagaspe P, Taillard J, et al. Maintenance of Wakefulness Test, obstructive sleep apnea syndrome, and driving risk. Ann Neurol. 2008;64(4):410–6.
54. Alonderis A, Barbé F, Bonsignore M, et al. Medico-legal implications of sleep apnoea syndrome: driving license regulations in Europ. Sleep Med. 2008;9(4):362–75.
55. Bonnet MH.ACNS clinical controversy: MSLT and MWT have limited clinical utility. J Clin Neurophysiol. 2006;23(1):50–8.

56. Bonnet MH, Arand DL. Impact of motivation on Multiple Sleep Latency Test and Maintenance of Wakefulness Test measurements. J Clin Sleep Med. 2005;1(4):386–90.
57. Philip P, Chaufton C, Taillard J, et al. Maintenance of Wakefulness Test scores and driving performance in sleep disorder patients and controls. Int J Psychophysiol. 2013;89(2):195–202.
58. Morrone E, D'Artavilla Lupo N, Trentin R, et al. Microsleep as a marker of sleepiness in obstructive sleep apnea patients. J Sleep Res. 2020;29(2):e12882.
59. Zhang C, Varvarigou V, Parks PD, et al. Psychomotor vigilance testing of professional drivers in the occupational health clinic: a potential objective screen for daytime sleepiness. Environ Med. 2012;54(3):296–302.
60. Ghosh D, Jamson SL, Baxter PD, Elliott MW. Continuous measures of driving performance on an advanced office-based driving simulator can be used to predict simulator task failure in patients with obstructive sleep apnoea syndrome. Thorax. 2012;67(9):815–21.
61. Schreier DR, Banks C, Mathis J. Driving simulators in the clinical assessment of fitness to drive in sleepy individuals: a systematic review. Sleep Med Rev. 2018;38:86–100.
62. Bratton DJ, Gaisl T, Schlatzer C, et al. Comparison of the effects of continuous positive airway pressure and mandibular advancement devices on sleepiness in patients with obstructive sleep apnoea: a network meta-analysis. Lancet Respir Med. 2015;3(11):869–78.
63. Tregear S, Reston J, Schoelles K. Nasal continuous positive airway pressure (nCPAP) treatment for obstructive sleep apnea, road traffic accidents and driving simulator performance: a meta-analysis. Sleep Med Rev. 2011;15(5):301–10.
64. Phillips B. Continuous positive airway pressure reduces risk of motor vehicle crash among drivers with obstructive sleep apnea: systematic review and meta-analysis. Sleep. 2010;33(10):1373–80.
65. Garbarino S, Guglielmi O, Campus C, et al. Screening, diagnosis, and management of obstructive sleep apnea in dangerous-goods truck drivers: to be aware or not? Sleep Med. 2016;25:98–104.
66. Sassani A, Findley LJ, Kryger M. Reducing motor-vehicle collisions, costs, and fatalities by treating obstructive sleep apnea syndrome. Sleep. 2004;27(3):453–8.
67. Engleman HM, Martin SE, Deary IJ, et al. Effect of continuous positive airway pressure treatment on daytime function in sleep apnoea/hypopnoea syndrome. Lancet. 1994;343(8897):572–5.
68. Phillips CL, Grunstein RR, Darendeliler MA. Health outcomes of continuous positive airway pressure versus oral appliance treatment for obstructive sleep apnea: a randomized controlled trial. Am J Respir Crit Care Med. 2013;187(8):879–87.
69. Alakuijala A, Maasilta P, Bachour A. The Oxford Sleep Resistance test (OSLER) and the Multiple Unprepared Reaction Time Test (MURT) detect vigilance modifications.in sleep apnea patients. J Clin Sleep Med. 2014;10(10):1075–82.
70. Burks SV, Anderson Matthew Bombyk JE, et al. Nonadherence with employer-mandated sleep apnea treatment and increased risk of serious truck crash sleep. 2016;39(5):967–75.
71. Bonsignore MR, Randerath W, Schiza S, et al. European Respiratory Society statement on sleep apnoea, sleepiness and driving risk. Eur Respir J. 2021;57(2):2001272.
72. Vakulin A, Baulk SD, Catcheside PG, et al. Driving simulator performance remains impaired in patients with severe OSA after CPAP treatment. J Clin Sleep Med. 2011;7(3):246–53.
73. Craig S, Pépin JL, Randerath W, et al. Investigation and management of residual sleepiness in CPAP-treated patients with obstructive sleep apnoea: the European view. Eur Respir Rev. 2022;31(164):210230.
74. Inoue Y, Takasaki Y, Yamashiro Y. Efficacy and safety of adjunctive modafinil treatment on residual excessive daytime sleepiness among nasal continuous positive airway pressure-treated Japanese patients with obstructive sleep apnea syndrome: a double-blind placebo-controlled study. J Clin Sleep Med. 2013;9(8):751–7.
75. Pépin JL, Georgiev O, Tiholov R, et al. Pitolisant for residual excessive daytime sleepiness in OSA patients adhering to CPAP: a randomized trial. Chest. 2021;159(4):1598–609.
76. Liao J, Shi Y, Gao X, et al. Efficacy of oral appliance for mild, moderate, and severe obstructive sleep apnea: a meta-analysis. Otolaryngology Head Neck Surg. 2024;170(5):1270–9.

77. Kumagai H, Tsuda H, Kawaguchi K, et al. Truck collisions attributed to falling asleep at the wheel in two commercial drivers prescribed oral appliance therapy for obstructive sleep apnea. J Clin Sleep Med. 2023;19(12):2117–22.
78. Bonsignore MR, Marrone O, Fanfulla F. Sleep apnea, sleepiness, and driving risk. Sleep Med Clin. 2019;14(4):431–9.
79. Adami A, Tonon D, Corica A, et al. Poor performance of screening questionnaires for obstructive sleep apnea in male commercial drivers. Sleep Breath. 2022;26(2):541–7.
80. Colvin LJ, Collop NA. Commercial motor vehicle driver obstructive sleep apnea screening and treatment in the United States: an update and recommendation overview. J Clin Sleep Med. 2016;12(1):113–25.
81. Gurubhagavatula I, Sullivan S, Meoli A, et al. Management of obstructive sleep apnea in commercial motor vehicle operators: recommendations of the AASM sleep and transportation safety awareness task force. J Clin Sleep Med. 2017;13(5):745–58.
82. Mukherjee S, Patel SR, Kales SN, et al. An official American thoracic society statement: the importance of healthy sleep. Recommendations and future priorities. Am J Respir Crit Care Med. 2015;191(12):1450–8.
83. Ghosh D, Mackay TW, Riha RL. European Union directive 2014/85/EU on driver licensing in obstructive sleep apnoea: early experiences with its application in the UK. Breathe (Sheff). 2016;12(3):e59–63.
84. Rainey D, Parenteau MA, Kales SN. Sleep and transportation safety: role of the employer. Sleep Med Clin. 2019;14(4):499–508.
85. Bhat A, Marciarille AM, Stevens D, et al. Drowsy driving considerations in non-commercial drivers for the sleep physician. J Clin Sleep Med. 2019;15(7):1069–71.

Part V
Topics

Chapter 14
CCHS and *PHOX2B*: What Should We Know About the Diagnosis and Management of Patients with CCHS Including *PHOX2B* Gene?

Yosuke Yamada, Hisaya Hasegawa, and Koichiro Tatsumi

Abstract Congenital central hypoventilation syndrome (CCHS) is a rare disease characterized by hypoventilation mainly during sleep, but hypoventilation can be present during both wakefulness and sleep in severe cases. There is an abnormality in the chemical regulation of the respiratory center in the medulla, which results in insufficient ventilatory responses to hypercapnia and hypoxemia, resulting in a state of severe hypoventilation that persists without dyspnea. The paired-like homeobox 2B (*PHOX2B*) gene is the disease-defining gene for CCHS. CCHS is frequently accompanied by Hirschsprung disease, neuroblastoma, and dysregulation of the autonomic nervous system. The basic treatment is to manage breathing, including during sleep, and in severe cases, when awake. Treatment options, such as diaphragm pacing, are now available for hypoventilation during wakefulness, which had been difficult to treat in the past in Japan. If respiratory management and other complications are properly managed, the prognosis is good. To further improve prognosis, it is important to continue to study more appropriate respiratory management and to address new issues such as the transition of pediatric patients to the adult care system.

Keywords Congenital central hypoventilation syndrome · Hypoventilation · Hypoventilation without dyspnea · *PHOX2B* gene · Diaphragm pacing

Y. Yamada (✉) · H. Hasegawa
Department of Neonatology, Tokyo Women's Medical University Adachi Medical Center, Tokyo, Japan
e-mail: yamada.yosuke@twmu.ac.jp; hasegawa.hisaya@twmu.ac.jp

K. Tatsumi
Department of Respirology, Graduate School of Medicine, Chiba University, Chiba, Japan
e-mail: tatsumi@faculty.chiba-u.jp

K. Chin (ed.), *The Current State of Sleep Disordered Breathing in Japan and Around the World*, Respiratory Disease Series: Diagnostic Tools and Disease Managements, https://doi.org/10.1007/978-981-96-6030-8_14

1 Introduction

Congenital central hypoventilation syndrome (CCHS) is a rare disease characterized by hypoventilation mainly during sleep, but hypoventilation can be present during both wakefulness and sleep in severe cases. There is an abnormality in the chemical regulation of the respiratory center in the medulla, which results in insufficient ventilatory responses to hypercapnia and hypoxemia, resulting in a state of severe hypoventilation that persists without dyspnea. It was first described in 1970 [1]. The incidence of CCHS is estimated to be approximately 1 per 50,000 to 200,000 live births, according to Western reports [2]. The onset of most cases is during the neonatal period, but cases of late-onset CCHS whose onset is between infancy and adulthood exist. Recent evidence suggests that the clinical manifestations of CCHS correspond to the spectrum of clinical problems attributable to neural crest dysfunction. CCHS is frequently accompanied by Hirschsprung disease, neuroblastoma, and dysregulation of the autonomic nervous system. The paired-like homeobox 2B (*PHOX2B*) gene is the disease-defining gene for CCHS. In approximately 90% of cases, 4–13 polyalanine repeat mutations (PARM) in the 20 polyalanine chains of the *PHOX2B* gene are detected. The basic treatment is to manage breathing, including during sleep, and in severe cases, when awake. If respiratory management and other complications are properly managed, the prognosis is good.

2 Overview

2.1 Pathophysiology

Normally, breathing during wakefulness is controlled by a chemical regulation mechanism that corresponds to blood carbon dioxide, oxygen concentration, pH, etc., a regulation mechanism mediated by lung stretch receptors, and a regulation mechanism from upper centers including the cerebrum. During non-REM sleep, it is primarily controlled by chemical regulatory mechanisms. The basic pathology of CCHS is thought to be a disturbance in the ventilatory response to blood carbon dioxide, oxygen concentration, and pH in the respiratory center [3]. Since Mellins et al.s [1] first report of CCHS in 1970, the etiology remained unclear. CCHS is associated with Hirschsprung disease, neuroblastoma, and other autonomic dysfunction, and because it has been reported in families, it was thought to be a genetic abnormality related to the autonomic nervous system. In 2003, it was revealed that *PHOX2B* gene abnormality was the cause of CCHS [4]. *PHOX2B* is a gene located on 4p12 that plays an important role in the differentiation and development of the autonomic nervous system of neural crest cells. Neural crest cells are expressed in brainstem neurons involved in the chemical regulation of respiration in the central nervous system, and in autonomic nerve ganglia in the peripheral nervous system. Approximately 90% of *PHOX2B* mutations are polyalanine repeat expansion mutations (PARM) of 4–13 alanines in the 20 polyalanine chain in exon3 and are classified from 24 PARM to 33 PARM according to the number of expansion mutations. The remaining approximately 10% have nonalanine expansion mutations (non-PARM) such as missense, nonsense, and frameshift mutations. In addition, it has become clear that the type of genetic mutation is related to clinical symptoms, and it has been found that the larger the PARM, the more severe the clinical hypoventilation is and the higher the incidence of some complications [4–6].

2.2 *Epidemiology*

According to reports from Europe and the United States, the incidence of CCHS is estimated to be approximately 1 per 50,000 to 200,000 live births [3]. The incidence of CCHS in Japan is estimated to be at least 1 per 150,000 live births [7]. There are undiagnosed cases, such as late-onset cases, and the prevalence of CCHS is thought to be higher. There is no difference in the prevalence of CCHS between ethnic groups.

2.3 *CCHS in Japan*

In a nationwide survey in Japan in 2006, 37 cases of CCHS were confirmed [8]. Patient characteristics were as follows: 18 were males, 19 were females, and the age range 4 months to 34 years. Complications included Hirschsprung disease in 13/37 and central nervous system disorders in 15/37. Prognoses were as follows: 3/37 died in hospital, 1/37 remained in hospital, 33/37 were on home mechanical ventilation (died 4/33, survived 29/33), and 0/37 were cured. Ventilation methods included tracheostomy (21/37), use of a nasal mask (9/37), use of a facemask (5/37), and diaphragmatic pacing (1/37). Of the 37 CCHS cases, 22 (59%) survived without disability, 8 (22%) survived with disability, and 7 (19%) died. In 2015, Shimokaze et al. [7]. reported 92 Japanese CCHS patients with *PHOX2B* mutations. The types of genetic mutations were 25 PARM in 19 cases, 26 PARM or more in 67 cases, and non-PARM in 6 cases.

Recently, with advances in early diagnosis and respiratory management, the prognosis and QOL of CCHS patients appear to be improving. As the prognosis improves, the number of CCHS patients reaching adulthood is increasing. For the transition of adult CCHS patients from the pediatric department to the adult department, efforts are being made to educate the adult department through symposiums, and creating guidelines for CCHS transitional care. The CCHS Family Network in Japan was established in 2008 by CCHS patients and their families. At first, it was a small group consisting of only a few families, but with the addition of medical professionals such as pediatricians and respiratory medicine, the group now includes many patients and families. The CCHS Family Network in Japan holds regular meetings to provide information on new treatments and management, and to support the transition of adult CCHS patients from the pediatric department to the adult department.

3 Diagnosis

3.1 Clinical History and Respiratory Symptoms of CCHS

Hypoventilation in CCHS is characterized by persistent hypoventilation without increased work of breathing. In other words, the patient is breathing calmly without tachypnea or retractions, but when SpO_2 and CO_2 are measured, they represent remarkable hypoventilation. Hypoventilation during sleep is the main symptom, but in severe cases, hypoventilation is also present during wakefulness. It is important to confirm hypoventilation in CCHS by continuously monitoring SpO_2 and $TcPCO_2$ ($EtCO_2$). Short-time monitoring or single evaluation by blood gas analysis is inadequate.

Symptoms in most patients of CCHS manifest in the neonatal period and require tracheal intubation immediately after birth due to severe cyanotic attacks or hypoventilation, which often results in difficulty in extubation. Even if patients do not require tracheal intubation, CCHS is suspected in patients who have remarkable hypoventilation without increased work of breathing during sleep. There is a type of CCHS called late-onset CCHS that is diagnosed after the neonatal period [9]. These patients often have a history of prolonged hypoventilation during respiratory infections, or require a longer time than usual to wean from anesthesia during surgery. In some cases, associated disorders of CCHS such as Hirschsprung disease are diagnosed first, and hypoventilation is noticed later.

3.2 Differential Diagnosis for CCHS

Because there are not many diseases with hypoventilation as a chief complaint, the differential diagnosis of CCHS varies widely; when CCHS is suspected, cardiovascular diseases, respiratory diseases other than CCHS, neuromuscular diseases, metabolic diseases, infectious diseases, and congenital malformations should be excluded. For differentiation, blood gas, X-ray, ultrasonography, head MRI, EEG, amino acid analysis, organic acid analysis, and other examinations should be performed as necessary [10]. When the above diseases are ruled out, or in parallel, respiratory examinations should be performed, and finally, *PHOX2B* gene testing should be performed (Fig. 14.1). The identification of autonomic disorders associated with CCHS may be useful in differentiating CCHS from other diseases. Autonomic abnormalities in CCHS include Hirschsprung disease, tumors of neural

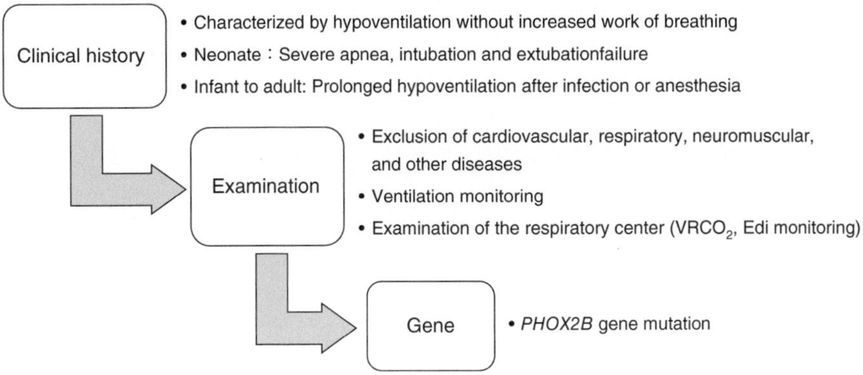

Fig. 14.1 Flowchart of diagnosis of CCHS. CCHS is suspected from episodes of characteristic hypoventilation and should be evaluated with ventilation monitoring. Definitive diagnosis is made by examination of the respiration and genetic testing after cardiovascular, respiratory, and neuromuscular diseases are ruled out. *VRCO₂* ventilatory response to CO_2, *Edi* electrical activity of diaphragm

crest cell origin such as neuroblastoma, gastroesophageal reflux disease, ocular symptoms such as loss of light reflex, and arrhythmias.

3.3 Diagnosis of CCHS

CCHS is diagnosed by confirming *PHOX2B* gene mutations or after excluding the differential diagnosis mentioned in Sect. 3.2 on central hypoventilation.

3.3.1 Respiratory Examinations in CCHS

Ventilation Monitoring

Ventilation monitoring can evaluate the characteristic hypoventilation of CCHS. This examination can be performed with a $TcPCO_2$ or $EtCO_2$ monitor that can assess the partial pressure of carbon dioxide in the blood. Figure 14.2 shows hypoventilation typical in CCHS during sleep. Since the patient often does not become completely apneic during sleep, the SpO_2 remains low with small ups and downs, and the $EtCO_2$ tends to rise. If increased work of breathing is not observed during this period, CCHS is strongly suspected. Since this characteristic hypoventilation can often be reproduced by monitoring for about 30 min to a few hours, caution should be taken not to expose the patient to hypoventilation unnecessarily for a long time.

Polysomnography

Polysomnography is an important examination for sleep-disordered breathing that can examine apnea or hypopnea events and analyze the cause (central or

	Monitoring time	Average	Min / Max
SpO_2	2 hr 27 min	90.2%	Min 77.0%
$TcPco_2$	2 hr 27 min	84.0 mmHg	Max 97.0 mmHg

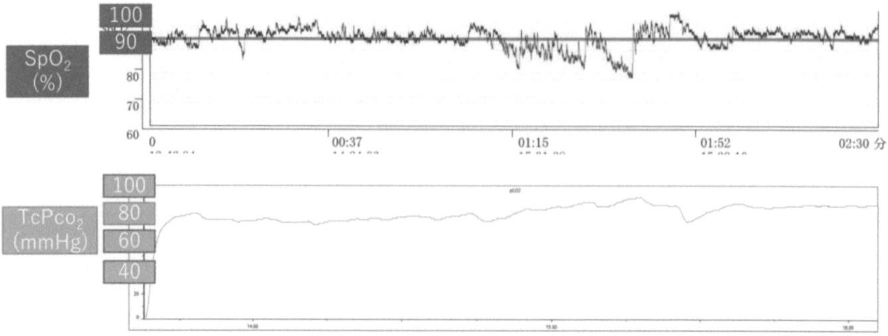

Fig. 14.2 Ventilation monitoring of CCHS. Ventilation monitoring is performed by recording continuous data on SpO_2 and $TcPCO_2$ ($EtCO_2$). CCHS is more strongly suspected when such severe hypoventilation without increased work of breathing is present

obstructive) of each event [1]. It is also useful in CCHS, but there are concerns that it is difficult to perform in the neonatal period and that patients whose hypoventilation is severe cannot tolerate monitoring for an extended time.

Ventilatory Response to CO_2 ($VRCO_2$)

$VRCO_2$ is an examination to quantitatively evaluate the ventilatory response to carbon dioxide gas, which is a chemical control of respiration of the respiratory center [11]. The patient rebreathes carbon dioxide in a closed circuit, and the increase in minute ventilation in response to an increase in partial pressure of carbon dioxide in the blood is measured. Other tests for chemical control of respiration are also available, and all of them report a remarkably lower response to carbon dioxide gas in CCHS compared to normal children [12].

Electrical Activity of Diaphragm Monitoring

Electrical activity of diaphragm (Edi) is a respiratory stimulus transmitted from the respiratory center to the diaphragm through the diaphragmatic nerve. Edi can be measured on ventilators equipped with NAVA mode, where the potential of the diaphragm is measured through a special gastric tube. Edi monitoring is an examination that monitors Edi and the partial pressure of carbon dioxide from wakefulness to sleep. Edi monitoring in CCHS reproduces the pathophysiology of CCHS itself. When the patient falls asleep, the inspiratory stimulus, Edi, decreases and respiration weakens, then the carbon dioxide concentration in the blood rises, resulting in hypoventilation. Furthermore, since respiratory activation does not occur in response to this hypoventilation, Edi does not increase and hypoventilation persists [13].

3.3.2 *PHOX2B* Gene Mutation

The type of gene anomalies in CCHS is classified into (1) with *PHOX2B* anomalies: polyalanine repeat expansion mutations (PARMs), non-PARMs (NPARMs) including missense, nonsense, and frameshift mutations in *PHOX2B*, (2) with other gene mutations and (3) no identified mutations.

Genotype-phenotype relationship in Japanese patients with CCHS has been explored by Sasaki A, Hayasaka K, and their colleagues at Yamagata University [7]. A mutation in *PHOX2B* would be closely linked with the development of CCHS. The gene function is associated with the development of the respiratory center and the differentiation and induction of the autonomic nervous system. The *PHOX2B* gene is mapped on chromosome 4p12 and encodes a highly conserved homeobox transcription factor of 314 amino acids with two short and stable polyalanine repeats of 9 and 20 residues. The *PHOX2B* genetic abnormalities are somewhat complicated. In Japanese cases of CCHS, *PHOX2B* gene mutation is heterozygous for PARMs, and the repeat of alanines ranges from 24 to 33 in >90% of patients with CCHS, and the remaining 10% of patients have heterozygous NPARMs that include missense, nonsense, and frameshift mutations in *PHOX2B*. Approximately 25% of the PARMs are inherited from the parents with somatic mosaicism or constitutive mutation, and the rest of ~75% is de novo mutation. Disease severity in the patients carrying PARMs increases as the length of the alanine repeats increases. The patients carrying long PARMs or most NPARMs present with severe phenotypes in the neonatal period. In contrast, the individuals carrying 24 or 25 PARM exhibit hypoventilation during the neonatal period or after the neonatal period.

In the largest Japanese survey of 92 patients regarding CCHS genotype-phenotype relationship, 19 cases carried 25 PARMs, 67 cases carried 26 or more PARMs, and 6 had NPARMs. The male-to-female ratio was ~3, no cases had Hirschsprung disease, 37% of cases developed hypoventilation after the neonatal period, and 42% of cases had mental retardation in 19 cases carrying 25 PARM. These cases with 25 PARM seemed to require additional genetic or epigenetic factors for CCHS development, and male sex was likely a predisposing factor. The patients carrying 25 PARM frequently had mental retardation likely because they were not able to receive appropriate ventilation support following a definitive diagnosis owing to subtle and or irregular hypoventilation.

In other 73 cases carrying 26 or more PARMs or NPARMs, the male-to-female ratio was equal, patients frequently complicated with Hirschsprung disease, and all patients presented with hypoventilation in the neonatal period. Clinical symptoms were severe in most patients carrying long PARMs and NPARMs. These findings suggest that the search for detailed *PHOX2B* genetic abnormalities in CCHS patients enables us to suggest the appropriate ventilator support patients require.

4 Respiratory Management

Lifelong ventilatory management is required, because there is no curative therapy for the disorder of the respiratory center of CCHS at present. Ventilation monitoring should be performed as a comprehensive assessment of respiration to determine whether respiratory management is necessary only during sleep or even during wakefulness. The main methods of respiratory care are tracheostomy positive pressure ventilation (TPPV), noninvasive positive pressure ventilation (NPPV), and diaphragm pacing (DP) (Table 14.1). Ventilator settings of mandatory ventilation on their own should be enough to guarantee sufficient ventilation because the respiratory center in CCHS is strongly impaired and spontaneous breathing is weak. The appropriateness of the settings should be confirmed by ventilation monitoring of the patient while on the ventilator. In addition, because CCHS requires lifelong respiratory management, ventilator settings should be reconsidered as the patient grows.

4.1 Comprehensive Respiratory Assessment

Because of the wide range of severity of hypoventilation in CCHS and the lack of subjective symptoms of hypoventilation, a comprehensive respiratory assessment should be performed on each patient. We have developed a three-pronged program called "respiratory dock" that includes an examination of the respiratory center, an examination of the respiratory system, and an assessment of ventilatory status. The respiratory center is evaluated by $VRCO_2$ and Edi monitoring, the respiratory system is examined by respiratory function test and laryngotracheobronchoscopy, and the ventilatory status is evaluated by ventilation monitoring in three states: during wakefulness without ventilator, during sleep with ventilator, and sleep without ventilator. The presence or absence of hypoventilation during wakefulness is particularly important in the assessment of ventilatory status. Around 40% of patients require continuous ventilator support due to hypoventilation during wakefulness [14]. Because patients with CCHS have no subjective symptoms of hypoventilation

Table 14.1 Main respiratory care in CCHS

Respiratory care	Advantages	Disadvantages
TPPV	Most reliable and stable airway management	Limitations in daily life, lower airway infection
NPPV	Fewer limitations in daily life	Difficult in ventilating during daytime, difficult using during childhood and infection
DP	Smallest device, easy to use outside house	Fewer experiences, lack long-term prognosis

TPPV tracheostomy positive pressure ventilation, *NPPV* noninvasive positive pressure ventilation, *DP* diaphragm pacing even during wakefulness, it is very important to perform ventilation monitoring during wakefulness without the ventilator.

4.2 Tracheostomy Positive Pressure Ventilation

TPPV is recommended during infancy. Infants sleep more frequently during the day, and sleeping time accounts for a larger proportion of the day. In addition, infants do not have a clear rhythm between wakefulness and sleep, and even when they appear to be wakeful, their level of consciousness may be low and hypoventilation may occur. And because patients of CCHS have no dyspnea, unless child patients are old enough to understand the need for ventilators, they are usually reluctant to wear nasal masks or use other devices. This can result in increased stress on child patients and decreased compliance with using ventilators by the parents. To prevent hypoventilation, the ventilator use must be ensured every time the patient sleeps, and easy to put on and take off. Since infancy is a period of development of the central nervous system, the accumulation of hypoventilation during this period has a significant impact on neurological prognosis. From these perspectives, TPPV that offers the best airway security and ventilation efficiency is considered appropriate during infancy. This is also described in the official statement of the American Thoracic Society [3] and the latest guideline 2020 [10], and there are reports from Japan that early tracheotomy is associated with a better neurological prognosis [15].

4.3 Noninvasive Positive Pressure Ventilation

NPPV is indicated from school age when the patients understand the significance of using a ventilator and the time and frequency of using a ventilator are reduced. If respiratory care of NPPV is performed appropriately, it can be expected to improve quality of life. To transition from TPPV to NIV, the patients should have no hypoventilation during wakefulness requiring respiratory care, have no major airway lesions that interfere with spontaneous breathing, and have acquired the mental development to use NPPV at any time. If respiratory care is necessary during wakefulness, it is difficult to transition to NIV. In this case, consider diaphragm pacing, as described in the next section. The developmental stage is most important in the transition to NPPV. Children with developmental concerns are more likely to be reluctant to wear masks, increasing the likelihood of inappropriate respiratory care. The practice of adequate mask ventilation for enough periods is necessary before the transition from TPPV to NPPV.

Although NPPV is rarely performed early in Japan, there have been several reports of respiratory management with NIV at an earlier stage in other countries. Kam et al. reported a case in which the patient was switched from TPPV to NIV at

3 years of age [16], and Migliori et al. reported two cases in which treatment was started with NIV at 1 month of age [17]. Ramesh et al. managed six cases with NIV with a median age of 1.5 months and reported good acceptance of mask ventilation and no major complications in most cases [18].

4.4 Diaphragm Pacing

DP is a new respiratory care in which electrodes are implanted in the phrenic nerve or diaphragm, and breathing is generated by stimulation from outside the body through these electrodes [19]. Pulse generators that emit external stimuli vary in size from product to product, but are considerably smaller and lighter than ventilators, allowing for artificial ventilation anytime, anywhere. Furthermore, breathing with DP is negative-pressure breathing similar to spontaneous breathing, unlike ventilator-assisted breathing. Therefore, a decrease in airway secretions and ventilator-associated pneumonia can be expected. In CCHS, the main indications are hypoventilation during wakefulness and weaning from the ventilator during sleep. In particular, DP for hypoventilation during wakefulness facilitates respiratory management during wakefulness, which has been difficult in the past and is expected to contribute to an improved prognosis.

Outside of Japan, DP is mostly the type in which electrodes are implanted in the phrenic nerve, and their effectiveness has been reported [20]. In Japan, the use of DP with electrodes implanted into the diaphragm began in 2020. Patients with PH due to hypoventilation during wakefulness have been reported to improve with respiratory care with DP during daytime [21], and some patients have been able to be weaned off the ventilator during sleep. DP precautions include upper airway obstruction when only DP is used in nontracheostomy patients. Because DP only contracts the diaphragm and the physiological movement to open the airway by contraction of the upper airway muscles does not occur, obstructive apnea may occur due to strong negative pressure in the chest cavity. Upper airway obstruction with DP is less likely to occur, and weaning from the ventilator during sleep is relatively easy in patients with tracheostomy.

5 Management of Associated Disorders

Complications of CCHS include those due to hypoventilation and those related to autonomic nerve dysfunction with *PHOX2B* gene mutation. Those related to autonomic nerve dysfunction require regular examination follow-up, and the guidelines also have recommendations for methods and frequency [10].

5.1 Complications Associated with Hypoventilation

Persistent hypoventilation has a variety of adverse effects, and important associated disorders due to hypoventilation include growth and developmental disorders in childhood, and pulmonary hypertension and heart failure in adulthood. In Japan, it is reported that inappropriate NPPV and late tracheostomy implementation result in a poor neurological prognosis [7, 15]. In adulthood, pulmonary hypertension has been observed in young adults in their 20–30 s [21]. Patients with hypoventilation during wakefulness, which has been difficult to treat, were at high risk for associated disorders due to hypoventilation. However, it is now possible to improve hypoventilation during wakefulness in such patients with the advent of DP, which is expected to improve their prognosis in the future. However, note the possibility that developmental disorder is not only due to hypoventilation but also due to CCHS itself which is a neurological disease affected by *PHOX2B* gene mutation.

5.2 Hirschsprung Disease

According to overseas data, about 20% of patients have Hirschsprung disease, and the incidence in NPARM is higher than that of PARM, ranging from 87% to 100%, depending on the report [3]. In Japan, the overall complication rate was 35% in a nationwide survey conducted in 2007 [8]. Among PARM, complications of Hirschsprung disease are very rare in 24 and 25PARM and are observed from 26PARM, with a higher complication rate in 27PARM and above. Because Hirschsprung disease is a major associated disorder of CCHS, the prognosis and quality of life (QOL), including frequent need for surgery, home central venous nutrition, and developmental effects, are influenced largely by the severity of Hirschsprung disease. Constipation is also a symptom of many CCHS patients, even if the diagnosis of Hirschsprung disease is not made.

5.3 Cardiovascular Disorders

Cardiovascular complications include sinus arrest, which requires attention if the patient experiences sinus arrest for more than 3 seconds. The complication rate is 19% in 26PARM and 83% in 27PARM. Overseas, cardiac pacemakers are frequently inserted, and it is reported that 67% of patients in 27PARM had pacemakers inserted [22]. In Japan, few cases of pacemakers have been reported. Sinus arrest is an important associated disorder because it can cause sudden death. The recommended examination time for Holter ECG is over 24 h.

5.4 *Neural Crest Tumors*

Neuroblastoma, a tumor of neural crest origin, is an associated disorder of CCHS. While the complication rate in patients with PARM is 1%, it is 50% in patients with NPARM [3]. Patients with more than 28 PARM tend to have neuroblastoma. Therefore, thoracoabdominal imaging is necessary in such cases.

5.5 *Other Autonomic Dysfunctions*

Ophthalmologic complications such as pupillary abnormalities, abnormal thermoregulation, and sweating disorders are common. Endocrine abnormalities such as hypoglycemia and thyroid problems have also been reported [10]. As the child patients begin to complain of symptoms from infancy onward, they present with a condition that may be considered dysautonomia. Not a few patients have difficulties in their daily lives.

6 Conclusion

The outline of CCHS including its progress and respiratory management in Japan was presented. Diagnosis and management can be difficult because hypoventilation in CCHS is atypical. However, the prognosis tends to improve with appropriate respiratory management. CCHS should be suspected when hypoventilation persists without increased work of breathing. Once a diagnosis is made, ventilation monitoring should be performed while awake and while asleep to determine the need for respiratory management and the setting of a respirator, and to prevent complications associated with hypoventilation as much as possible. Treatment options, such as diaphragm pacing, are now available for hypoventilation during wakefulness, which had been difficult to treat in the past in Japan. Since there is a wide variety of associated autonomic dysfunctions, appropriate follow-up is necessary. To further improve prognosis, it is important to continue to study appropriate respiratory management and to address new issues such as the transition of pediatric patients to the adult care system.

References

1. Mellins RB, et al. Failure of automatic control of ventilation (Ondine's curse): report of an infant born with this syndrome and review of the literature. Medicine (Baltimore). 1970;49:487–504.
2. Vanderlaan M, et al. Epidemiologic survey of 196 patients with congenital central hyperventilation syndrome. Pediatr Pulmonol. 2004;37:217–29.

3. Weese-Mayer DE, et al. An official ATS clinical policy statement: congenital central hypoventilation syndrome genetic basis, diagnosis, and management. Am J Respir Crit Care Med. 2010;181:626–44.
4. Amiel J, et al. Polyalanine expansion and frameshift mutations of the paired-like homeobox gene *PHOX2B* in congenital central hypoventilation syndrome. Nat Genet. 2003;33:459–61.
5. Sasaki A, et al. Molecular analysis of congenital central hypoventilation syndrome. Hum Genet. 2003;114:22–6.
6. Weese-Mayer DE, et al. Idiopathic congenital central hypoventilation syndrome: analysis of genes pertinent to early autonomic nervous system embryologic development and identification of mutations in *PHOX2B*. Am J Med Genet A. 2003;123:267–78.
7. Shimokaze T, et al. Genotype-phenotype relationship in Japanese patients with congenital central hypoventilation syndrome. J Hum Genet. 2015;60:473–7.
8. Hasegawa H, et al. Japanese Society of Pediatric Pulmonology Working Group (JSPPWG). Epidemiologic survey of patients with congenital central hypoventilation syndrome in Japan. Pediatr Int. 2012;54:123–6.
9. Trochet D, et al. *PHOX2B* germline and somatic mutations in late-onset central hypoventilation syndrome. Am J Respir Crit Care Med. 2008;177:906–11.
10. Trang H, et al. Guidelines for diagnosis and management of congenital central hypoventilation syndrome. Orphanet J Rare Dis. 2020;15:252.
11. Yamada Y, et al. Ventilatory response to CO_2 with read's rebreathing method in normal infants. Pediatr Pulmonol. 2021;56:2259–64.
12. Carroll MS, et al. Residual chemosensitivity to ventilatory challenges in genotyped congenital central hypoventilation syndrome. J Appl Physiol. 1985;2014(116):439–50.
13. Yamada Y, et al. Evaluation of respiratory center function in congenital central hypoventilation syndrome by monitoring electrical activity of the diaphragm. Pediatr Int. 2021;63:168–71.
14. Weese-Mayer DE, et al. Congenital central hypoventilation syndrome from past to future: model for translational and transitional autonomic medicine. Pediatr Pulmonol. 2009;44:521–35.
15. Irahara K, et al. Relation between psychological development and respiratory management in patients with congenital central hypoventilation syndrome in Japan. No To Hattatsu. 2015;47:343–7. Japanese
16. Kam K, et al. Congenital central hypoventilation syndrome; safety of early transition to non-invasive ventilation. Pediatr Pulmonol. 2014;49:410–3.
17. Migilori C, et al. Early use of nasal-BiPAP in two infants with congenital central hypoventilation syndrome. Acta Pediatr. 2003;92:823–6.
18. Ramesh P, et al. Mask ventilation in the early management of congenital central hypoventilation syndrome. Arch Dis Child Fetal Neonatal Ed. 2008;93:F400–3.
19. Le Pimpec-Barthes F, et al. Diaphragm pacing: the state of the art. J Thorac Dis. 2016;8:S376–86.
20. Nicholson KJ, et al. Thoracoscopic placement of phrenic nerve pacers for diaphragm pacing in congenital central hypoventilation syndrome. J Ped Surgery. 2015;50:78–81.
21. Yamada Y, et al. Diaphragm pacing for congenital central hypoventilation syndrome: a novel case of pacing implanted into the diaphragm. Pediatr Int. 2022;64:e14915.
22. Gronli JO, et al. Congenital central hypoventilation syndrome: *PHOX2B* genotype determines risk for sudden death. Pediatr Pulmonol. 2008;43:77–86.

Chapter 15
Sleep-Disordered Breathing Associated with Neuromuscular Diseases: What Should We Know About Sleep-Disordered Breathing in Patients with Neurological Disorders?

Hideaki Nakayama

Abstract Neuromuscular diseases (NMDs) are frequently associated with sleep-disordered breathing (SDB), encompassing various types such as central sleep apnea, sleep-related hypoventilation, and obstructive sleep apnea. SDB is often observed in the progression of NMD before the manifestation of daytime breathing symptoms. Although the pathogenesis of SDB in NMD is not fully understood, factors related to NMD and anatomical considerations such as obesity and micrognathia are believed to play a role. Although polysomnography with evaluation of SDB is recommended for diagnosis, there are limited facilities where polysomnography can be performed and it may be difficult due to the patient's condition; therefore, alternative testing methods are needed. Treatment is often conducted in the same manner as for SDB; however, depending on the case, ventilatory support may be required or tracheostomy may be considered. This chapter provides an overview of NMD and SDB, focusing on adult patients with major NMDs: amyotrophic lateral sclerosis, myotonic dystrophy, and multiple system atrophy.

Keywords Obstructive apnea · Central apnea · Hypoventilation · Stridor · Floppy epiglottis

H. Nakayama (✉)
Department of Somnology, Tokyo Medical University, Tokyo, Japan
e-mail: hidenaka@tokyo-med.ac.jp

K. Chin (ed.), *The Current State of Sleep Disordered Breathing in Japan and Around the World*, Respiratory Disease Series: Diagnostic Tools and Disease Managements, https://doi.org/10.1007/978-981-96-6030-8_15

1 Introduction

Neuromuscular diseases (NMDs) are conditions that cause movement disorders due to lesions in the brain, spinal cord, peripheral nerves, or muscles. Respiratory dysfunction can occur because of respiratory muscle weakness or abnormal and uncoordinated breathing pattern generation, attributed to the involvement of the central nervous system (CNS) nuclei responsible for respiratory control during sleep and waking. This section reviews sleep-disordered breathing (SDB) in patients with NMD.

2 Respiratory Events Seen During Sleep in NMD

The types of respiratory events observed during sleep in patients with NMD are listed in Table 15.1.

1. Obstructive apnea/hypopnea
   Obstructive apnea/hypopnea is characterized by upper airway closure or narrowing during sleep while respiratory effort continues.
2. Central apnea/hypopnea
   Central apnea/hypopnea is characterized by a cessation or reduction of airflow due to absent or reduced respiratory effort.
3. Hypoventilation
   Nocturnal hypoventilation is associated with an abnormal increase in the arterial PCO_2 during sleep.
4. Diaphragmatic (or pseudo-central) events
   Diaphragmatic events reflect hypopneas that are neither obstructive nor central, but rather are likely due to diaphragmatic weakness and occur during phasic REM sleep (Fig. 15.1). When REM atonia worsens with diaphragmatic dysfunction, there may be a loss of excursion of both the chest and abdominal signals (relatively chest > abdominal) on polysomnography (PSG), appearing as pseudo-central events. Diaphragmatic events may be the most common respiratory events during sleep in NMD and can be misdiagnosed as obstructive or central

Table 15.1 Causes of respiratory events associated with neuromuscular disease

Respiratory events	Causes
Obstructive apnea/hypopnea	Anatomical: Obesity, small jaw or macroglossia Neurologic: Pharyngeal hypotonia or bulbar symptoms
Central apnea/hypopnea	High loop gain, heart failure, or damage of respiratory control
Hypoventilation	Low lung volumes, muscle weakness, decreased ventilatory response to hypercarbia
Diaphragmatic (pseudo-central) events	Diaphragm weakness, REM-related atonia

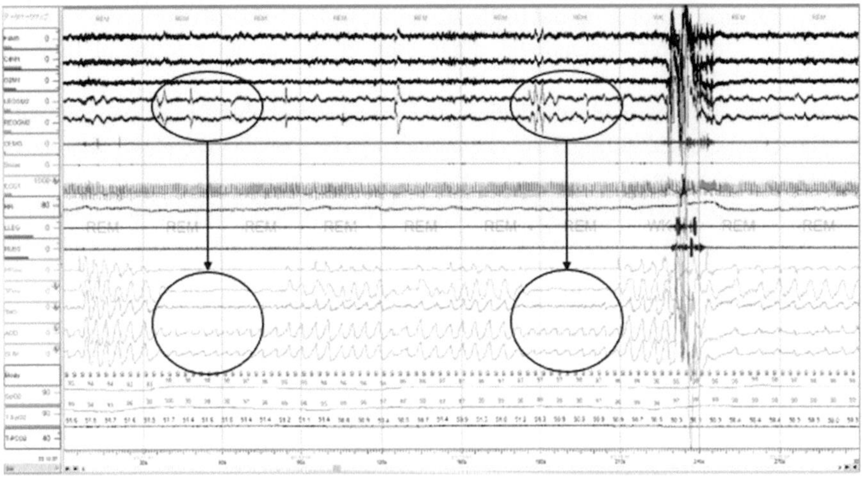

Fig. 15.1 Diaphragmatic respiratory events during phasic REM sleep in patients with neuromuscular disease

events [2]. These are considered as early warning signs of respiratory muscle weakness in NMD [3].

These four respiratory events do not always present in isolation and instead may coexist. According to the International Classification of Sleep Disorders, Third Edition (ICSD3) [4], SDB is classified into obstructive sleep apnea (OSA) disorder, central sleep apnea syndrome (CSAS), and sleep-related hypoventilation. OSA is defined as five or more predominantly obstructive events (apneas and hypopneas) per hour of sleep with sleep-related complaints (sleepiness, choking, etc.) or 15 or more predominantly obstructive events per hour of sleep. CSAS is defined as five or more predominantly central events per hour of sleep, with or without Cheyne-Stokes respiration, due to various etiologies. Sleep-related hypoventilation for adults is defined as an increase in the arterial PCO_2 or surrogate to a value $\geq$55 mmHg for $\geq$10 min, or a $\geq$ 10 mmHg increase in the arterial PCO_2 or surrogate relative to the awake supine value, to a value exceeding 50 mmHg for 10 min or more. End-tidal PCO_2 or transcutaneous PCO_2 is recommended as a surrogate for arterial PCO_2. The diagnostic criteria can be met for more than one of these disorders. Some of these disorders may manifest and be recognized through treatment.

3 Diagnostic Measures of SDB in Adults with NMD

In the 2007 American Academy of Sleep Medicine (AASM) clinical practice guideline [16], PSG was strongly recommended for the diagnosis of SDB in patients with significant cardiorespiratory disease, potential respiratory muscle weakness due to neuromuscular conditions, awake hypoventilation or suspicion of sleep-related hypoventilation, chronic opioid medication use, history of stroke, or severe insomnia. PSG is the gold standard for diagnosing OSA and other forms of SDB in patients with NMD.

However, PSG is often impractical and poorly accessible for all patients with NMD. In the clinical setting, PSG may not always be possible; therefore, alternative measures are required.

Home sleep apnea testing (HSAT) is one of these measures. A recent study compared the diagnostic accuracy, feasibility, and patient preference between HSAT and PSG for the detection of SDB in NMD [41]. For an apnea-hypopnea index (AHI) ≥15/h, HSAT sensitivity and specificity were 50% and 88%, respectively. For an oxygen desaturation index (ODI) ≥5/h, HSAT sensitivity and specificity were 95% and 78%, respectively. Although the HSAT underestimated the AHI from PSG by −10.7/h, HSAT was preferred to PSG by 61% of the participants. HSAT is thought to be a viable diagnostic approach for OSA in NMD when PSG is not feasible; however, it should be recognized that HSAT does not accurately distinguish between upper airway obstruction and other forms of SDB such as central sleep apnea (CSA) and hypoventilation.

Nocturnal pulse oximetry is another method. It is widely accepted as an important screening tool for assessing the degree of nocturnal hypoventilation and the need for noninvasive ventilation (NIV) in patients with nocturnal hypoventilation. This is because oxygen saturation and the level of arterial PCO_2 are likely to be inversely correlated unless gas exchange of the lung is impaired; thus, when oxygen saturation decreases, the level of arterial PCO_2 may increase in subjects with hypoventilation. Transcutaneous or end-tidal PCO_2 monitoring through capnography is also used to evaluate hypoventilation.

4 Treatment of SDB in NMD

SDB in NMD is often treated with continuous positive airway pressure (CPAP) and an oral appliance (OA), as in typical OSA. NIV, such as bilevel positive airway pressure (BiPAP) or adaptive servoventilation (ASV), may be used in patients with hypoventilation or CSA [2].

5 The Prevalence of SDB Seen in NMD

Table 15.2 shows the frequency and type of SDB depending on the location and cause of NMD. The prevalence of SDB is unclear because epidemiological studies have not yet been conducted in patients with NMD. Therefore, this is estimated primarily through case series. The frequency of SDB in patients with a stroke is extremely high at 60–80%. Stroke may occur as a result of OSA, and it is also reported that CSA is more frequent in the acute phase of stroke than in the chronic phase [15]. In Charcot-Marie-Tooth disease, which is a peripheral neuropathy, OSA

Table 15.2 Frequency and types of sleep-related breathing disorders in neuromuscular disease categorized according to disease site

Main damage sites and etiology	Diseases	SDB prevalence	Major SDB type
Nerve			
Central nerve system			
Cerebrovascular	Stroke	60–81%	OSA,CSAS
Degenerative	Multiple system atrophy	15–37%	OSA, CSAS, stridor
	Parkinsonism	26–60%	OSA
	Amyotrophic lateral sclerosis	17–76%	SRH
Peripheral nerve system	Charcot-Marie-tooth disease	40%	OSA
Neuromuscular junction	Myasthenia gravis	32–56%	OSA
Muscles			
Hereditary	DMD	57%	OSA,SRH
	Myotonic dystrophy	55%	OSA, CSAS,SRH
Metabolic	Acid maltase deficiency(Pompe disease)	55%	OSA, SRH

Abbreviations: *OSA* obstructive sleep apnea, *CSAS* central sleep apnea syndrome, *SRH* sleep-related hypoventilation

accounts for approximately 40% of cases [2], and in myasthenia gravis, it accounts for 30–50% of cases [1].

SDB occurs in approximately 50% of myopathy cases, and OSA and hypoventilation have been reported [1]. The majority (26–60%) of patients with Parkinson's disease have OSA [11].

The relationship between NMD and SDB could include the simple coexistence of the two conditions, or SDB occurring against a background of NMD. The risk factors for OSA in NMD are generally similar to those in the general population (including obesity and male sex). For the latter, the pathophysiological features of some NMD may predispose patients to obstructive events, such as pharyngeal hypotonia, neuropathy, or bulbar dysfunction [11].

Next, we describe SDB in patients with amyotrophic lateral sclerosis (ALS), myotonic dystrophy, and multiple system atrophy (MSA).

6 SDB in Three Major NMDs

6.1 ALS

ALS is a progressive neurodegenerative disease characterized by the degeneration of neurons in the cortex, brainstem nuclei, and ventral horn of the spinal cord. It is characterized by rapidly progressive muscle weakness, muscle atrophy and fascicu lations, spasticity, dysarthria, dysphagia, and respiratory compromise. In ALS, the loss of motor neurons in the brainstem and spinal cord results in pharyngeal, laryngeal, diaphragmatic, and intercostal muscle weakness, which predisposes patients to respiratory dysfunction. Bulbar dysfunction has been observed in some cases. Respiratory failure is the most common cause of death in ALS [11].

Breathing abnormalities during sleep frequently precede daytime respiratory dysfunction owing to the physiological vulnerability of respiration during sleep. SDB is reported to be present in 17–76% of patients with ALS. It encompasses sleep-related hypoventilation, OSA, and CSAS. Among these, sleep-related hypoventilation is the most common form of SDB in ALS. SDB is often observed in individuals with normal respiratory function [5].

Sleep-related hypoventilation is caused by diaphragmatic weakness and palsy of the respiratory accessory muscles. This condition may exacerbate, particularly during REM sleep.

Bulbar dysfunction does not appear to increase the risk of OSA in ALS. However, upper airway hypotonia and muscle weakness can lead to an excessive reduction in the airway lumen, resulting in OSA [11].

In one study, excessive daytime sleepiness was found in 23% of the patients [11].

Patients with ALS almost invariably require ventilatory support. Numerous studies have shown that NIV significantly improves survival, quality of life, and cognitive performance in patients with ALS, even in the face of disease progression [21].

NIV provides a median improvement in survival of more than 13 months [7]. While early NIV could reduce respiratory decline and decrease respiratory effort in ALS, patients with minimal respiratory symptoms are unlikely to continue long-term NIV. One study reported an adherence of approximately 3 h/day to early NIV [14].

However, compared with ALS patients with normal to moderately impaired bulbar function, NIV did not prolong survival in patients with poor bulbar function [26].

6.2 *Myotonic Dystrophy*

Myotonic dystrophy is one of the most common muscular dystrophies observed in adults. It is an autosomal dominant condition caused by a trinucleotide cytosine-thymine-guanine (CTG) repeat expansion in the DPMK gene on chromosome 19. This condition is characterized by progressive muscle weakness and myotonia, along with the involvement of multiple organ systems, including the respiratory, cardiac, endocrine, ophthalmologic, and central nervous systems. Respiratory failure is the primary cause of mortality [9].

Breathing is affected by sleep and wakefulness [40]. Moreover, 55–69% of patients with myotonic dystrophy have sleep apnea, with most cases being obstructive [8, 25]. Central apnea and nocturnal hypoventilation were also observed. The natural history and time course of respiratory function decline in this condition are poorly understood [9].

Excessive daytime sleepiness is a common problem for people with myotonic dystrophy, affecting 33–80% of the population [17, 42].

Respiratory sleep abnormalities in myotonic dystrophy are likely multifactorial [9]. While respiratory muscle weakness may play a role, central respiratory drive and upper airway collapse are likely to be involved [12]. There is increasing evidence of the dysregulation of ventilation at the central level. Respiratory dysfunction, predominantly a restrictive ventilatory pattern, is common in myotonic dystrophy and is associated with alveolar hypoventilation, chronic hypercapnia, and sleep disturbances in SDB.

NIV is used to treat respiratory insufficiency in patients with respiratory muscle weakness and SDB [9].

Treatments for sleep disorders such as CPAP for OSA, NIV for nocturnal hypoventilation associated with neuromuscular weakness, and modafinil for excessive daytime sleepiness associated with narcolepsy have been reported [40].

The 207th European Neuromuscular Center Workshop (2014) recommends the initiation of NIV when there is at least one daytime or nighttime symptom suggestive of chronic respiratory insufficiency in combination with:

- Daytime hypercapnia, $PaCO_2 \geq 45$ mmHg or.
- Vital capacity <50% predicted based on the best of three measures and maximum inspiratory pressure < 60 cm H_2O or.
- Evidence of nocturnal hypoventilation [9].

One study showed that 120 patients with myotonic dystrophy were categorized into four groups: OSA (18%), hypoventilation (27%), predominant sleepiness (30%), and normal groups. Patients in the OSA group were treated with CPAP, with 13 of the 27 (48%) patients continuing it. Patients in the hypoventilation group were offered NIV, and 12 of 33 (36%) patients continued it. Twelve of 36 (33%) patients with predominant sleepiness continued modafinil. Therefore, even if the treatment was selected based on respiratory dysfunction and/or sleepiness, treatment adherence was insufficient [40].

6.3 MSA

MSA is a sporadic neurodegenerative disorder characterized clinically by a combination of parkinsonian, autonomic, cerebellar, or pyramidal signs and pathologically by cell loss, gliosis, and glial cytoplasmic inclusions in several CNS structures. MSA is an alpha-synucleinopathy along with other neurodegenerative diseases such as Parkinson's disease and dementia with Lewy bodies [38]. Two phenotypes can be distinguished clinically based on the predominant motor symptoms: the parkinsonian variant (MSA-P) and the cerebellar variant (MSA-C). In Asian populations, 70–80% of MSA cases are of the MSA-C type, and in Caucasian populations, 67–84% are of the MSA-P type. This classification is based on the most prominent symptoms at the time an individual is evaluated. The median survival time is

9.8 years from the onset of symptoms. The most common causes of death are bronchopneumonia and sudden death [19, 39].

Patients with MSA commonly experience SDB, which includes OSA, CSAS, irregular and apneustic breathing, and stridor [11]. OSA is prevalent, ranging from 37% to 65% [36, 30]. Recently, the natural history of SDB in patients with MSA was reported. The severity of SDB in 24 patients with MSA showed a significant increase in the mean AHI from 19.4 to 34.4/h over a mean interval of 2.4 years, while 29% had spontaneous remission [24]. Stridor is another characteristic finding of SDB seen in MSA, defined as a loud and high-pitched sound during the inspiratory phase [29]. Stridor originates from vocal cord vibrations. Stridor during sleep occurs in 13–23% of patients as noticed by caregivers or medical staff. When patients with MSA were studied using video-PSG, stridor during sleep was more common, occurring in 30–42% of cases [13, 28, 36]. Stridor in MSA-C is more common than that in MSA-P and occurs at all stages of the disease [27]. Stridor initially presents during sleep, and as the disease progresses, it may also occur during wakefulness. The presence of stridor during sleep is considered a life-threatening characteristic, as it is associated with decreased survival and higher rates of sudden death during sleep [10]. Excessive daytime sleepiness has been reported in approximately 30% of Caucasian and Asian patients with MSA [22, 33, 37].

The cause of these breathing abnormalities in MSA is thought to be related not only to anatomical and/or physiological upper airway narrowing, but also to the neurodegenerative process damaging the brainstem structures controlling respiration [6]. OSA typically results from the narrowing of the upper airway, primarily involving the soft palate and the root of the tongue. In MSA, the sites of obstruction evaluated under drug-induced sleep endoscopy are diverse. In one study, the pharyngeal obstruction pattern seen was observed in approximately 30% of cases. Laryngeal involvement of the vocal cords was observed in approximately half of the cases [30]. A floppy epiglottis is seen and can cause laryngeal obstruction when sucked into the laryngeal inlet during inspiration [34]. It is reported that patients with MSA exhibit more irregular breathing patterns and that these irregularities are independently associated with the severity of OSA in patients with MSA [23]. This suggests that impaired ventilatory control in patients with MSA may contribute not only to CSAS, irregular breathing, and Cheyne-Stokes respiration but also to the development of OSA. Three of 24 patients with MSA developed CSA from OSA during their clinical course [24]. Thus, some of these SDB types change throughout the disease, possibly because of the complicated respiratory regulatory system abnormalities associated with disease progression. In some patients, CSA events, which may have been masked by OSA events, can appear after tracheostomy and CPAP therapy [11].

And the etiology of stridor in patients with MSA also remains unclear. There are two possible mechanisms underlying this phenomenon. One mechanism is that stridor results from a dystonic contraction of the laryngeal muscles that adduct the vocal cords. Another mechanism is that stridor is caused by paralysis of the sole muscles that abduct the vocal cords. The mechanism involved is debatable. This may depend on the patient, or in some instances, both mechanisms may be involved [11]. Stridor can occur either alone or in combination with OSA or CSA.

As in OSA, CPAP and OA are the treatments of choice. Three studies on MSA patients suffering from SDB showed that most patients accept PAP (69–72%) with an average nightly use of 4 h or more [18].

In a retrospective follow-up of 29 patients with MSA who were on CPAP, half of the patients stopped CPAP at 13 months. A floppy epiglottis was more frequently observed in patients who discontinued PAP in one study [32].

Laryngoscopy was performed under propofol sedation in 17 patients with MSA and SDB. The response to CPAP varied in 9 patients with a floppy epiglottis. CPAP did not improve SDB in patients with severe floppy epiglottis and aggravated the severity of floppy epiglottis in two cases. However, in the remaining seven patients with mild floppy epiglottis, CPAP improved upper airway obstruction. Thereafter, Mikami reported the treatment of OA in three patients with MSA who presented with floppy epiglottis and found that in two of them, AHI was reduced (baseline to OA 83.4 to 33.7, 32.6 to 18.8). The remaining one who was obese with a BMI $\geq$30 kg/m^2 had no effect [20]. In some cases, OA can improve SDB in patients with MSA and floppy epiglottis.

There are two main options for treating stridor in patients with MSA: tracheostomy and CPAP. Both CPAP and tracheostomy were found to increase the survival of patients with MSA and stridor [10]. CPAP therapy should be considered first because tracheostomy is an invasive surgical procedure. However, tracheostomy should be considered if CPAP is not tolerated, and may be a first-line intervention if stridor is present during wakefulness because of the high risk of respiratory failure and death [27].

Of the 45 patients who were followed up, 25 underwent therapeutic intervention for SDB. Regrettably, 10 died: 7 sudden deaths, and 3 developed anoxic encephalopathy. Of the 7 sudden deaths, 6 occurred during sleep; 2 were treated with tracheostomy, and 3 were treated with CPAP [31].

Although the cause of sudden death during sleep remains elusive, respiratory arrest, cardiac arrest, arrhythmias, or lung aspiration may be potential factors [11, 35].

An increase in survival may be achieved through interventions like CPAP, BiPAP, ASV, and/or tracheostomy. It is crucial to consider ventilatory support when managing frequent CSA following tracheostomy.

7 Conclusion

A wide variety of SDBs is frequently observed in individuals with NMD. Anatomical factors, such as obesity and bone structure, may play a role, and SDB may manifest due to specific factors underlying NMD. A diagnosis should be made using PSG while evaluating hypoventilation as much as possible. Treatment should be tailored to the specific SDB type. Although some treatments have demonstrated effectiveness, patient adherence is not always optimal. Further studies are required to investigate SDB in patients with NMD.

References

1. Aboussouan LS. Sleep-disordered breathing in neuromuscular disease. Am J Respir Crit Care Med. 2015;191:979–89.
2. Aboussouan LS, Mireles-Cabodevila E. Sleep-disordered breathing in neuromuscular disease: diagnostic and therapeutic challenges. Chest. 2017;152:880–92.
3. Albdewi MA, Liistro G, El Tahry R. Sleep-disordered breathing in patients with neuromuscular disease. Sleep Breath. 2018;22:277–86.
4. American Academy of Sleep Medicine. International classification of sleep disorders: diagnostic and coding manual. Darien, American Academy of Sleep Medicine; 2014.
5. Atalaia A, De Carvalho M, Evangelista T, et al. Sleep characteristics of amyotrophic lateral sclerosis in patients with preserved diaphragmatic function. Amyotroph Lateral Scler. 2007;8:101–5.
6. Benarroch EE. Brainstem in multiple system atrophy: clinicopathological correlations. Cell Mol Neurobiol. 2003;23:519–26.
7. Berlowitz DJ, Howard ME, Fiore JF Jr, et al. Identifying who will benefit from non-invasive ventilation in amyotrophic lateral sclerosis/motor neurone disease in a clinical cohort. J Neurol Neurosurg Psychiatry. 2016;87:280–6.
8. Bianchi ML, Losurdo A, Di Blasi C, et al. Prevalence and clinical correlates of sleep disordered breathing in myotonic dystrophy types 1 and 2. Sleep Breath. 2014;18:579–89.
9. Boentert M, Cao M, Mass D, et al. Consensus-based care recommendations for pulmonologists treating adults with myotonic dystrophy type 1. Respiration. 2020;99:360–8.
10. Cortelli P, Calandra-Buonaura G, Benarroch EE, et al. Stridor in multiple system atrophy: consensus statement on diagnosis, prognosis, and treatment. Neurology. 2019;93:630–9.
11. Gaig C, Iranzo A. Sleep-disordered breathing in neurodegenerative diseases. Curr Neurol Neurosci Rep. 2012;12:205–17.
12. Hawkins AM, Hawkins CL, Abdul Razak K, et al. Respiratory dysfunction in myotonic dystrophy type 1: a systematic review. Neuromuscul Disord. 2019;29:198–212.
13. Iranzo A, Santamaria J, Tolosa E. Continuous positive air pressure eliminates nocturnal stridor in multiple system atrophy. Barcelona multiple system atrophy study group. Lancet. 2000;356:1329–30.
14. Jacobs TL, Brown DL, Baek J, et al. Trial of early noninvasive ventilation for ALS: a pilot placebo-controlled study. Neurology. 2016;87:1878–83.
15. Johnson KG, Johnson DC. Frequency of sleep apnea in stroke and TIA patients: a meta-analysis. J Clin Sleep Med. 2010;6:131–7.
16. Kapur VK, Auckley DH, Chowdhuri S, et al. Clinical practice guideline for diagnostic testing for adult obstructive sleep apnea: an American Academy of sleep medicine clinical practice guideline. J Clin Sleep Med. 2017;13:479–504.
17. Laberge L, Begin P, Montplaisir J, et al. Sleep complaints in patients with myotonic dystrophy. J Sleep Res. 2004;13:95–100.
18. Lajoie AC, Gu Y, Lim A, et al. Adherence to continuous positive airway pressure for the treatment of obstructive sleep apnea in neurodegenerative diseases: a systematic review. Sleep Med Rev. 2023;71:101836.
19. Low PA, Reich SG, Jankovic J, et al. Natural history of multiple system atrophy in the USA: a prospective cohort study. Lancet Neurol. 2015;14:710–9.
20. Mikami T, Kobayashi T, Hasebe D, et al. Oral appliance therapy for obstructive sleep apnea in multiple system atrophy with floppy epiglottis: a case series of three patients. Sleep Breath. 2022;27:213–9. https://doi.org/10.1007/s11325-022-02607-0.
21. Morelot-Panzini C, Bruneteau G, Gonzalez-Bermejo J. NIV in amyotrophic lateral sclerosis: the 'when' and 'how' of the matter. Respirology. 2019;24:521–30.
22. Moreno-Lopez C, Santamaria J, Salamero M, et al. Excessive daytime sleepiness in multiple system atrophy (SLEEMSA study). Arch Neurol. 2011;68:223–30.

23. Nakayama H, Hokari S, Ohshima Y, et al. Breathing irregularity is independently associated with the severity of obstructive sleep apnea in patients with multiple system atrophy. J Clin Sleep Med. 2018;14:1661–7.
24. Ohshima Y, Nakayama H, Matsuyama N, et al. Natural course and potential prognostic factors for sleep-disordered breathing in multiple system atrophy. Sleep Med. 2017;34:13–7.
25. Pincherle A, Patruno V, Raimondi P, et al. Sleep breathing disorders in 40 Italian patients with myotonic dystrophy type 1. Neuromuscul Disord. 2012;22:219–24.
26. Radunovic A, Annane D, Rafiq MK, et al. Mechanical ventilation for amyotrophic lateral sclerosis/motor neuron disease. Cochrane Database Syst Rev. 2017;2018:CD004427.
27. Ralls F, Cutchen L. Respiratory and sleep-related complications of multiple system atrophy. Curr Opin Pulm Med. 2020;26:615–22.
28. Rekik S, Martin F, Dodet P, et al. Stridor combined with other sleep breathing disorders in multiple system atrophy: a tailored treatment? Sleep Med. 2018;42:53–60.
29. Shiba K, Isono S, Nakazawa K. Paradoxical vocal cord motion: a review focused on multiple system atrophy. Auris Nasus Larynx. 2007;34:443–52.
30. Shimohata T, Shinoda H, Nakayama H, et al. Daytime hypoxemia, sleep-disordered breathing, and laryngopharyngeal findings in multiple system atrophy. Arch Neurol. 2007;64:856–61.
31. Shimohata T, Ozawa T, Nakayama H, et al. Frequency of nocturnal sudden death in patients with multiple system atrophy. J Neurol. 2008;255:1483–5.
32. Shimohata T, Tomita M, Nakayama H, et al. Floppy epiglottis as a contraindication of CPAP in patients with multiple system atrophy. Neurology. 2011;76:1841–2.
33. Shimohata T, Nakayama H, Tomita M, et al. Daytime sleepiness in Japanese patients with multiple system atrophy: prevalence and determinants. BMC Neurol. 2012;12:130.
34. Shimohata T, Nakayama H, Aizawa N, et al. Discontinuation of continuous positive airway pressure treatment in multiple system atrophy. Sleep Med. 2014;15:1147–9.
35. Shimohata T, Aizawa N, Nakayama H, et al. Mechanisms and prevention of sudden death in multiple system atrophy. Parkinsonism Relat Disord. 2016;30:1–6.
36. Vetrugno R, Provini F, Cortelli P, et al. Sleep disorders in multiple system atrophy: a correlative video-polysomnographic study. Sleep Med. 2004;5:21–30.
37. Wang H, Tang X, Zhou J, et al. Excessive daytime sleepiness is associated with non-motor symptoms of multiple system atrophy: a cross-sectional study in China. Front Neurol. 2021;12:798771.
38. Wenning GK, Colosimo C, Geser F, et al. Multiple system atrophy. Lancet Neurol. 2004;3:93–103.
39. Wenning GK, Geser F, Krismer F, et al. The natural history of multiple system atrophy: a prospective European cohort study. Lancet Neurol. 2013;12:264–74.
40. West SD, Lochmuller H, Hughes J, et al. Sleepiness and sleep-related breathing disorders in myotonic dystrophy and responses to treatment: a prospective cohort study. J Neuromuscul Dis. 2016;3:529–37.
41. Westenberg JN, Petrof BJ, Noel F, et al. Validation of home portable monitoring for the diagnosis of sleep-disordered breathing in adolescents and adults with neuromuscular disorders. J Clin Sleep Med. 2021;17:1579–90. https://doi.org/10.5664/jcsm.9254.
42. Yu H, Laberge L, Jaussent I, et al. Daytime sleepiness and REM sleep characteristics in myotonic dystrophy: a case-control study. Sleep. 2011;34:165–70.

Chapter 16
Blood Pressure, Nocturia, and Obstructive Sleep Apnea: Is Obstructive Sleep Apnea a Factor that Increases Sleep Blood Pressure?

Yasuharu Tabara

Abstract Blood pressure (BP) during sleep (i.e., nocturnal BP) is an independent risk factor for cardiovascular outcomes. Given that factors associated with nocturnal BP differ from those associated with awake BP, studies need to clarify the complete physiological background for nocturnal BP elevation to achieve 24-h BP control. Evidence suggests that obstructive sleep apnea is associated with nocturnal BP, though its effect on BP is not strong enough to increase mean levels of nocturnal BP. Nocturia, a manifestation of salt sensitivity, has been strongly associated with both sleep apnea and nocturnal BP, indicating that the association between obstructive sleep apnea and nocturnal BP may be partly mediated by nocturia. Instead, we found that sleep apnea was significantly associated with morning BP, though their relationship has received less attention. The association between sleep apnea and morning BP deserves further investigation to reduce cardiovascular disease risk.

Keywords Obstructive sleep apnea · Nocturia · Nocturnal blood pressure · Home blood pressure

Y. Tabara (✉)
Graduate School of Public Health, Shizuoka Graduate University of Public Health, Shizuoka, Japan

Center for Genomic Medicine, Kyoto University Graduate School of Medicine, Sakyo-ku, Kyoto, Japan
e-mail: tabara@s-sph.ac.jp

K. Chin (ed.), *The Current State of Sleep Disordered Breathing in Japan and Around the World*, Respiratory Disease Series: Diagnostic Tools and Disease Managements, https://doi.org/10.1007/978-981-96-6030-8_16

1 Introduction

Obstructive sleep apnea (OSA) may exert some influence over blood pressure (BP), particularly nocturnal and morning BP at home. Although nocturia is a manifestation often observed in patients with OSA, recent studies have clarified that nocturia is also strongly associated with nocturnal BP. Nonetheless, to accurately determine the pathophysiological importance of OSA in development of cardiovascular disease, a complete understanding of the relationship between OSA, nocturia, and nocturnal BP is required. This chapter summarizes the current understanding of these relationships based on the results of epidemiological studies.

2 Measuring BP

Hypertension is usually diagnosed based on BP measurements obtained at the clinic (office BP), with a systolic/diastolic BP of 140/90 mmHg being widely used as the diagnostic threshold of hypertension. However, office BP is often confounded by the white-coat effect and does not necessarily represent an individual's true BP. Another important concern is that office BP is less reproducible and is measured infrequently, which may become an obstacle in controlling the BP of patients with hypertension. Therefore, several guidelines on the management of hypertension [1–4] suggest using BP measured at home (home BP), particularly home BP measured in the morning, for the diagnosis and treatment of hypertension in addition to office BP. In fact, the Ohasama study had been the first to report that home BP had better prognostic significance than did office BP [5], with several subsequent epidemiological studies validating the superiority of home BP for assessing cardiovascular disease risk [6, 7].

Home BP can be measured easily and inexpensively using commercially available BP monitors (Table 16.1). The availability of repeated measurements provides important information in the treatment of hypertension, such as long-term and seasonal changes in BP. Although ambulatory BP monitoring using a specific device is an objective standard when assessing out-of-office BP, it is unsuitable for repeated measurements and difficult to use in routine clinical practice due to the complexity of teaching patients how to use of monitor and evaluate BP values recoded in the

Table 16.1 Measurement conditions of home blood pressure

Measure at morning and evening
Morning: within 1 h after waking up, after urination, before taking medications, before breakfast, after a few minutes of rest in a sitting position
Evening: before going to bed, after a few minutes of rest in a sitting position
Use a cuff-oscillometric device with an upper arm cuff
Measure one to three times per occasion

monitor. The availability of web-based digital therapeutics systems [8] may further facilitate the use of home BP measurements in the diagnosis and treatment of hypertension.

3 Nocturnal BP Measurement

Aside from BP measured while awake, BP measured during sleep has been known to be independently associated with cardiovascular disease outcomes [9, 10]. Given that BP typically decreases by 10–20% during sleep (Fig. 16.1), individuals who exhibit a minimal BP drop or elevated BP during sleep have been considered to be at risk for cardiovascular disease. An ambulatory BP monitoring device is typically used for sleep BP measurements. However, considering that BP measurements obtained using this device are not limited to those during sleep, such values are usually referred to as nocturnal BP. Recently, a timer-equipped home BP monitor has been used to measure BP at night. Although the methods for measuring nighttime BP using the home BP monitor have not been standardized and can differ from one study to another [11], the obtained values may be closer to BP at sleep than that measured by ambulatory BP monitor. Therefore, it is proposed that nocturnal BP measured using a timer-equipped device be called "nocturnal home BP" to distinguish it from nocturnal BP measured using an ambulatory monitoring device [12]. Given that nocturnal home BP is equivalent to nocturnal BP [13–15], the former, which can be measured repeatedly, should be more widely used for nighttime BP assessment. Association analysis for subclinical cardiovascular disease risk factors suggests that measurements obtained over three nights were desirable for the assessment of nocturnal home BP [16].

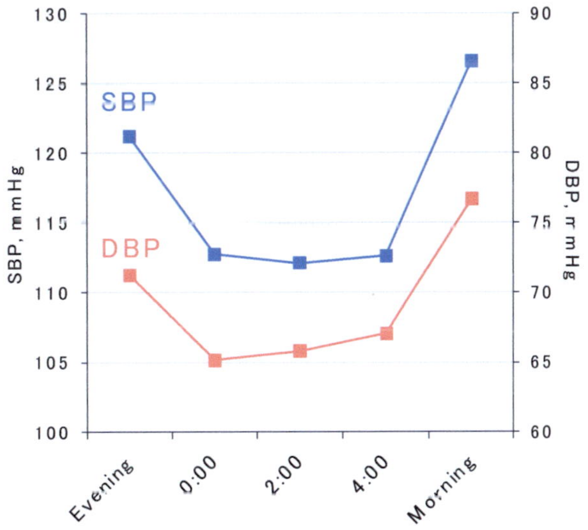

Fig. 16.1 Changes in BP during sleep. The graph was depicted using the dataset of the Nagahama study. Sleep BP was measured automatically at 0:00, 2:00, and 4:00 using a time-equipped cuff oscillometric device. Sleep BP was determined by referring to the actigram. *BP* blood pressure, *SBP* systolic *BP*, *DBP* diastolic BP

4 Factors Associated with Nocturnal BP

To reduce BP burden on cardiovascular disease, BP must remain low over a 24-h period, not just during waking hours. However, factors that increase nocturnal BP have yet to be fully elucidated. Previous studies have suggested that OSA can be a factor that increases nocturnal BP [17]. Indeed, evidence has shown that BP increased dramatically in response to apneic events, though OSA did not exert an effect strong enough to increase mean BP at night. We also reported that oxygen desaturation index measured using a finger-type pulse oximetry showed negligible impact, if any, on sleep BP levels and nocturnal BP decline after analyzing the dataset of the Nagahama study [18], a longitudinal epidemiological study based on the Nagahama city residents. In our analysis of sleep BP, we used a subset of the Nagahama study population that consisted of 5854 participants. Sleep BP was measured on multiple days using a timer-equipped BP monitor that was programmed to automatically measure BP at 0:00, 2:00, and 4:00. Among the BP values recorded on the BP monitor, those measured during sleep were identified using actigrams obtained using an ActiWatch attached to the participant's nondominant wrist. The actigram was also used to calculate the oxygen desaturation index considering that objective measurements of sleep duration improve accuracy at which the severity of sleep apnea is assessed using the oxygen desaturation index. Given the setting and large population size of our previous study, our finding suggesting that sleep apnea had little effect on sleep BP was sufficient to deny sleep apnea as a major factor in elevating sleep BP.

Instead, our findings identified nocturnal urination frequency as a strong determinant of nocturnal BP [19]. Although BP during sleep is 10–20% lower than that while awake, the drop in BP during sleep decreases linearly with increasing nocturnal urination frequency independent of awake BP and use of antihypertensive drugs. This association was also independent of lower sleep efficiency [18], suggesting a physiological relationship between nocturia and sleep BP. In the late 1900s, experimental epidemiological studies had clarified that salt sensitivity was a factor strongly associated with nocturnal BP [20–22]. Essential hypertensive patients who were salt-sensitive showed a lower nocturnal BP drop, especially after salt loading, than did non-salt-sensitive patients [20]. In addition, salt-sensitive patients showed a higher nocturnal BP after salt loading than did non-salt-sensitive patients, though similar nocturnal BP levels were observed in both groups under salt-restricted conditions [21]. This association can be explained, in part, by decreased renal function, which causes natriuresis to persist during sleep [22]. Our finding of an independent association between circulating levels of B-type natriuretic peptide, a simple marker of systemic fluid retention, and the decrease in nocturnal BP drop [19, 23] supports the importance of natriuresis as a factor for nocturnal BP.

5 OSA and Nocturnal Urination Frequency

Aside from salt sensitivity, OSA has been known to be associated with nocturnal urination frequency based on cross-sectional studies on patients with sleep-disordered breathing [24–26] and those of the general population [27, 28]. An interventional study reported that continuous positive airway pressure treatment reduced the frequency of nighttime urination [29], suggesting that the relationship between OSA and nocturia is not just an epiphenomenon. A plausible explanation for this relationship could be that the apnea-induced decrease in intrathoracic pressure increases venous return to the atrium, which in turn promotes secretion of natriuretic peptides from the atrium [30]. Our previous analysis of the Nagahama study dataset showed a linear relationship between nocturnal urination frequency and likelihood of OSA, with the odds ratio for nocturnal urination of more than three times reaching 2.79 in men and 7.46 in women after adjusting for possible confounding factors, including B-type natriuretic peptide and renal function [31]. The risk score for OSA, developed based on the results of the Naghama study, which consisted of easily assessed factors such as age, sex, body mass index, BP, observation of sleep apnea, sleep duration, and nocturnal urination frequency, showed a strong association with OSA, with an area under the curve of 0.842 [31].

6 Interpreting the Relationship Between OSA, Nocturia, and Nocturnal BP

As summarized in Fig. 16.2, salt sensitivity should be considered a factor that lies farthest upstream. Salt-sensitive individuals accumulate more body fluid than do nonsensitive individuals, even after consuming the same amount of salt, partially due to reduced renal function. As such, natriuresis that could not be completed during awake period persists during sleep, which increases urine production throughout the night. Given that a high BP is needed for glomeruli to filter sodium, increases in urine production at the night, which is referred to as nocturia, show a positive association with nocturnal BP. Therefore, nocturia is a manifestation but not a direct cause of nocturnal BP elevation. Similarly, high B-type natriuretic peptide levels are an epiphenomenon but not a direct cause of nocturnal BP elevation. OSA is associated with nocturia via the increase in intrathoracic pressure. Conversely, the shift in body fluid into the upper body caused by lying down and consequent narrowing of the respiratory tract had been suggested as another mechanism for the relationship between OSA and nocturia [32]. Regardless, OSA would not be influential enough to increase mean nocturnal BP, except in patients with severe OSA. Low sleep efficiency was a factor that directly increases nocturnal BP [18]. Seasonal variations in BP have been well documented, with lower BP levels having been observed during hotter seasons. Very interestingly, however, our study showed that sleep BP was higher in summer [33].

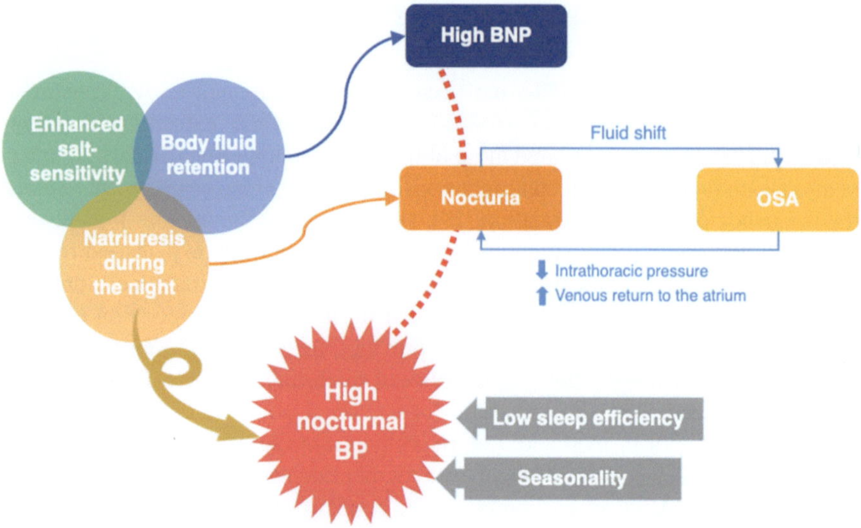

Fig. 16.2 Schematic diagram of the relationship between BP, nocturia, and OSA. *BP* blood pressure, *OSA* obstructive sleep apnea, *BNP* B-type natriuretic peptide

7 Is OSA an Innocent Bystander in Its Relationship with BP?

As described earlier, OSA exerted limited influence on nocturnal BP, if any. However, OSA was positively associated with morning BP [34] in the Nagahama population with normal BP. The phenomenon of home morning hypertension with office normotension has been referred to as "masked hypertension," given that the potentially increased BP at home cannot be reflected by the BP measured at the clinic. Several studies have reported that masked hypertension was an independent risk factor for cardiovascular outcomes [35] due in part to that home BP is less biased than office BP. BP measured at home, particularly that measured in the morning, has been more closely associated with poor cardiovascular outcomes than that measured in the office [5, 36].

One reason for the poor BP control in the morning among hypertensive patients receiving treatment is that the concentrations of drugs administered in the morning reach trough levels during this period. However, in cases with masked hypertension, who usually remain untreated, identifying other reasons that may be involved in morning BP elevation is necessary to avoid unfavorable outcomes. Therefore, several studies have focused on identifying factors associated with masked hypertension. Candidate factors that may be associated with masked hypertension include left ventricular hypertrophy [37] and atherosclerotic changes in the large arteries

[37, 38]. Other conventional factors associated with masked hypertension include older age, male sex, obesity, smoking habits, diabetes, and high normal office BP [39]. Apart from these factors, we had revealed a significant association between OSA and morning BP [34]. The results of an experimental study using a canine model also showed that OSA increased daytime but not nighttime BP [40] probably due to increased central nervous system activity. Furthermore, studies have shown that OSA was independently associated with increased morning BP relatively to evening BP [41] and that continuous positive airway pressure therapy reduced morning BP [42]. Given these findings, we are certain that a link exists between OSA and morning BP, emphasizing the importance of OSA in the prevention of hypertension with an understanding that its effects are stronger on morning BP than on nighttime BP.

8 What Should We Know About a Correlation Among Nocturia, OSA, and BP?

Nocturia is a good marker to identify individuals who need detailed assessment of OSA and nocturnal BP. Plausible physiological mechanisms underlying the relationship between nocturia and OSA and nocturia and nocturnal BP have been well documented, though it is unlikely that there is a physiological link between OSA and nocturnal BP. OSA may have some influence on morning BP.

9 Conclusion

Both OSA and hypertension are established risk factors for cardiovascular diseases. To fully elucidate the risk of these diseases in a large number of patients, understanding the potential relationship between OSA and hypertension is indispensable (Table 16.2). I hope this chapter furthers your understanding on the relationship between OSA and hypertension, which may be useful in daily clinical practice and disease prevention programs.

Table 16.2 Factors associated with sleep and morning BP in the general population

	Nocturia	Low sleep efficiency	OSA	Summer	Carotid hypertrophy
Sleep BP	↑	↑		↓	↑
Morning BP			↑	↑	↑

BP blood pressure, *OSA* obstructive sleep apnea

References

1. Umemura S, Arima H, Arima S, Asayama K, Dohi Y, Hirooka Y, Horio T, Hoshide S, Ikeda S, Ishimitsu T, Ito M, Ito S, Iwashima Y, Kai H, Kamide K, Kanno Y, Kashihara N, Kawano Y, Kikuchi T, Kitamura K, Kitazono T, Kohara K, Kudo M, Kumagai H, Matsumura K, Matsuura H, Miura K, Mukoyama M, Nakamura S, Ohkubo T, Ohya Y, Okura T, Rakugi H, Saitoh S, Shibata H, Shimosawa T, Suzuki H, Takahashi S, Tamura K, Tomiyama H, Tsuchihashi T, Ueda S, Uehara Y, Urata H, Hirawa N. The Japanese Society of Hypertension Guidelines for the management of hypertension (JSH 2019). Hypertens Res. 2019;42:1235–481. https://doi.org/10.1038/s41440-019-0284-9.
2. Imai Y, Kario K, Shimada K, Kawano Y, Hasebe N, Matsuura H, Tsuchihashi T, Ohkubo T, Kuwajima I, Miyakawa M. Japanese society of hypertension committee for guidelines for self-monitoring of blood pressure at home. The Japanese society of hypertension guidelines for self-monitoring of blood pressure at home (Second Edition). Hypertens Res. 2012;35:777–95. https://doi.org/10.1038/hr.2012.56.
3. Mancia G, Kreutz R, Brunström M, Burnier M, Grassi G, Januszewicz A, Muiesan ML, Tsioufis K, Agabiti-Rosei E, Algharably EAE, Azizi M, Benetos A, Borghi C, Hitij JB, Cifkova R, Coca A, Cornelissen V, Cruickshank JK, Cunha PG, Danser AHJ, de Pinho RM, Delles C, Dominiczak AF, Dorobantu M, Doumas M, Fernández-Alfonso MS, Halimi JM, Járai Z, Jelaković B, Jordan J, Kuznetsova T, Laurent S, Lovic D, Lurbe E, Mahfoud F, Manolis A, Miglinas M, Narkiewicz K, Niiranen T, Palatini P, Parati G, Pathak A, Persu A, Polonia J, Redon J, Sarafidis P, Schmieder R, Spronck B, Stabouli S, Stergiou G, Taddei S, Thomopoulos C, Tomaszewski M, Van de Borne P, Wanner C, Weber T, Williams B, Zhang ZY, Kjeldsen SE, Authors/Task Force Members. 2023 ESH guidelines for the management of arterial hypertension the task force for the management of arterial hypertension of the European Society of Hypertension Endorsed by the International Society of Hypertension (ISH) and the European renal association (ERA). J Hypertens. 2023. In press; https://doi.org/10.1097/HJH.0000000000003480.
4. Whelton PK, Carey RM, Aronow WS, Casey DE Jr, Collins KJ, Dennison Himmelfarb C, DePalma SM, Gidding S, Jamerson KA, Jones DW, Mac Laughlin EJ, Muntner P, Ovbiagele B, Smith SC Jr, Spencer CC, Stafford RS, Taler SJ, Thomas RJ, Williams KA Sr, Williamson JD, Wright JT Jr. 2017 ACC/AHA/AAPA/ABC/ACPM/AGS/APhA/ASH/ASPC/NMA/PCNA guideline for the prevention, detection, evaluation, and management of high blood pressure in adults: a report of the American College of Cardiology/American Heart Association task force on clinical practice guidelines. J Am Coll Cardiol. 2018;71:e127–248. https://doi.org/10.1016/j.jacc.2017.11.006.
5. Ohkubo T, Imai Y, Tsuji I, Nagai K, Kato J, Kikuchi N, Nishiyama A, Aihara A, Sekino M, Kikuya M, Ito S, Satoh H, Hisamichi S. Home blood pressure measurement has a stronger predictive power for mortality than does screening blood pressure measurement: a population-based observation in Ohasama, Japan. J Hypertens. 1998;16:971–5. https://doi.org/10.1097/00004872-199816070-00010.
6. Sega R, Facchetti R, Bombelli M, Cesana G, Corrao G, Grassi G, Mancia G. Prognostic value of ambulatory and home blood pressures compared with office blood pressure in the general population: follow-up results from the Pressioni Arteriose Monitorate e Loro Associazioni (PAMELA) study. Circulation. 2005;111:1777–83. https://doi.org/10.1161/01.CIR.0000160923.04524.5B.
7. Agarwal R, Andersen MJ. Prognostic importance of clinic and home blood pressure recordings in patients with chronic kidney disease. Kidney Int. 2006;69:406–11. https://doi.org/10.1038/sj.ki.5000081.
8. Kario K, Nomura A, Harada N, Okura A, Nakagawa K, Tanigawa T, Hida E. Efficacy of a digital therapeutics system in the management of essential hypertension: the HERB-DH1 pivotal trial. Eur Heart J. 2021;42:4111–22. https://doi.org/10.1093/eurheartj/ehab559.

9. Kario K, Hoshide S, Mizuno H, Kabutoya T, Nishizawa M, Yoshida T, Abe H, Katsuya T, Fujita Y, Okazaki O, Yano Y, Tomitani N, Kanegae H, JAMP Study Group. Nighttime blood pressure phenotype and cardiovascular prognosis: practitioner-based nationwide JAMP study. Circulation. 2020;142:1810–20. https://doi.org/10.1161/CIRCULATIONAHA.120.049730.
10. Yang WY, Melgarejo JD, Thijs L, Zhang ZY, Boggia J, Wei FF, Hansen TW, Asayama K, Ohkubo T, Jeppesen J, Dolan E, Stolarz-Skrzypek K, Malyutina S, Casiglia E, Lind L, Filipovský J, Maestre GE, Li Y, Wang JG, Imai Y, Kawecka-Jaszcz K, Sandoya E, Narkiewicz K, O'Brien E, Verhamme P, Staessen JA. International database on ambulatory blood pressure in relation to cardiovascular outcomes (IDACO) investigators. Association of office and ambulatory blood pressure with mortality and cardiovascular outcomes. JAMA. 2019;322:409–20. https://doi.org/10.1001/jama.2019.9811.
11. Kollias A, Ntineri A, Stergiou GS. Association of night-time home blood pressure with night-time ambulatory blood pressure and target-organ damage: a systematic review and meta-analysis. J Hypertens. 2017;35:442–52. https://doi.org/10.1097/HJH.0000000000001189.
12. Asayama K, Fujiwara T, Hoshide S, Ohkubo T, Kario K, Stergiou GS, Parati G, White WB, Weber MA, Imai Y. International expert Group of Nocturnal Home Blood Pressure. Nocturnal blood pressure measured by home devices: evidence and perspective for clinical application. J Hypertens. 2019;37:905–16. https://doi.org/10.1097/HJH.0000000000001987.
13. Hosohata K, Kikuya M, Asayama K, Metoki H, Imai Y, Ohkubo T. Comparison of nocturnal blood pressure based on home versus ambulatory blood pressure measurement: the Ohasama study. Clin Exp Hypertens. 2020;42:685–91. https://doi.org/10.1080/10641963.2020.1779281.
14. Ushio H, Ishigami T, Araki N, Minegishi S, Tamura K, Okano Y, Uchino K, Tochikubo O, Umemura S. Utility and feasibility of a new programmable home blood pressure monitoring device for the assessment of nighttime blood pressure. Clin Exp Nephrol. 2009;13:480–5. https://doi.org/10.1007/s10157-009-0192-4.
15. Ishikawa J, Hoshide S, Eguchi K, Ishikawa S, Shimada K, Kario K. Japan morning surge-home blood pressure study investigators group. Nighttime home blood pressure and the risk of hypertensive target organ damage. Hypertension. 2012;60:921–8. https://doi.org/10.1161/HYPERTENSIONAHA.112.198101.
16. Kollias A, Andreadis E, Agaliotis G, Kolyvas GN, Achimastos A, Stergiou GS. The optimal night-time home blood pressure monitoring schedule: agreement with ambulatory blood pressure and association with organ damage. J Hypertens. 2018;36:243–9. https://doi.org/10.1097/HJH.0000000000001562.
17. Kuwabara M, Hamasaki H, Tomitani N, Shiga T, Kario K. Novel triggered nocturnal blood pressure monitoring for sleep apnea syndrome: distribution and reproducibility of hypoxia-triggered nocturnal blood pressure measurements. J Clin Hypertens. 2017;19:30–7. https://doi.org/10.1111/jch.12878.
18. Matsumoto T, Tabara Y, Murase K, Setoh K, Kawaguchi T, Nagashima S, Kosugi S, Nakayama T, Wakamura T, Hirai T, Matsuda F, Chin K, Nagahama Study Group. Association between sleep disturbance and nocturnal blood pressure profiles by a linear mixed model analysis: the Nagahama study. Sleep Med. 2019;61:104–9. https://doi.org/10.1016/j.sleep.2019.01.049.
19. Matsumoto T, Tabara Y, Murase K, Setoh K, Kawaguchi T, Nagashima S, Kosugi S, Nakayama T, Wakamura T, Hirai T, Matsuda F, Chin K, Nagahama study group. Nocturia and increase in nocturnal blood pressure: the Nagahama study. J Hypertens. 2018;36:2185–92. https://doi.org/10.1097/HJH.0000000000001802.
20. Uzu T, Kazembe FS, Ishikawa K, Nakamura S, Inenaga T, Kimura G. High sodium sensitivity implicates nocturnal hypertension in essential hypertension. Hypertension. 1996;28:139–42. https://doi.org/10.1161/01.hyp.28.1.139.
21. Uzu T, Ishikawa K, Fujii T, Nakamura S, Inenaga T, Kimura G. Sodium restriction shifts circadian rhythm of blood pressure from nondipper to dipper in essential hypertension. Circulation. 1997;96:1859–62. https://doi.org/10.1161/01.cir.96.6.1859.

22. Fujii T, Uzu T, Nishimura M, Takeji M, Kuroda S, Nakamura S, Inenaga T, Kimura G. Circadian rhythm of natriuresis is disturbed in nondipper type of essential hypertension. Am J Kidney Dis. 1999;33:29–35. https://doi.org/10.1016/s0272-6386(99)70254-4.
23. Tabara Y, Igase M, Miki T, Ohyagi Y, Matsuda F, Kohara K, J-SHIPP Study Group. B-type natriuretic peptide is a determinant of the nocturnal increase in blood pressure independently of arterial hypertrophy and hypoxia. J Hypertens. 2016;34:2393–401. https://doi.org/10.1097/HJH.0000000000001104.
24. Oztura I, Kaynak D, Kaynak HC. Nocturia in sleep-disordered breathing. Sleep Med. 2006;7:362–7. https://doi.org/10.1016/j.sleep.2005.10.004.
25. Kang SH, Yoon IY, Lee SD, Kim JW. The impact of sleep apnoea syndrome on nocturia according to age in men. BJU Int. 2012;110:E851–6. https://doi.org/10.1111/j.1464-410X.2012.11342.x.
26. Romero E, Krakow B, Haynes P, Ulibarri V. Nocturia and snoring: predictive symptoms for obstructive sleep apnea. Sleep Breath. 2010;14:337–43. https://doi.org/10.1007/s11325-009-0310-2.
27. Martin SA, Appleton SL, Adams RJ, Taylor AW, Catcheside PG, Vakulin A, McEvoy RD, Antic NA, Wittert GA. Nocturia, other lower urinary tract symptoms and sleep dysfunction in a community-dwelling cohort of men. Urology. 2016;97:219–26. https://doi.org/10.1016/j.urology.2016.06.022.
28. Parthasarathy S, Fitzgerald M, Goodwin JL, Unruh M, Guerra S, Quan SF. Nocturia, sleep-disordered breathing, and cardiovascular morbidity in a community-based cohort. PLoS One. 2012;7:e30969. https://doi.org/10.1371/journal.pone.0030969.
29. Wang T, Huang W, Zong H, Zhang Y. The efficacy of continuous positive airway pressure therapy on nocturia in patients with obstructive sleep apnea: a systematic review and meta-analysis. Int Neurourol J. 2015;19:178–84. https://doi.org/10.5213/inj.2015.19.3.178.
30. Umlauf MG, Chasens ER, Greevy RA, Arnold J, Burgio KL, Pillion DJ. Obstructive sleep apnea, nocturia and polyuria in older adults. Sleep. 2004;27:139–44. https://doi.org/10.1093/sleep/27.1.139.
31. Hamada S, Tabara Y, Murase K, Matsumoto T, Setoh K, Wakamura T, Kawaguchi T, Kosugi S, Nakayama T, Hirai T, Matsuda F, Chin K, Nagahama Study Group. Night-time frequency of urination as a manifestation of sleep-disordered breathing: the Nagahama study. Sleep Med. 2021;77:288–94. https://doi.org/10.1016/j.sleep.2020.09.007.
32. Kasai T, Bradley TD, Friedman O, Logan AG. Effect of intensified diuretic therapy on overnight rostral fluid shift and obstructive sleep apnoea in patients with uncontrolled hypertension. J Hypertens. 2014;32:673–80. https://doi.org/10.1097/HJH.0000000000000047.
33. Tabara Y, Matsumoto T, Murase K, Nagashima S, Hirai T, Kosugi S, Nakayama T, Wakamura T, Chin K, Matsuda F, Nagahama study group. Seasonal variation in nocturnal home blood pressure fall: the Nagahama study. Hypertens Res. 2018;41:198–208. https://doi.org/10.1038/s41440-017-0003-3.
34. Tabara Y, Matsumoto T, Murase K, Setoh K, Kawaguchi T, Nakayama T, Wakamura T, Hirai T, Chin K, Matsuda F, Nagahama study group. Sleep-related factors associated with masked hypertension: the Nagahama study. J Hypertens. 2023;41:1298–305. https://doi.org/10.1097/HJH.0000000000003466.
35. Booth JN 3rd, Diaz KM, Seals SR, Sims M, Ravenell J, Muntner P, Shimbo D. Masked hypertension and cardiovascular disease events in a prospective cohort of blacks: the Jackson heart study. Hypertension. 2016;68:501–10. https://doi.org/10.1161/HYPERTENSIONAHA.116.07553.
36. Niiranen TJ, Hänninen MR, Johansson J, Reunanen A, Jula AM. Home-measured blood pressure is a stronger predictor of cardiovascular risk than office blood pressure: the Finn-home study. Hypertension. 2010;55:1346–51. https://doi.org/10.1161/HYPERTENSIONAHA.109.149336.
37. Redmond N, Booth JN 3rd, Tanner RM, Diaz KM, Abdalla M, Sims M, Muntner P, Shimbo D. Prevalence of masked hypertension and its association with subclinical cardiovascu-

lar disease in African Americans: results from the Jackson heart study. J Am Heart Assoc. 2016;5:e002284. https://doi.org/10.1161/JAHA.115.002284.
38. Hänninen MR, Niiranen TJ, Puukka PJ, Kesäniemi YA, Kähönen M, Jula AM. Target organ damage and masked hypertension in the general population: the Finn-home study. J Hypertens. 2013;31:1136–43. https://doi.org/10.1097/HJH.0b013e32835fa5dc.
39. Sheppard JP, Fletcher B, Gill P, Martin U, Roberts N, McManus RJ. Predictors of the home-clinic blood pressure difference: a systematic review and meta-analysis. Am J Hypertens. 2016;29:614–25. https://doi.org/10.1093/ajh/hpv157.
40. Brooks D, Horner RL, Kozar LF, Render-Teixeira CL, Phillipson EA. Obstructive sleep apnea as a cause of systemic hypertension. Evidence from a canine model. J Clin Invest 1997; 99:106–109. doi:https://doi.org/10.1172/JCI119120.
41. Johansson JK, Niiranen TJ, Puukka PJ, Jula AM. Factors affecting the difference between morning and evening home blood pressure: the Finn-home study. Blood Press. 2011;20:27–36. https://doi.org/10.3109/08037051.2010.518675.
42. Hoshide S, Yoshida T, Mizuno H, Aoki H, Tomitani N, Kario K. Association of night-to-night adherence of continuous positive airway pressure with day-to-day morning home blood pressure and its seasonal variation in obstructive sleep apnea. J Am Heart Assoc. 2022;11:e024865. https://doi.org/10.1161/JAHA.121.024865.

Correction to: Obstructive Sleep Apnea and Lifestyle Diseases: Clinical Question Is There a Correlation Between Sleep Apnea and Lifestyle Diseases?

Takeshi Matsumoto and Kazuo Chin

Correction to:
Chapter 4 in: K. Chin (ed.), *The Current State of Sleep Disordered Breathing in Japan and Around the World*, Respiratory Disease Series: Diagnostic Tools and Disease Managements, https://doi.org/10.1007/978-981-96-6030-8_4

Owing to an unfortunate error on the part of Springer Nature the authorship of Preface and *Chapter 4, Obstructive Sleep Apnea and Lifestyle Diseases: Clinical Question Is There a Correlation Between Sleep Apnea and Lifestyle Diseases?* was wrong in the initially published version. This has now corrected. Springer Nature would like to apologize to the chapter authors and to the editors of the book.

The updated version of this chapter can be found at
https://doi.org/10.1007/978-981-96-6030-8_4

K. Chin (ed.), *The Current State of Sleep Disordered Breathing in Japan and Around the World*, Respiratory Disease Series: Diagnostic Tools and Disease Managements, https://doi.org/10.1007/978-981-96-6030-8_17

MIX
Papier aus verantwortungsvollen Quellen
Paper from responsible sources
FSC® C105338

If you have any concerns about our products,
you can contact us on
ProductSafety@springernature.com

In case Publisher is established outside the EU,
the EU authorized representative is:
Springer Nature Customer Service Center GmbH
Europaplatz 3, 69115 Heidelberg, Germany

Printed by Libri Plureos GmbH
in Hamburg, Germany